T0383348

The Neuroscience of
PAIN, STRESS, AND EMOTION

The Neuroscience of
PAIN, STRESS, AND EMOTION
Psychological and Clinical Implications

Edited by

MUSTAFA AL'ABSI

University of Minnesota Medical School, Minneapolis, Duluth, MN, USA

MAGNE ARVE FLATEN

Department of Psychology, Norwegian University of Science and Technology, Trondheim, Norway

Amsterdam • Boston • Heidelberg • London
New York • Oxford • Paris • San Diego
San Francisco • Singapore • Sydney • Tokyo
Academic Press is an imprint of Elsevier

Academic Press is an imprint of Elsevier
125 London Wall, London EC2Y 5AS, UK
525 B Street, Suite 1800, San Diego, CA 92101-4495, USA
225 Wyman Street, Waltham, MA 02451, USA
The Boulevard, Langford Lane, Kidlington, Oxford OX5 1GB, UK

Notices
Knowledge and best practice in this field are constantly changing. As new research and
experience broaden our understanding, changes in research methods, professional practices,
or medical treatment may become necessary.

Practitioners and researchers may always rely on their own experience and knowledge in
evaluating and using any information, methods, compounds, or experiments described herein.
In using such information or methods they should be mindful of their own safety and the
safety of others, including parties for whom they have a professional responsibility.

To the fullest extent of the law, neither the Publisher nor the authors, contributors, or editors,
assume any liability for any injury and/or damage to persons or property as a matter of
products liability, negligence or otherwise, or from any use or operation of any methods,
products, instructions, or ideas contained in the material herein.

ISBN: 978-0-12-800538-5

British Library Cataloguing-in-Publication Data
A catalogue record for this book is available from the British Library

Library of Congress Cataloging-in-Publication Data
A catalog record for this book is available from the Library of Congress

For information on all Academic Press publications visit
our website at http://store.elsevier.com

  Working together
to grow libraries in
developing countries

www.elsevier.com • www.bookaid.org

Publisher: Mara Conner
Acquisition Editor: Mara Conner
Editorial Project Manager: Kathy Padilla
Production Project Manager: Chris Wortley
Designer: Mark Rogers

Typeset by TNQ Books and Journals
www.tnq.co.in

CONTENTS

Part 3: Clinical Implications

CONTRIBUTORS

Mustafa al'Absi
University of Minnesota Medical School, Minneapolis, Duluth, MN, USA

Martina Amanzio
Department of Psychology, University of Turin, Turin, Piedmont, Italy

Emily J. Bartley
University of Florida, Pain Research and Intervention Center of Excellence, Gainesville, FL, USA

Fabrizio Benedetti
Department of Neuroscience, University of Turin Medical School, Turin, Piedmont, Italy

Emma E. Biggs
Research Group Health Psychology, University of Leuven, Leuven, Belgium; Department of Cognitive Neuroscience, Maastricht University, Maastricht, The Netherlands

Tavis S. Campbell
Department of Psychology, University of Calgary, Calgary, AB, Canada

Blaine Ditto
Department of Psychology, McGill University, Montreal, QC, Canada

Roger B. Fillingim
University of Florida, Pain Research and Intervention Center of Excellence, Gainesville, FL, USA

Magne Arve Flaten
Department of Psychology, Norwegian University of Science and Technology, Trondheim, Norway

Kristin Horsley
Department of Psychology, McGill University, Montreal, QC, Canada

Maria Hrozanova
Department of Neuroscience, Norwegian University of Science and Technology, Trondheim, Norway

Francis J. Keefe
Duke Medical Center, Duke University, Durham, NC, USA

Ann Meulders
Research Group Health Psychology, University of Leuven, Leuven, Belgium; Center for Excellence on Generalization Research in Health and Psychopathology, University of Leuven, Leuven, Belgium

Robert Murison
Department of Biological and Medical Psychology, University of Bergen, Bergen, Norway

Motohiro Nakajima
University of Minnesota Medical School, Minneapolis, Duluth, MN, USA

Akiko Okifuji
Department of Anesthesiology, University of Utah, Salt Lake City, UT, USA

Sara Palermo
Department of Neuroscience, University of Turin Medical School, Turin, Piedmont, Italy

Paul Pauli
Department of Psychology, Biological Psychology, Clinical Psychology and Psychotherapy, University of Würzburg, Würzburg, Germany

Donald D. Price
Division of Neuroscience, Department of Oral and Maxillofacial Surgery, University of Florida, Gainesville, FL, USA

Jamie L. Rhudy
Department of Psychology, The University of Tulsa, Tulsa, OK, USA

Tore C. Stiles
Department of Psychology, Norwegian University of Science and Technology, Trondheim, Norway

Dennis C. Turk
Department of Anesthesiology, University of Washington, Seattle, WA, USA

Lene Vase
Department of Psychology and Behavioural Sciences, School of Business and Social Sciences, Aarhus University, Aarhus, Denmark

Johan W.S. Vlaeyen
Research Group Health Psychology, University of Leuven, Leuven, Belgium; Center for Excellence on Generalization Research in Health and Psychopathology, University of Leuven, Leuven, Belgium; Department of Clinical Psychological Science, Maastricht University, Maastricht, The Netherlands

Matthias J. Wieser
Department of Psychology, Biological Psychology, Clinical Psychology and Psychotherapy, University of Würzburg, Würzburg, Germany

FOREWORD

In the course of my 35 years as a pain researcher and clinician I have had the opportunity to attend numerous international scientific meetings that featured plenary talks in which the biopsychosocial model of pain was discussed. Though many of the presenters were well known and their talks well organized, all too often I have left these sessions with a feeling of disappointment. For example, a prominent psychologist might give an overview of the biopsychosocial model and then spend most of his or her time talking about studies of the psychology of pain. Likewise, a world-renowned basic scientist giving a plenary talk might briefly mention the biopsychosocial model, but then focus his or her talk on novel basic science findings on the biology of pain with little attempt to relate these findings to psychological or social aspects of pain.

One of the hallmarks of the biopsychosocial model is its insistence that pain (and other phenomena such as stress) is best understood when biological, psychological, and social viewpoints are integrated. This book exemplifies this approach as few others have. It is written by two international experts whose own research programs on pain and stress represent a gold standard against which others are compared. The systematic and programmatic nature of their work is impressive, with one study building logically upon another. Dr Magne Flaten, for example, has conducted a series of important studies on the role of expectations (placebo, nocebo) in pain and pain regulation. Dr Mustafa al'Absi is widely recognized for his program of neurobiological research linking pain to stress, appetite, and addiction.

In this book, Drs Flaten and al'Absi have assembled a set of well-written chapters provided by authors, each of whom is a world-class expert in his or her field. Each chapter provides an up-to-date overview of a key topic in the pain and stress area. Readers will find many of the chapters to be true gems. To mention a few of these: Robert Mursin provides a superb overview of the neurobiology of stress. A key message is the importance that early learning and social status have in the development of stress and pain-regulation processes. A chapter by Jamie Rhudy critically appraises recent studies of pain and emotion and highlights emerging findings that suggest that problems with emotional modulation may be a risk factor for persistent pain. Drs Flaten and al'Absi's own chapter on pain and placebo is one of the best in this book because it brings together state-of-the-art studies dealing with biological processes (endogenous opioids) and psychological processes (instructions, expectations) that are critical to our current understanding of placebo effects on pain. This chapter is nicely complemented by a chapter by Drs Amanzio, Plaermo, and Benedetti on nocebo and pain. This research team is internationally recognized for the development of novel methodologies for studying both placebo and nocebo processes and linking these responses to underlying biochemical and anatomical findings. Finally, Blaine Ditto and his colleagues provide an excellent overview of studies of pain, blood pressure, and hypertension. This chapter is one of the best I've seen on this topic since it includes novel insights into how blood pressure-related hypoalgesia can modulate both pain and stress.

Clinicians working in the areas of pain and stress will find this book extremely helpful because it provides research that will help them understand clinical phenomena they deal with every day. For a clinician, understanding the biological processes by which stress influences pain, or the neurobiology of stress and addiction in patients suffering from chronic pain, is important for several reasons. First, it enables the practitioner to better understand the varied ways that different individuals cope with persistent pain or stress. Second, it provides information that can be used to educate patients in ways that help them reconceptualize pain and stress and better understand what they can do to manage problematic responses. Finally, understanding the current literature on pain and stress can help clinicians better tailor their interventions so as to best address a given patient's concerns.

Researchers interested in pain and stress will find this book to be invaluable. Each chapter highlights important emerging areas of research and pinpoints key directions for future research. Those looking to develop their own research agenda and program of research will want this book in their personal library.

If you are looking for a book that truly integrates the biological, psychological, and social perspectives on pain and stress I encourage you to get this book. Readers eager to learn about the latest research linking the different elements of the biopsychosocial model (biological to psychological, psychological to social, biological to social) will enjoy this book immensely. The book exemplifies the best of the biopsychosocial model and demonstrates how the promise of this model is now being fulfilled. If you've been disappointed by prior plenary talks, review papers, and chapters on the biopsychosocial model of pain and stress I encourage you to give this book a read. This book will not disappoint you. Instead, it will enlighten, energize, and excite you.

Francis J. Keefe, PhD
Professor, Psychiatry and Behavioral Sciences, Duke Medical Center
Professor of Psychology and Neuroscience, Duke University

PART 1

Introduction and Background on Pain and Stress

CHAPTER 1

Neuroscience of Pain and Emotion

Matthias J. Wieser, Paul Pauli
Department of Psychology, Biological Psychology, Clinical Psychology and Psychotherapy,
University of Würzburg, Würzburg, Germany

NEUROANATOMY OF PAIN AND EMOTION

The International Association for the Study of Pain defines pain as an "unpleasant sensory and emotional experience associated with actual or potential tissue damage, or described in terms of such damage" (International Association for the Study of Pain, 1994, pp. 209–214). This definition implies that pain and nociception have to be differentiated, with the latter referring to the physiological processes triggered by tissue damage. Although nociception normally results in pain, this is not mandatory, and vice versa, pain may be experienced without nociception. This definition also clarifies that negative emotions are a constituent of the pain experience, and therefore a close interaction or overlap between brain processes related to pain and emotions has to be expected. As a matter of fact, it may be argued that pain is an emotion, an emotion that requires the presence of a bodily sensation with qualities like those reported during tissue-damaging stimulation (Price, 1999).

The pain–emotion interaction is also emphasized by the fact that both pain and emotions are adaptive responses to survival-relevant challenges in the environment. Whereas pain's main functional significance is to alert the organism that its body integrity is threatened in order to attend to the source of pain and possibly avoid it, emotion's functional significance lies in the detection of motivationally relevant stimuli that may trigger avoidance or approach behavior. Both pain and emotions thus have an adaptive value that ensures the survival of the organism.

Nociceptive Pathways

Human nociception is the process of encoding specific somatosensory information in the periphery and its transduction to the brain. Nociceptors are peripheral neurons that respond to noxious stimulation and detect

The Neuroscience of Pain, Stress, and Emotion
http://dx.doi.org/10.1016/B978-0-12-800538-5.00001-7

potentially damaging stimuli (Basbaum & Jessell, 2000). Nociceptors can be specific to a particular type of stimulus (e.g., mechanical, chemical, or temperature) or can respond to a variety of noxious stimulations. The latter nociceptive neurons are referred to as polymodal nociceptors and are more abundant in the human body in comparison to the stimulation-specific nociceptors (Ringkamp & Meyer, 2008). The nociceptive signal is trans-duced to the central nervous system (CNS) by two main types of nociceptive fibers constituting the starting point of the nociceptive signal cascade and found throughout the body tissue: the thinly myelinated Aδ neurons, which transmit information about acute and localized pain at fast conduction speed, and the unmyelinated C fibers, which signal more widespread pain with slower conduction speeds (Campbell & Meyer, 2006).

After nociceptive stimulation, the Aδ and C fibers transmit the noci-ceptive signals to the CNS. The peripheral Aδ and C fibers terminate in the dorsal horn of the spinal cord. In turn, second-order neurons are activated, and the axons of these neurons cross the midline of the spinal cord directly to the ventral surface of the spinal cord. Ascending pain signals are then sent to the brain via the spinothalamic tract, whose fibers project to the intralaminar and ventroposterior nuclei of the thalamus (Ringkamp & Meyer, 2008). Then two supraspinal neuronal systems can be differentiated with regard to their primary role within the processing of nociceptive information: the lateral system, mainly encoding sensory discriminative components of pain, and the medial system encoding the affective, motivational component of the resulting pain percept (Apkarian, 2013; Price, 2000).

It is important to note that these ascending nociceptive pathways can be modulated by descending pathways starting in the brain. These mainly alter the transmission of nociceptive inputs at the spinal dorsal horn (Kwon, Altin, Duenas, & Alev, 2014). The periaqueductal gray (PAG) and the rostroventral medulla (RVM) are two regions known to play a role in the endogenous control of pain via the inhibitory PAG–RVM–dorsal horn pathway (Fields & Basbaum, 1994). Receiving inputs from frontal and insular cortices, hypothalamus, and amygdala, the PAG has a critical role in the descending modulation of pain by interacting with the RVM and the dorsolateral pontine tegmentum (Fields & Basbaum, 1994). The PAG, parabrachial nucleus, and nucleus tractus solitaries provide input to the RVM, which has direct connections to the laminae of the dorsal horn (Millan, 1999, 2002).

Central Representation of Pain

In the brain, pain is represented in neuronal networks that encompass a number of subcortical and cortical structures that code various aspects of pain (Apkarian, Bushnell, Treede, & Zubieta, 2005; Peyron, Laurent, & Garcia-Larrea, 2000). Functional imaging studies most consistently revealed the following main brain areas constituting the brain network for acute pain (see Figure 1): primary and secondary somatosensory cortices, insular cortex (INS), anterior cingulate cortex (ACC), prefrontal cortex (PFC), and thalamus (Th) (Apkarian et al., 2005; Price, 2000). The somatosensory cortex receives input from the lateral nuclei of the Th, whereas the ACC receives input mainly from the medial portions of the Th via the INS and further provides the PFC with nociceptive information. The cerebellum receives direct input from the spinothalamic tract and is one of the subcortical pain–coding structures together with the caudate putamen, amygdala, and PAG. Accordingly, sensory and discriminatory aspects of pain are encoded in somatosensory, lateral thalamic, and cerebellar portions of the brain, whereas affective and cognitive components of pain are represented dominantly in the cingulate, insular, and prefrontal areas (Apkarian et al., 2005; Bushnell, Čeko, & Low, 2013).

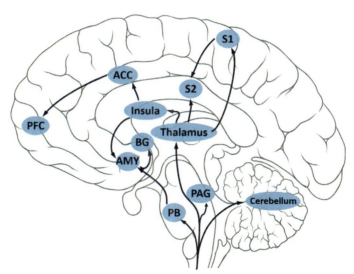

Figure 1 The brain network for acute pain. ACC, anterior cingulate cortex; AMY, amygdala; BG, basal ganglia; PAG, periaqueductal gray; PB, parabrachial nucleus; PFC, prefrontal cortex; S1 and S2, primary and secondary somatosensory cortices. (*Adapted from Bushnell et al. (2013).*)

This network, which has been referred to as the "pain matrix" (e.g., Tracey & Mantyh, 2007) and was inspired by the so-called neuromatrix of pain (Melzack, 1999, 2001), proposes a specific neuroanatomical representation of pain (as mentioned above). However, this concept has been challenged with regard to its pain specificity (Iannetti & Mouraux, 2010; Legrain, Iannetti, Plaghki, & Mouraux, 2011), concluding that various somatosensory and emotional states have common neural representations. Yet, a series of functional magnetic resonance imaging (fMRI) studies encompassing a large data set (more than 100 participants) and incorporating various experimental pain approaches revealed activity in the ventrolateral Th, S2, and dorsal posterior INS to be specific for pain and distinguishable from other salient events such as social rejection. These findings identified—at least to some degree—a brain signature that specifically corresponds to the sensory and affective representation of pain (Wager et al., 2013).

Given the unbeatable time resolution of electroencephalography (EEG) and magnetoencephalography (MEG), it is no surprise that studies employing these techniques were able to disentangle the dual pain sensation that is typically elicited by a single brief painful stimulus and which is based on the difference of about 1 sec in conduction times of $A\delta$ and C fibers (see above). These studies found two sequential brain activations in EEG and MEG recordings from S1 versus S2 and ACC (e.g., Bromm & Treede, 1987; Iannetti, Zambreanu, Cruccu, & Tracey, 2005; Ploner, Gross, Timmermann, & Schnitzler, 2002; Ploner, Holthusen, Noetges, & Schnitzler, 2002; Timmermann et al., 2001; Tran et al., 2002). The first early $A\delta$-fiber-mediated brain activation can be further subdivided into an early (100–200 ms after stimulus onset) and a late EEG/MEG response beyond 200 ms latency (Treede, Meier, Kunze, & Bromm, 1988).

Taken together, these results demonstrate that the perception and processing of pain and pain-related information are not tied to a single core neural structure. Rather, the neural substrates of pain share substantial commonalities with other highly salient sensory or emotional experiences. Nevertheless, it seems that sensory and affective qualities of (thermal) pain are represented by a set of regions throughout the brain that are now collectively known as the "neurological pain signature" (NPS) (Apkarian, 2013; Wager et al., 2013), which—at least for thermal pain—seems to be dissociated from a general salience signal and correlates better with pain perception than temperature itself.

Emotional Networks in the Brain

Although everyone seems to know what an emotion is, we do not have an unequivocally accepted definition, but a consensus on four key criteria (see Sander, 2013): (1) Emotions are multicomponent phenomena; (2) emotions are two-step processes involving emotion elicitation mechanisms that produce emotional responses; (3) emotions have relevant objects; and (4) emotions have a brief duration.

Studies on the emotional networks in the brain refer to two taxonomies of emotions: On one hand, categorical classes of few emotions, for example, six evolutionarily shaped basic emotions such as joy, fear, anger, sadness, disgust, and surprise (Ekman, 1992; Ekman & Friesen, 1975), and on the other hand, dimensions of valence and arousal (see Lang, 2010). As a consequence, studies on emotional networks in the brain examined brain responses either triggered by distinct basic emotions via facial expressions (e.g., Morris et al., 1998) or elicited by emotional stimuli varying in valence and arousal (e.g., Lang et al., 1998).

The so-called *valence hypothesis* was to some extent already discussed by Aristotle in his book Rethoric, who defined emotions (pathos) "as that which leads one's condition to become so transformed that his judgement is affected, and which is accompanied by pleasure and pain" (cited after Sander, 2013). Please note that this definition incorporates pain as the prototype of negative effect. Several hundred years later Wundt (1905) also suggested that the dimensions of valence, arousal, and tension underlie emotions (cited after Sander, 2013). A study by Anderson et al. (2003) using odors varying in valence and arousal indicated that the orbitofrontal cortex codes the stimulus's valence, while amygdala activity is associated with the stimulus's arousal. Yet, Lang, Bradley, and Cuthbert (2008) developed an extensive set of picture stimuli varying in valence and arousal allowing one to systematically examine verbal–cognitive, motoric–behavioral, and physiological–neural responses to these emotional stimuli. Using such picture stimuli, we (Gerdes et al., 2010), among others, examined brain activations related to the elicited valence and arousal. On one hand, negatively valenced stimuli were found to trigger amygdala, hippocampus, and medial occipital lobe activations, and especially right amygdala and left caudate body activity increased with the arousal qualities of these unpleasant pictures. On the other hand, positively valenced pictures triggered activations in the left occipital regions and in the medial temporal lobe, and an increase in arousal of these pictures was associated with activity in the right caudate head extending to the nucleus accumbens and the left dorsolateral PFC. Thus, the amygdala seems to play a major role in the processing of unpleasant stimuli, particularly highly arousing unpleasant stimuli. This conclusion was confirmed by Sabatinelli et al. (2011), who conducted a meta-analysis that included 157 studies examining brain responses to emotional scenes and emotional faces. They also identified the amygdala as the region with most overlap between studies involved in the processing of these emotional stimuli varying in valence, followed by regions of the medial PFC, inferior frontal/orbitofrontal cortex, inferior temporal cortex, and extrastriate occipital cortex.

As pain can be considered unpleasant and highly arousing, these brain imaging results related to the valence hypothesis suggest that the amygdala and the PFC are involved in the processing of unpleasant stimuli in general and in the processing of pain, too. Interestingly, laterality research also revealed that the frontal regions of the right hemisphere play a special role in the processing of negative emotions and pain (Pauli, Wiedemann, & Nickola, 1999a,b).

Models of *emotion categories* are mostly locationist models when it comes to the neural underpinnings. Thus, a limited number of phylogenetically shaped discrete emotion categories (Ekman et al., 1987; Panksepp, 1998) are hypothesized to result from activity of distinct brain areas or networks that are inherited or shared with other mammals (Panksepp & Watt, 2011). Early meta-analyses of emotion category–brain location studies from Murphy, Nimmo-Smith, and Lawrence (2003) and Phan, Wager, Taylor, and Liberzon (2002) agreed that the right and left amygdale were preferentially activated with fear and that the rostral ACC was associated with sadness. Also, both analyses suggest disgust to be related to activations in the basal ganglia. Whereas Murphy et al. also reported disgust-specific activity in the INS, Phan et al. found that INS activity was associated with negative emotions generally. At first glance, these effects speak in favor of at least a certain degree of functionally specialized brain areas for different emotion categories. However, even for the most consistent finding, a fear–amygdala correspondence, Phan et al. (2002) and Murphy et al. (2003) reported that only 60% and 40% of studies involving fear, respectively, showed increased activation in the amygdala (for further analysis of the other brain–emotion associations, see Barrett, 2006). In the same vein, a more recent meta-analytic review (Lindquist, Wager, Kober, Bliss-Moreau, & Barrett, 2012) comparing the locationist approach with the psychological constructionist approach found little evidence that discrete emotion categories can be consistently and specifically localized to distinct brain areas. This meta-analysis favors the constructionist model, meaning that "emotions emerge when people make meaning out of sensory input from the body and from the world using knowledge of prior experience" based on basic psychological operations that are not specific to emotions (Lindquist et al., 2012, p. 129). Thus, if pain would be an emotion, this model assumes that pain is the consequence of the processing of nociceptive system input based on previous experiences.

Fear is of special interest for pain research since animal as well as human models of fear are based on classical conditioning, and most of these fear conditioning studies use unconditioned stimuli (US; e.g., mildly painful electric stimuli) that elicit pain as the unconditioned response (UR). The conditioned stimulus, mostly an acoustic or visual cue, after association with the US, elicits fear as the conditioned response (CR). Since the CR and the UR are expected to be similar, the brain responses elicited by cued fear stimuli might be related to actual pain experiences. Confirming animal studies (LeDoux, 1996, 1998) indicating that the amygdala is crucial for such fear conditioning, we (Andreatta et al., 2012, 2015) and others (e.g., Büchel & Dolan, 2000) observed that a cue or a context that becomes associated with a painful US elicits amygdala activity. However, a 2015 meta-analysis (Fullana et al., 2015) on 27 fear conditioning studies indicated no amygdala activity but revealed an extended fear network that includes the central autonomic–interoceptive network, i.e., anterior INS, dorsal ACC, dorsal midbrain including PAG and parabrachial nucleus, ventro-medial Th, hypothalamus, and pontomedullary junction.

PAIN AND EMOTION INTERACTIONS

As reviewed above, pain and emotions share neural representations in the brain (see Wager & Atlas, 2013), mostly in the anterior INS and ACC. Consequently, one may assume mutual influences via directly shared representations and intracortical cross talk. However, as we will see below, the most compelling neural basis of emotional influences on pain so far is via the activation of the descending pain modulatory system.

Emotional Modulation of Pain

The extensive literature on the effects of emotions on pain consistently shows that pain is reduced by positive and increased by negative emotions (for excellent reviews, see Bushnell et al., 2013; Roy, 2015; Wiech & Tracey, 2009; but see the paragraph on stress-induced hypoalgesia below).

This conclusion is mainly based on experiments using various affective stimuli to modulate the participants' emotions and measuring their effect on pain processing. Our discussion of the brain processes mediating these effects of emotions on pain will focus on studies using affective pictures (emotional scenes or emotional faces) to modulate emotions, as this is the most frequently used experimental approach allowing a comparison of results. The interested reader in search for studies using other emotion-induction modalities is referred to the review by Roy (2015). This review also summarizes studies that induced positive and negative emotions by the application of odors (e.g., Villemure, Slotnick, & Bushnell, 2003), tastes (Lewkowski, Ditto, Roussos, & Young, 2003), affective pictures (e.g., Kenntner-Mabiala & Pauli, 2005; Meagher, Arnau, & Rhudy, 2001; Rhudy & Meagher, 2001; Rhudy, Williams, McCabe, Nguyen, & Rambo, 2005), pain-related pictures (Godinho et al., 2012), films (e.g., Weisenberg, Raz, & Hener, 1998), music (Roy, Lebuis, Hugueville, Peretz, & Rainville, 2012; Roy, Peretz, & Rainville, 2008), hypnotic suggestions (e.g., Rainville, Duncan, Price, Carrier, & Bushnell, 1997), or sentences (e.g., Zelman, Howland, Nichols, & Cleeland, 1991). The majority of these studies reported that unpleasant emotions increase pain ratings and decrease pain perception threshold and pain tolerance. In contrast but somewhat less strong, pleasant emotions generally reduce pain ratings and increase pain perception threshold and pain tolerance. As we will discuss below, these general emotion effects seem to rely on the descending pain pathways, as concomitant affective modulations of the lower limb nociceptive flexion reflex (NFR) strongly suggest (Bartolo et al., 2013; Rhudy et al., 2005; Roy et al., 2012; Roy, Lebuis, Peretz, & Rainville, 2011; Roy, Piché, Chen, Peretz, & Rainville, 2009).

Visual Emotional Stimuli and Pain Processing

First, functional imaging studies investigated where in the brain emotions modulate pain processing. These studies showed that the increased perception of pain during the presentation of negative compared to neutral or positive affective pictures resulted in enhanced activity of sensory and affective pain-associated areas like the paracentral lobule and Th, the anterior INS, and the parahippocampal gyrus and amygdale (Roy et al., 2009). Since activity in the right INS covaried with the modulation of pain perception, this study supports theories postulating that the INS serves as an integrative node for information from ascending interoceptive signals with more general information within the broader emotional–motivational context (Craig, 2003). In sum, fMRI studies suggest that the emotional modulation of pain seems to result mainly in changes in the affective component of pain, reflected by variations of activity in the "medial pain system" comprising the PFC, ACC, and PAG, which encode the affective-motivational component of pain (Bushnell et al., 2013; Loggia, Mogil, & Bushnell, 2008).

Second, somatosensory-evoked potentials (SEPs) were used to examine when emotions modulate pain processing. In such studies from our group we examined how the SEPs triggered by mildly painful electric stimuli were modulated by simultaneously presented affective pictures inducing negative, neutral, or positive emotions (Kenntner-Mabiala, Andreatta, Wieser, Mühlberger, & Pauli, 2008; Kenntner-Mabiala & Pauli, 2005; Kenntner-Mabiala, Weyers, & Pauli, 2007). As expected, the affective valence of the pictures modulated pain ratings such that the very same pain stimulus was rated the most intense and unpleasant when negative pictures were shown concurrently and least intense and unpleasant during positive pictures. Most important, we also observed that the N150 of the SEP varied as a function of the affective valence in concordance with the pain ratings with lowest amplitudes when pleasant and highest amplitudes when unpleasant pictures were presented. The P260 of the SEP, however, was not modulated by the pictures' valence, but in concordance with the pictures' arousal with reduced amplitudes for arousing (positive and negative valence) compared to neutral pictures (Kenntner-Mabiala & Pauli, 2005). These results were overall replicated in a second study in which additionally attention was manipulated to focus on the sensory or affective aspects of the pain stimuli or on the picture stimuli (Kenntner-Mabiala et al., 2008). Attentional modulation effects were found only for sensory pain ratings, with lower pain ratings when attention was focused on pictures compared to attention focused on pain. A similar effect was observed for the P260, which was further modulated by the pictures' arousal. The N150 instead was modulated by valence only, thus replicating (Kenntner-Mabiala & Pauli, 2005). Based on these and another study from our lab, we conclude that attention and emotion have distinct effects on pain processing as reflected in SEPs, with emotions induced before and during pain processing modulating the N150, while attention modulates the P260 (Kenntner-Mabiala et al., 2008; Kenntner-Mabiala & Pauli, 2005). Importantly, we did not find comparable effects of emotions on SEPs triggered by nonpainful somatosensory stimuli. These SEP studies on the affective modulation of pain processing allow no conclusion about the involved brain areas, but demonstrate that emotions affect rather early stages of pain processing.

Third, in a series of studies it was shown that emotions induced by affective pictures also modulate spinal nociceptive reflexes, i.e., the RIII withdrawal reflex or lower limb nociceptive flexion response (NFR) (Bartolo et al., 2013; Rhudy et al., 2005; Rhudy, Williams, McCabe, Russell, & Maynard, 2008; Roy et al., 2012; Roy et al., 2011, 2009). This polysynaptic reflex causes a flexion of the stimulated leg (approximately 90–180 ms after stimulation), which is consistent with the conduction velocity of Aδ nociceptive afferents (Sandrini et al., 2005). Importantly, the reflex's amplitude increases with perceived pain, suggesting that modulation of NFR amplitude by emotions may reflect spinal nociceptive processes (Sandrini et al., 2005). These findings strongly suggest that valence-dependent effects of emotion on pain are mediated by descending modulatory circuits that alter afferent nociceptive signals at various stages of pain processing (Tracey & Mantyh, 2007). This idea of a spinal modulation of pain by emotions is also supported by the aforementioned affective modulation of the N150 component of nociceptive SEPs (Kenntner-Mabiala et al., 2008; Kenntner-Mabiala & Pauli, 2005), which occurs in parallel with the NFR's temporal window. In addition, it was reported that heart rate accelerations and skin conductance responses (Rhudy et al., 2005) to nociceptive stimuli are also modulated by emotions, indicating emotion effects on autonomic pain responses. Importantly, Roy et al. (2009) measured both the affective modulation effects on spinal nociceptive responses (NFR) and fMRI responses, and this study revealed that the emotional modulation of the NFR amplitude correlated with pain-evoked activity in structures receiving direct or indirect nociceptive inputs, such as the brain stem, Th, cerebellum, amygdala, and medial PFC. Again, this suggests descending modulatory circuits that alter afferent nociceptive signals at various stages of pain processing.

Fourth, the arousal induced by emotional pictures also has to be considered regarding its effect on pain processing. High-arousing positive emotional stimuli cause more pronounced decreases in pain than low-arousing stimuli, and highly compared to moderately arousing negative stimuli result in stronger pain increases (Rhudy et al., 2005, 2008). Thus, picture valence determines the direction of pain modulation (either increase or decrease), while the level of arousal determines the strength of this modulation. However, these pain-enhancing effects of negative pictures have to be distinguished from hypoalgesia induced by strong aversive stimulations or stress-induced analgesia. First, there are quantitative differences. The arousal induced by unpleasant picture stimuli is far less than the arousal induced by the stimuli used to trigger stress hypoalgesia in humans (e.g., Trier social stress test, threat of electric shocks) or animals (e.g., confrontation with predator). Second, there exist qualitative differences. The experimental paradigms employed in human studies of stress-induced analgesia do not manipulate purely emotional processes. For example, Rhudy and Meagher (2000) showed that anxiety induced by the announcement of possible electric shocks (instructed fear) lowers pain thresholds, like negatively valenced pictures do, while fear triggered by the experience of painful electric shocks prior to pain assessment increases pain thresholds. However, since participants in the fear group experienced pain stimuli before pain threshold assessment, the latter effect might be explained by the engagement of diffuse noxious inhibitory controls (Millan, 2002) rather than the negative emotion "fear" per se. Similarly, stress induction by a cognitively demanding task (Yilmaz et al., 2010) introduces confounding factors, i.e., distraction if pain is tested during the task or fatigue if pain is tested after the task. As a consequence, cognitive and not emotional effects on pain are revealed.

In sum, most of the results regarding effects of emotional picture stimuli on pain processing may be explained by the *emotional priming hypothesis* (Lang, 1995). This hypothesis suggests that emotional background stimuli (e.g., emotional pictures) prime the organism for responses to stimuli of congruent valence. In human studies, such emotional priming effects are visible for verbal, autonomic, and central responses as well as reflexes (Lang, 2010; Lang & Bradley, 2010). In the case of a pain stimulus, its processing is primed, i.e., facilitated, if the organism is in a negative emotional state and inhibited if the organism is in a positive emotional state. However, we cannot conclude that these effects are pain-specific since emotions also modulate responses to other sensory stimulations that are threatening but not painful, such as breathlessness (Von Leupoldt, Mertz, Kegat, Burmester, & Dahme, 2006; Von Leupoldt et al., 2010) or loud aversive noise bursts (e.g., Schupp, Cuthbert, Bradley, Birbaumer, & Lang, 1997).

Emotional Faces and Pain Processing

Only recently have researchers started to investigate the effects of emotional facial expressions, including facial expressions of pain, on pain processing (for a review, see Wieser, Gerdes, Reicherts, & Pauli, 2014). Especially the social importance of nonverbal communication makes facial expressions (of pain) an interesting model for studying effects on concurrent pain processing (Williams, 2002). Until now, the modulation of pain by this crucial feature in nonverbal emotion communication has rarely been studied, presumably because facial expressions, compared to other affective pictures, do not elicit strong emotional states or arousal in the observer (e.g., Alpers, Adolph, & Pauli, 2011; Bradley, Codispoti, Cuthbert, & Lang, 2001; Britton, Taylor, Sudheimer, & Liberzon, 2006). As discussed above, such low-arousing emotional stimuli cannot be expected to have strong effects on pain processing. However, as revealed by the meta-analysis of Sabatinelli et al. (2011), the processing of faces is associated with activity in some of the same brain areas that are activated by pain or that are known to belong to the higher-order output relays on the PAG in the descending pain system. Indeed, one of the few studies available on this topic demonstrated that emotional faces in general compared to neutral facial expressions increase pain perception accompanied by alterations in pain-related brain oscillations (Senkowski, Kautz, Hauck, Zimmermann, & Engel, 2011).

Since faces may express distinct emotions, facial stimuli were also used to investigate how distinct emotional categories alter pain processing. Regarding the effects of faces expressing sadness, two previous reports observed an increase in perceived pain (Yoshino et al., 2012, 2010), and one study showed that viewing blocks of sad faces compared with blocks of happy or neutral faces causes participants to report higher pain unpleasantness and higher pain intensity (Bayet, Bushnell, & Schweinhardt, 2014). Thus, the social signal of sadness expressed in another person's face seems to enhance pain perception in the observer. Similarly, facial pain compared to neutral expressions were found to augment pain perception (Mailhot, Vachon-Presseau, Jackson, & Rainville, 2012).

These findings, again, may be explained by the emotional priming hypotheses postulating that the facial expression of others induces an emotional state that facilitates or inhibits the processing of stimuli of congruent or incongruent valence, respectively. Thus, sad or painful facial expressions induce negative affect in the observer, and this emotion facilitates pain processing. An alternative, more specific theoretical explanation for the interaction of viewing others' facial expression of pain and one's own sensation of pain is offered by the Perception–Action Model (PAM) of empathy (Preston & de Waal, 2002). The PAM proposes that the capacity to feel the internal state of someone else activates corresponding representations in an observer. Indeed, it was found that observing others' facial expression of pain also amplifies one's own facial and neural responses to pain, revealing a vicarious effect of facial pain expression (Mailhot et al., 2012; Vachon-Presseau et al., 2011, 2013, 2012). Similar effects of facial mimicry were found for other facial expressions (Weyers, Mühlberger, Hefele, & Pauli, 2006). Additional support for the PAM derives from neuroimaging studies indicating that emotions observed in others are mapped onto a self-reference framework supposed to serve the rapid understanding of the others' feelings, goals, and intentions (Jackson, Brunet, Meltzoff, & Decety, 2006; Jackson, Rainville, & Decety, 2006; Wicker et al., 2003). Consequently, the PAM would predict selective pain enhancement by watching pain faces of others compared to other negative facial expressions, whereas the motivational priming hypothesis would assume a general enhancement of pain by negative facial expressions, but not necessarily selectivity of pain faces. Studies directly comparing both theories are lacking as of now.

Influence of Pain on Emotion

The effects of pain on emotion processing have been investigated rarely, although from a clinical perspective the high prevalence of mood disorders in chronic pain suggests effects in this direction (Bair, Robinson, Katon, & Kroenke, 2003; Campbell, Clauw, & Keefe, 2003). A first study by Godinho, Frot, Perchet, Magnin, and Garcia-Larrea (2008), on the one hand, found that pleasant pictures, when paired with pain, are rated less pleasant and elicit attenuated visual-evoked responses in the EEG. On the other hand, this study observed no enhanced responses to unpleasant pictures when paired with pain. In a later study of our own, we asked participants to display evaluative facial responses congruent and incongruent to pictures of emotional facial expressions during painful or non-painful pressure stimulation (Gerdes, Wieser, Alpers, Strack, & Pauli, 2012). Normally, voluntary facial muscle reactions registered by means of electromyogram are facilitated (i.e., fewer errors and faster responses) in response to pictures displaying muscle-congruent facial expressions, i.e., facilitated reactions of the corrugator supercilii muscle in response to negative facial expressions and facilitated reactions of the zygomaticus major in response to positive facial expressions. Such effects are interpreted as motor-compatibility and automatic evaluation of affective stimuli. In our study, pressure pain generally slowed compatible as well as incompatible muscle responses (zygomaticus and corrugator) and resulted in fewer erroneous incompatible (corrugator) responses to happy faces.

However, pain did not affect muscle responses to angry faces and affective ratings. Thus, our results confirm Godinho et al. (2008), pointing to the notion that pain particularly reduces responses to pleasant stimuli, but seems to have no exacerbating effect on the processing of negative emotional stimuli. This observation may be partly explained by the pain-reducing effects of distraction, which may dampen the actual facilitatory effects of pain for unpleasant emotions.

In a further study, we investigated the effect of tonic pressure pain on the electrocortical correlates of face processing (Wieser, Gerdes, Greiner, Reicherts, & Pauli, 2012). Here, fearful, happy, and neutral faces were presented while participants received tonic pressure stimulation. Face-evoked brain potentials revealed no affective but an attentional modulation by pain: early and late indices of attention allocation toward faces (P100 and LPP of the ERP) were diminished during the tonic pain compared to the control condition. This finding corroborates reports of an attentional interruptive function of pain (Eccleston & Crombez, 1999), which has been demonstrated for visual processing (Bingel, Rose, Glascher, & Buchel, 2007) and attentional (e.g., Seminowicz & Davis, 2006; Tiemann, Schulz, Gross, & Ploner, 2010) and memory processes (Forkmann et al., 2013).

In sum, these studies suggest that experimental pain alters perception and processing of positive affective stimuli (scenes and faces), although most effects were observed with regard to attentional mechanisms. However, little is known about how pain alters the processing of facial displays of pain specifically. Given the match between observed and experienced pain, one may argue that selective enhancement and mutual influences have to be expected. The hypothesis was addressed by a study by us investigating how a painful stimulation influences the perception of facial expressions of pain, as well as, vice versa, how a facial expression of pain modulates pain perception (Reicherts, Gerdes, Pauli, & Wieser, 2013). To this end, participants received painful thermal stimuli while passively watching dynamic facial expressions (pain, fear, joy, and a neutral expression). To compare the influence of complex visual with low-level stimulation, a central fixation cross was presented as the control condition. Participants were asked to rate the intensity of the thermal stimuli and also to rate the valence and the arousal triggered by the facial expressions. In addition, facial electromyography was recorded as an index of emotion and pain perception. Results indicate that faces in general compared to the low-level control condition decreased pain ratings, suggesting a general attention modulation of pain by complex (social) stimuli. In addition, the facial responses to the painful stimulation were found to correlate with the pain intensity ratings. Most important, painful thermal stimuli increased the perceived arousal of simultaneously presented fear, and especially pain, expressions of others; and vice versa, pain expressions of others compared to all other facial expressions led to higher pain ratings. Thus, we found independent effects of attention and facial expressions on pain ratings and, vice versa, a selective enhancement of arousal ratings of pain faces by pain.

These findings allow an important conclusion about a bidirectional relation between emotion and pain, especially between pain-expressing faces and pain processing. First, extending previous findings (Mailhot et al., 2012; Vachon-Presseau et al., 2011, 2012, 2013), pain-specific modulations of pain perception were revealed, such that the highest pain ratings of painful thermal stimuli were obtained while participants watched faces of pain compared to other facial expressions. Importantly, our study revealed that the effect was larger for pain compared to fear faces, suggesting that the facial expression of pain enhances pain perception, not only owing to its negative valence but also to its pain relevance. This finding cannot be explained unequivocally by the motivational priming hypothesis. Results probably suggest that not only the valence of a facial expression enhances pain perception, but that the expressed pain itself primes the sensorimotor system, which might drive a potentiating proalgesic mechanism (Godinho et al., 2012). As mentioned above, another potential mechanism of pain modification in addition to the affective priming hypotheses has been put forward as the PAM of empathy (Preston & de Waal, 2002). This model would postulate that the observation of others' pain activates a similar neural network implicated in the first-person experience of the very same phenomenon (Jackson, Meltzoff, & Decety, 2005). Accordingly, the perceived pain expression of others is mapped on the observer's own neural representations and as such facilitates and primes own-pain perceptions. This shared-representations account has been supported by neuroimaging studies (Jackson, Rainville, et al., 2006). However, it has to be noted that the overlapping brain responses to pain and to facial expressions of pain may not indicate shared representations of actual pain and observed pain, but a much more unspecific response to salient stimuli (Iannetti, Salomons, Moayedi, Mouraux, & Davis, 2013).

Neural Bases of Pain–Emotion Interactions

As elaborated above, emotions are strong modulators of pain. Empirical evidence both from neuroimaging/neurophysiology and from psycho-physiological paradigms demonstrates that the affective modulation of pain becomes effective on spinal as well as supraspinal levels (Roy, 2015). On the one hand, effects of emotions on pain appear to be implemented by descending pain-modulatory systems, which involve pathways from the cerebral cortex down to the spinal cord. These networks originate in the PAG and project to brain-stem nuclei, including the RVM and the locus coeruleus, and further down to the dorsal horn of the spinal cord (Figure 2). Effects are either inhibitory or excitatory on spinal cord nociceptive afferent projection neurons. As outputs from higher-order forebrain regions such as the ACC, PFC, and amygdala reach the PAG, it seems plausible that these descending systems could be activated by various psychological factors such

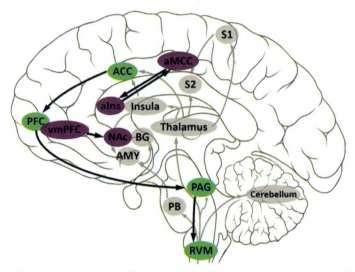

Figure 2 The brain network for emotion–pain interactions (see text). Spinal modulations of pain by emotions are mediated via the descending pain modulatory system (green regions). Supraspinal modulations of pain by emotions are mainly mediated via the ventromedial prefrontal cortex (vmPFC), nucleus accumbens (NAc), anterior insula (aIns), and anterior midcingulate cortex (aMCC) (shown in purple). Gray regions show parts of the ascending pain pathways as depicted in Figure 1. ACC, anterior cingulate cortex; AMY, amygdala; BG, basal ganglia; PAG, periaqueductal gray; PB, parabrachial nucleus; PFC, prefrontal cortex; RVM, rostroventral medulla; S1 and S2, primary and secondary somatosensory cortices. (*Adapted from Bushnell et al. (2013).*)

as cognitive and emotional processes (Fields, 2004; Mason, 2012; Ossipov, Dussor, & Porreca, 2010). On the other hand, it has to be noted that ascending nociceptive signals—as soon as they enter the cerebral cortex— are subjected to a multisensory integration process in which various external stimuli, including emotional stimuli, can influence the perception of pain, i.e., its localization, intensity, and unpleasantness (Haggard, Iannetti, & Longo, 2013). Similar mechanisms are postulated as responsible for manipulations of attentional focus on the pain's sensory dimension (Bushnell et al., 2013; Villemure & Bushnell, 2009).

The supraspinal modulation of pain by higher-order cognition in a top-down manner is nicely supported by studies in which the threat value of nociceptive stimuli is manipulated by suggesting that they may cause injury. This manipulation increases pain perception through preactivation of the anterior midcingulate cortex (aMCC) and anterior INS, during anticipation of the nociceptive stimulation, and of the aMCC during the actual pain stimulation (Wiech & Tracey, 2009). In the same vein, hypnotic suggestions to reappraise painful thermal stimuli as more or less unpleasant specifically affect ratings of pain unpleasantness, an effect presumably linked to an up- or downregulation of aMCC activity (Rainville et al., 1997). Also in line with these results are studies showing that the very same reappraisal strategies proven to be efficient in reducing negative emotions (Gross, 2002) also are successfully used to downregulate pain (Lapate et al., 2012). The strikingly similar effects of reappraisal on pain and negative emotions point to the notion that both may rely upon the same lateral-prefrontal and medial-prefrontal subcortical pathways (Atlas, Bolger, Lindquist, & Wager, 2010; Leknes et al., 2013; Roy, Shohamy, & Wager, 2012).

Woo, Roy, Buhle, and Wager (2015) were able to demonstrate that the nucleus accumbens and the ventromedial PFC constitute a system that mediates the effects of self-regulation on pain rating and is dissociable from the NPS. The fMRI responses of the NPS triggered by pain were not affected by self-regulation strategies and did not mediate the effects of self-regulation on pain ratings, suggesting that another brain region or a set of regions may have this role instead. Together with studies on placebo analgesia (e.g., Eippert et al., 2009) these findings provide compelling evidence that higher-order brain areas exert influences on pain experience, but that fundamentally distinct brain mechanisms can result in similar modulations of the experience of pain (Ploner, Bingel, & Wiech, 2015) (Figure 2).

Since the influence of pain on emotion processing has been almost neglected in experimental brain research, we can only speculate about involved brain regions. First studies point to reduced processing of positive affective stimuli under pain, while others found only reduced processing of emotional material in general owing to the attentional demand of acute pain. As mentioned above, the neural bases for such emotion–pain interaction may constitute a network of the amygdala (Simons et al., 2014), the anterior INS (Craig, 2003), and subregions of the ACC (Vogt, 2005). Particularly the anterior part of the midcingulate gyrus (aMCC) is consistently activated by negative affect and pain and characterized by substantial connections with subcortical regions involved in negative affect and pain (the spinothalamic system, PAG, amygdala, nucleus accumbens, and substantia nigra) (Shackman et al., 2011; Vogt, 2005). This makes the aMCC an ideal candidate as a mediator structure for pain–emotion interactions.

CONCLUSIONS

Emotions have strong modulatory effects on pain, which may be summarized according to their physiological and psychological mechanisms within the influential model of pain processing by Price (2000). According to this model, the experience of pain is represented in the brain via interactions between sensory, cognitive, and affective/motivational systems (Roy, 2015). Emotion effects on these pain representations may be due to spinal modulations of nociceptive pathways through descending modulatory pathways and/or supraspinal modulations via higher-order brain areas. Please also note that psychological effects on pain may be partly mediated through influences of higher-order brain areas such as the medial PFC on target structures of the descending system (e.g., PAG) and that both processes may be involved in the reappraisal of pain, anticipation of pain, and placebo analgesia. On an experimental level, a clear differentiation of spinal and supraspinal mechanisms contributing to the effects of emotions on pain remains a challenge (Apkarian, 2013; Ploner et al., 2015).

As a consequence, when we aim to further elucidate and identify the neural underpinnings of the emotion–pain interaction, it seems warranted to measure pain at all possible levels of the pain-processing hierarchy in a multimethod approach (reflex recordings, measures of autonomic activity, fMRI, EEG, facial muscle EMG recordings, etc.). As a first step, accounting for the network rather than the single faculty perspective, the multivariate pattern analysis approaches to the neural signature of pain may be also applied to psychophysiological and behavioral pain-processing measures. With regard to the underlying neural mechanisms, we think that the time has come not only to investigate different types of pain modulation in isolation but also to systematically compare them, which may help to find more precise definitions of key neural mechanisms underlying pain modulation at all levels of the neural hierarchy (Ploner et al., 2015). In the long term, the better understanding of the psychological and neural mechanisms affecting pain processing will lead to a better understanding of pain itself and probably improve our understanding of chronic pain and development of treatments.

REFERENCES

Alpers, G. W., Adolph, D., & Pauli, P. (2011). Emotional scenes and facial expressions elicit different psychophysiological responses. *International Journal of Psychophysiology, 80*(3), 173–181.

Anderson, A. K., Christoff, K., Stappen, I., Panitz, D., Ghahremani, D. G., Glover, G., et al. (2003). Dissociated neural representations of intensity and valence in human olfaction. *Nature Neuroscience, 6*(2), 196–202.

Andreatta, M., Fendt, M., Muhlberger, A., Wieser, M. J., Imobersteg, S., Yarali, A., et al. (2012). Onset and offset of aversive events establish distinct memories requiring fear and reward networks. *Learning and Memory, 19*(11), 518–526.

Andreatta, M., Glotzbach-Schoon, E., Muhlberger, A., Schulz, S. M., Wiemer, J., & Pauli, P. (2015). Initial and sustained brain responses to contextual conditioned anxiety in humans. *Cortex, 63*, 352–363.

Apkarian, A. V. (2013). A brain signature for acute pain. *Trends in Cognitive Sciences, 17*(7), 309–310. http://dx.doi.org/10.1016/j.tics.2013.05.001.

Apkarian, A. V., Bushnell, M. C., Treede, R.-D., & Zubieta, J.-K. (2005). Human brain mechanisms of pain perception and regulation in health and disease. *European Journal of Pain, 9*(4), 463–484. http://dx.doi.org/10.1016/j.ejpain.2004.11.001.

Atlas, L. Y., Bolger, N., Lindquist, M. A., & Wager, T. D. (2010). Brain mediators of predictive cue effects on perceived pain. *The Journal of Neuroscience, 30*(39), 12964–12977.

Bair, M. J., Robinson, R. L., Katon, W., & Kroenke, K. (2003). Depression and pain comorbidity: a literature review. *Archives of Internal Medicine, 163*(20), 2433.

Bartolo, M., Serrao, M., Gamgebeli, Z., Alpaidze, M., Perrotta, A., Padua, L., et al. (2013). Modulation of the human nociceptive flexion reflex by pleasant and unpleasant odors. *Pain®, 154*(10), 2054–2059.

Barrett, L. F., & Wager, T. D. (2006). The structure of emotion: evidence from neuroimaging studies. *Current Directions in Psychological Science, 15*, 79–83.

Basbaum, A. I., & Jessell, T. M. (2000). The perception of pain. *Principles of Neural Science, 4*, 472–491.

Bayet, S., Bushnell, M. C., & Schweinhardt, P. (2014). Emotional faces alter pain perception. *European Journal of Pain, 18*(5), 712–720.

Bingel, U., Rose, M., Glascher, J., & Buchel, C. (2007). fMRI reveals how pain modulates visual object processing in the ventral visual stream. *Neuron, 55*(1), 157–167.

Bradley, M. M., Codispoti, M., Cuthbert, B. N., & Lang, P. J. (2001). Emotion and motivation I: defensive and appetitive reactions in picture processing. *Emotion, 1*(3), 276–298.

Britton, J. C., Taylor, S. F., Sudheimer, K. D., & Liberzon, I. (2006). Facial expressions and complex IAPS pictures: common and differential networks. *Neuroimage, 31*(2), 906–919.

Bromm, B., & Treede, R. D. (1987). Human cerebral potentials evoked by CO_2 laser stimuli causing pain. *Experimental Brain Research, 67*(1), 153–162.

Büchel, C., & Dolan, R. J. (2000). Classical fear conditioning in functional neuroimaging. *Current Opinion in Neurobiology, 10*(2), 219–223.

Bushnell, M. C., Čeko, M., & Low, L. A. (2013). Cognitive and emotional control of pain and its disruption in chronic pain. *Nature Reviews Neuroscience, 14*(7), 502–511.

Campbell, L. C., Clauw, D. J., & Keefe, F. J. (2003). Persistent pain and depression: a biopsychosocial perspective. *Biological Psychiatry, 54*(3), 399–409. http://dx.doi.org/10.1016/s0006-3223(03)00545-6.

Campbell, J. N., & Meyer, R. A. (2006). Mechanisms of neuropathic pain. *Neuron, 52*(1), 77–92.

Craig, A. D. (2003). A new view of pain as a homeostatic emotion. *Trends in Neurosciences, 26*(6), 303–307.

Eccleston, C., & Crombez, G. (1999). Pain demands attention: a cognitive-affective model of the interruptive function of pain. *Psychological Bulletin, 125,* 356–366.

Eippert, F., Bingel, U., Schoell, E. D., Yacubian, J., Klinger, R., Lorenz, J., et al. (2009). Activation of the opioidergic descending pain control system underlies placebo analgesia. *Neuron, 63*(4), 533–543.

Ekman, P. (1992). An argument for basic emotions. *Cognition and Emotion, 6,* 169–200.

Ekman, P., & Friesen, W.-V. (1975). *Unmasking the face: A guide to recognizing emotions from facial clues.* Englewood Cliffs, NJ: Prentice Hall.

Ekman, P., Friesen, W. V., O'Sullivan, M., Chan, A., Diacoyanni-Tarlatzis, I., Heider, K., et al. (1987). Universals and cultural differences in the judgments of facial expressions of emotion. *Journal of Personality and Social Psychology, 53*(4), 712.

Fields, H. L. (2004). State-dependent opioid control of pain. *Nature Reviews Neuroscience, 5*(7), 565–575. http://dx.doi.org/10.1038/nrn1431.

Fields, H. L., & Basbaum, A. I. (1994). Central nervous system mechanisms of pain modulation. In P. D. Wall, & R. Melzack (Eds.), *Textbook of pain* (pp. 243–257). New York: Churchill Livingston.

Forkmann, K., Wiech, K., Ritter, C., Sommer, T., Rose, M., & Bingel, U. (2013). Pain-specific modulation of hippocampal activity and functional connectivity during visual encoding. *The Journal of Neuroscience, 33*(6), 2571–2581.

Fullana, M. A., Harrison, B. J., Soriano-Mas, C., Vervliet, B., Cardoner, N., Àvila-Parcet, A., et al. (2015). Neural signatures of human fear conditioning: an updated and extended meta-analysis of fMRI studies. *Molecular Psychiatry.*

Gerdes, A. B. M., Wieser, M. J., Alpers, G. W., Strack, F., & Pauli, P. (2012). Why do you smile at me while I'm in pain? – pain selectively modulates voluntary facial muscle responses to happy faces. *International Journal of Psychophysiology, 85,* 161–167.

Gerdes, A. B. M., Wieser, M. J., Mühlberger, A., Weyers, P., Alpers, G. W., Plichta, M., et al. (2010). Brain activations to emotional pictures are differentially associated with valence and arousal ratings. *Frontiers in Human Neuroscience, 4,* 175. http://dx.doi.org/10.3389/fnhum.2010.00175.

Godinho, F., Faillenot, I., Perchet, C., Frot, M., Magnin, M., & Garcia-Larrea, L. (2012). How the pain of others enhances our pain: searching the cerebral correlates of 'compassional hyperalgesia'. *European Journal of Pain, 16*(5), 748–759.

Godinho, F., Frot, M., Perchet, C., Magnin, M., & Garcia-Larrea, L. (2008). Pain influences hedonic assessment of visual inputs. *European Journal of Neuroscience, 27*(9), 2219–2228.

Gross, J. J. (2002). Emotion regulation: affective, cognitive, and social consequences. *Psychophysiology, 39*(3), 281–291.

Haggard, P., Iannetti, G. D., & Longo, M. R. (2013). Spatial sensory organization and body representation in pain perception. *Current Biology, 23*(4), R164–R176.

Iannetti, G. D., & Mouraux, A. (2010). From the neuromatrix to the pain matrix (and back). *Experimental Brain Research, 205*(1), 1–12. http://dx.doi.org/10.1007/s00221-010-2340-1.

Iannetti, G. D., Salomons, T. V., Moayedi, M., Mouraux, A., & Davis, K. D. (2013). Beyond metaphor: contrasting mechanisms of social and physical pain. *Trends in Cognitive Sciences, 17*(8), 371–378.

Iannetti, G. D., Zambreanu, L., Cruccu, G., & Tracey, I. (2005). Operculoinsular cortex encodes pain intensity at the earliest stages of cortical processing as indicated by amplitude of laser-evoked potentials in humans. *Neuroscience, 131*(1), 199–208.

International Association for the Study of Pain. (1994). Pain terms: a current list with definitions and notes on usage. In H. Merskey, & N. Bogduk (Eds.), *Classification of chronic pain: Descriptions of chronic pain syndromes and definitions of pain terms* (2nd ed.). Seattle: IASP-Press.

Jackson, P. L., Brunet, E., Meltzoff, A. N., & Decety, J. (2006). Empathy examined through the neural mechanisms involved in imagining how I feel versus how you feel pain. *Neuropsychologia, 44*(5), 752–761.

Jackson, P. L., Meltzoff, A. N., & Decety, J. (2005). How do we perceive the pain of others? A window into the neural processes involved in empathy. *Neuroimage, 24*(3), 771–779.

Jackson, P. L., Rainville, P., & Decety, J. (2006). To what extent do we share the pain of others? Insight from the neural bases of pain empathy. *Pain, 125*(1–2), 5–9.

Kenntner-Mabiala, R., Andreatta, M., Wieser, M. J., Mühlberger, A., & Pauli, P. (2008). Distinct effects of attention and affect on pain perception and somatosensory evoked potentials. *Biological Psychology, 78*(1), 114–122.

Kenntner-Mabiala, R., & Pauli, P. (2005). Affective modulation of brain potentials to painful and non-painful stimuli. *Psychophysiology, 42*, 559–567.

Kenntner-Mabiala, R., Weyers, P., & Pauli, P. (2007). Independent effects of emotion and attention on sensory and affective pain perception. *Cognition and Emotion, 21*(8), 1615–1629.

Kwon, M., Altin, M., Duenas, H., & Alev, L. (2014). The role of descending inhibitory pathways on chronic pain modulation and clinical implications. *Pain Practice, 14*(7), 656–667.

Lang, P. J. (1995). The emotion probe: studies of motivation and attention. *American Psychologist, 50*(5), 372–385.

Lang, P. J. (2010). Emotion and motivation: toward consensus definitions and a common research purpose. *Emotion Review, 2*(3), 229–233.

Lang, P. J., & Bradley, M. M. (2010). Emotion and the motivational brain. *Biological Psychology, 84*(3), 437–450.

Lang, P. J., Bradley, M. M., & Cuthbert, B. N. (2008). *International affective picture system (IAPS): Affective ratings of pictures and instruction manual.* Technical Report A-8. Gainesville, FL: University of Florida.

Lang, P. J., Bradley, M. M., Fitzsimmons, J. R., Cuthbert, B. N., Scott, J. D., Moulder, B., et al. (1998). Emotional arousal and activation of the visual cortex: an fMRI analysis. *Psychophysiology, 35*(2), 199–210.

Lapate, R. C., Lee, H., Salomons, T. V., van Reekum, C. M., Greischar, L. L., & Davidson, R. J. (2012). Amygdalar function reflects common individual differences in emotion and pain regulation success. *Journal of Cognitive Neuroscience, 24*(1), 148–158.

LeDoux, J. E. (1996). *The emotional brain: The mysterious underpinnings of emotional life.* New York, NY: Simon & Schuster.

LeDoux, J. E. (1998). Fear and the brain: where have we been, and where are we going? *Biological Psychiatry, 44*(12), 1229–1238.

Legrain, V., Iannetti, G. D., Plaghki, L., & Mouraux, A. (2011). The pain matrix reloaded: a salience detection system for the body. *Progress in Neurobiology, 93*(1), 111–124.

Leknes, S., Berna, C., Lee, M. C., Snyder, G. D., Biele, G., & Tracey, I. (2013). The importance of context: when relative relief renders pain pleasant. *Pain, 154*(3), 402–410.

Lewkowski, M. D., Ditto, B., Roussos, M., & Young, S. N. (2003). Sweet taste and blood pressure-related analgesia. *Pain, 106*(1), 181–186.

Lindquist, K. A., Wager, T. D., Kober, H., Bliss-Moreau, E., & Barrett, L. F. (2012). The brain basis of emotion: a meta-analytic review. *Behavioral and Brain Sciences, 35*(03), 121–143.

Loggia, M. L., Mogil, J. S., & Bushnell, M. C. (2008). Experimentally induced mood changes preferentially affect pain unpleasantness. *The Journal of Pain, 9*(9), 784–791. http://dx.doi.org/10.1016/j.jpain.2008.03.014.

Mailhot, J.-P., Vachon-Presseau, E., Jackson, P. L., & Rainville, P. (2012). Dispositional empathy modulates vicarious effects of dynamic pain expressions on spinal nociception, facial responses and acute pain. *European Journal of Neuroscience, 35*(2), 271–278.

Mason, P. (2012). Medullary circuits for nociceptive modulation. *Current Opinion in Neurobiology, 22*(4), 640–645. http://dx.doi.org/10.1016/j.conb.2012.03.008.

Meagher, M. W., Arnau, R. C., & Rhudy, J. L. (2001). Pain and emotion: effects of affective picture modulation. *Psychosomatic Medicine, 63*(1), 79–90.

Melzack, R. (1999). From the gate to the neuromatrix. *Pain, 82*, S121–S126.

Melzack, R. (2001). Pain and the neuromatrix in the brain. *Journal of Dental Education, 65*(12), 1378–1382.

Millan, M. J. (1999). The induction of pain: an integrative review. *Progress in Neurobiology, 57*(1), 1–164.

Millan, M. J. (2002). Descending control of pain. *Progress in Neurobiology, 66*(6), 355–474.

Morris, J. S., Friston, K. J., Buechel, C., Frith, C. D., Young, A. W., Calder, A. J., et al. (1998). A neuromodulatory role for the human amygdala in processing emotional facial expressions. *Brain, 121*(1), 47–57.

Murphy, F., Nimmo-Smith, I., & Lawrence, A. (2003). Functional neuroanatomy of emotions: a meta-analysis. *Cognitive, Affective, & Behavioral Neuroscience, 3*(3), 207–233. http://dx.doi.org/10.3758/cabn.3.3.207.

Ossipov, M. H., Dussor, G. O., & Porreca, F. (2010). Central modulation of pain. *Journal of Clinical Investigation, 120*(11), 3779–3787.

Panksepp, J. (1998). *Affective neuroscience: The foundations of human and animal emotions.* New York, NY: Oxford University Press.

Panksepp, J., & Watt, D. (2011). What is basic about basic emotions? Lasting lessons from affective neuroscience. *Emotion Review, 3*(4), 387–396. http://dx.doi.org/10.1177/1754073911410741.

Pauli, P., Wiedemann, G., & Nickola, M. (1999a). Pain sensitivity, cerebral laterality, and negative affect. *Pain, 80*(1–2), 359–364. http://dx.doi.org/10.1016/s0304-3959(98)00231-0.

Pauli, P., Wiedemann, G., & Nickola, M. (1999b). Pressure pain thresholds asymmetry in left- and right-handers: associations with behavioural measures of cerebral laterality. *European Journal of Pain, 3*(2), 151–156. http://dx.doi.org/10.1053/eujp.1999.0108.

Peyron, R., Laurent, B., & Garcia-Larrea, L. (2000). Functional imaging of brain responses to pain. A review and meta-analysis (2000). *Neurophysiologie Clinique, 30*(5), 263–288.

Phan, K. L., Wager, T., Taylor, S. F., & Liberzon, I. (2002). Functional neuroanatomy of emotion: a meta-analysis of emotion activation studies in PET and fMRI. *Neuroimage, 16*(2), 331–348.

Ploner, M., Bingel, U., & Wiech, K. (2015). Towards a taxonomy of pain modulations. *Trends in Cognitive Sciences, 19*(4), 180–182. http://dx.doi.org/10.1016/j.tics.2015.02.007.

Ploner, M., Gross, J., Timmermann, L., & Schnitzler, A. (2002). Cortical representation of first and second pain sensation in humans. *Proceedings of the National Academy of Sciences, 99*(19), 12444–12448.

Ploner, M., Holthusen, H., Noetges, P., & Schnitzler, A. (2002). Cortical representation of venous nociception in humans. *Journal of Neurophysiology, 88*(1), 300–305.

Preston, S. D., & de Waal, F. B. (February 2002). Empathy: its ultimate and proximate bases. *Behavioral and Brain Sciences, 25*(1), 1–20.

Price, D. D. (1999). *Psychological mechanisms of pain and analgesia.* Seattle, WA: IASP Press.

Price, D. D. (2000). Psychological and neural mechanisms of the affective dimension of pain. *Science, 288,* 1769–1772.

Rainville, P., Duncan, G. H., Price, D. D., Carrier, B., & Bushnell, M. C. (1997). Pain affect encoded in human anterior cingulate but not somatosensory cortex. *Science, 277*(5328), 968–971.

Reicherts, P., Gerdes, A. B., Pauli, P., & Wieser, M. J. (2013). On the mutual effects of pain and emotion: facial pain expressions enhance pain perception and vice versa are perceived as more arousing when feeling pain. *Pain, 154*(6), 793–800.

Rhudy, J. L., & Meagher, M. W. (2000). Fear and anxiety: divergent effects on human pain thresholds. *Pain, 84*(1), 65–75.

Rhudy, J. L., & Meagher, M. W. (2001). The role of emotion in pain modulation. *Current Opinion in Psychiatry, 14,* 241–245.

Rhudy, J. L., Williams, A. E., McCabe, K. M., Nguyen, M., & Rambo, P. (2005). Affective modulation of nociception at spinal and supraspinal levels. *Psychophysiology, 42*(5), 579–587.

Rhudy, J. L., Williams, A. E., McCabe, K. M., Russell, J. L., & Maynard, L. J. (2008). Emotional control of nociceptive reactions (ECON): do affective valence and arousal play a role? *Pain, 136*(3), 250–261.

Ringkamp, M., & Meyer, R. (2008). Physiology of nociceptors. In T. A, R. H. Masland, T. D. Albright, R. H. Masland, P. Dallos, D. Oertel, et al. (Eds.), *The senses: A comprehensive reference.* New York: Academic Press.

Roy, M. (2015). Cerebral and spinal modulation of pain by emotions and attention. *Pain, Emotion and Cognition,* 35–52. Springer.

Roy, M., Lebuis, A., Hugueville, L., Peretz, I., & Rainville, P. (2012). Spinal modulation of nociception by music. *European Journal of Pain, 16*(6), 870–877.

Roy, M., Lebuis, A., Peretz, I., & Rainville, P. (2011). The modulation of pain by attention and emotion: a dissociation of perceptual and spinal nociceptive processes. *European Journal of Pain, 15*(6), 641.e1–641.e10.

Roy, M., Peretz, I., & Rainville, P. (2008). Emotional valence contributes to music-induced analgesia. *Pain, 134*(1), 140–147.

Roy, M., Piché, M., Chen, J.-I., Peretz, I., & Rainville, P. (2009). Cerebral and spinal modulation of pain by emotions. *Proceedings of the National Academy of Sciences, 106*(49), 20900–20905. http://dx.doi.org/10.1073/pnas.0904706106.

Roy, M., Shohamy, D., & Wager, T. D. (2012). Ventromedial prefrontal-subcortical systems and the generation of affective meaning. *Trends in Cognitive Sciences, 16*(3), 147–156.

Sabatinelli, D., Fortune, E. E., Li, Q., Siddiqui, A., Krafft, C., Oliver, W. T., et al. (2011). Emotional perception: meta-analyses of face and natural scene processing. *Neuroimage, 54*(3), 2524–2533.

Sander, D. (2013). Models of emotion: the affective neuroscience approach. In J. L. Armony, & P. Vuilleumier (Eds.), *The Cambridge handbook of human affective neuroscience* (pp. 5–56). Cambridge: Cambridge University Press.

Sandrini, G., Serrao, M., Rossi, P., Romaniello, A., Cruccu, G., & Willer, J. C. (2005). The lower limb flexion reflex in humans. *Progress in Neurobiology, 77*(6), 353–395.

Schupp, H. T., Cuthbert, B. N., Bradley, M. M., Birbaumer, N., & Lang, P. J. (1997). Probe P3 and blinks: two measures of affective startle modulation. *Psychophysiology, 34*(1), 1–6.

Seminowicz, D. A., & Davis, K. D. (2006). Cortical responses to pain in healthy individuals depends on pain catastrophizing. *Pain, 120*(3), 297–306.

Senkowski, D., Kautz, J., Hauck, M., Zimmermann, R., & Engel, A. K. (2011). Emotional facial expressions modulate pain-induced beta and gamma oscillations in sensorimotor cortex. *The Journal of Neuroscience, 31*(41), 14542–14550.

Shackman, A. J., Salomons, T. V., Slagter, H. A., Fox, A. S., Winter, J. J., & Davidson, R. J. (2011). The integration of negative affect, pain and cognitive control in the cingulate cortex. *Nature Reviews Neuroscience, 12*(3), 154–167.

Simons, L. E., Moulton, E. A., Linnman, C., Carpino, E., Becerra, L., & Borsook, D. (2014). The human amygdala and pain: evidence from neuroimaging. *Human Brain Mapping, 35*(2), 527–538. http://dx.doi.org/10.1002/hbm.22199.

Tiemann, L., Schulz, E., Gross, J., & Ploner, M. (2010). Gamma oscillations as a neuronal correlate of the attentional effects of pain. *Pain, 150*(2), 302–308.

Timmermann, L., Ploner, M., Haucke, K., Schmitz, F., Baltissen, R., & Schnitzler, A. (2001). Differential coding of pain intensity in the human primary and secondary somatosensory cortex. *Journal of Neurophysiology, 86*(3), 1499–1503.

Tracey, I., & Mantyh, P. W. (2007). The cerebral signature for pain perception and its modulation. *Neuron, 55*(3), 377–391.

Tran, T. D., Inui, K., Hoshiyama, M., Lam, K., Qiu, Y., & Kakigi, R. (2002). Cerebral activation by the signals ascending through unmyelinated C-fibers in humans: a magnetoencephalographic study. *Neuroscience, 113*(2), 375–386.

Treede, R. D., Meier, W., Kunze, K., & Bromm, B. (1988). Ultralate cerebral potentials as correlates of delayed pain perception: observation in a case of neurosyphilis. *Journal of Neurology, Neurosurgery & Psychiatry, 51*(10), 1330–1333.

Vachon-Presseau, E., Martel, M. O., Roy, M., Caron, E., Jackson, P. L., & Rainville, P. (2011). The multilevel organization of vicarious pain responses: effects of pain cues and empathy traits on spinal nociception and acute pain. *Pain, 152*(7), 1525–1531.

Vachon-Presseau, E., Roy, M., Martel, M. O., Albouy, G., Chen, J., Budell, L., et al. (2012). Neural processing of sensory and emotional-communicative information associated with the perception of vicarious pain. *Neuroimage, 63*(1), 54–62.

Vachon-Presseau, E., Roy, M., Martel, M.-O., Albouy, G., Sullivan, M. J., Jackson, P. L., et al. (2013). The two sides of pain communication: effects of pain expressiveness on vicarious brain responses revealed in chronic back pain patients. *The Journal of Pain, 14*(11), 1407–1415.

Villemure, C., & Bushnell, M. C. (2009). Mood influences supraspinal pain processing separately from attention. *Journal of Neuroscience, 29*(3), 705–715. http://dx.doi.org/10.1523/jneurosci.3822-08.2009.

Villemure, C., Slotnick, B. M., & Bushnell, M. C. (2003). Effects of odors on pain perception: deciphering the roles of emotion and attention. *Pain, 106*(1–2), 101–108.

Vogt, B. A. (2005). Pain and emotion interactions in subregions of the cingulate gyrus. *Nature Reviews Neuroscience, 6*(7), 533–544.

Von Leupoldt, A., Mertz, C., Kegat, S., Burmester, S., & Dahme, B. (2006). The impact of emotions on the sensory and affective dimension of perceived dyspnea. *Psychophysiology, 43*(4), 382–386.

Von Leupoldt, A., Vovk, A., Bradley, M. M., Keil, A., Lang, P. J., & Davenport, P. W. (2010). The impact of emotion on respiratory - related evoked potentials. *Psychophysiology, 47*(3), 579–586.

Wager, T. D., & Atlas, L. Y. (2013). How is pain influenced by cognition? neuroimaging weighs. *Perspectives on Psychological Science, 8*(1), 91–97.

Wager, T. D., Atlas, L. Y., Lindquist, M. A., Roy, M., Woo, C.-W., & Kross, E. (2013). An fMRI-based neurologic signature of physical pain. *New England Journal of Medicine, 368*(15), 1388–1397.

Weisenberg, M., Raz, T., & Hener, T. (1998). The influence of film-induced mood on pain perception. *Pain, 76*(3), 365–375.

Weyers, P., Mühlberger, A., Hefele, C., & Pauli, P. (2006). Electromyographic responses to static and dynamic avatar emotional facial expressions. *Psychophysiology, 43*(5), 450–453.

Wicker, B., Keysers, C., Plailly, J., Royet, J. P., Gallese, V., & Rizzolatti, G. (2003). Both of us disgusted in my insula: the common neural basis of seeing and feeling disgust. *Neuron, 40*(3), 655–664.

Wiech, K., & Tracey, I. (2009). The influence of negative emotions on pain: behavioral effects and neural mechanisms. *Neuroimage, 47*(3), 987–994.

Wieser, M. J., Gerdes, A. B. M., Greiner, R., Reicherts, P., & Pauli, P. (2012). Tonic pain grabs attention, but leaves the processing of facial expressions intact-Evidence from event-related brain potentials. *Biological Psychology, 90*(3), 242–248.

Wieser, M. J., Gerdes, A. B. M., Reicherts, P., & Pauli, P. (2014). Mutual influences of pain and emotional face processing. *Frontiers in Psychology, 5.*

Williams, A. C. d. C. (2002). Facial expression of pain: an evolutionary account. *Behavioral and Brain Sciences, 25*, 439–488.

Woo, C. W., Roy, M., Buhle, J. T., & Wager, T. D. (2015). Distinct brain systems mediate the effects of nociceptive input and self-regulation on pain. *PLoS Biology, 13*(1), e1002036.

Wundt, W. (1905). *Grundriss der Psychologie (Fundamentals of psychology)* (7th rev. ed.). Leipzig: Engelman.

Yilmaz, P., Diers, M., Diener, S., Rance, M., Wessa, M., & Flor, H. (2010). Brain correlates of stress-induced analgesia. *Pain, 151*(2), 522–529.

Yoshino, A., Okamoto, Y., Onoda, K., Shishida, K., Yoshimura, S., Kunisato, Y., et al. (2012). Sadness enhances the experience of pain and affects pain-evoked cortical activities: an MEG study. *The Journal of Pain, 13*(7), 628–635.

Yoshino, A., Okamoto, Y., Onoda, K., Yoshimura, S., Kunisato, Y., Demoto, Y., et al. (2010). Sadness enhances the experience of pain via neural activation in the anterior cingulate cortex and amygdala: an fMRI study. *Neuroimage, 50*(3), 1194–1201.

Zelman, D. C., Howland, E. W., Nichols, S. N., & Cleeland, C. S. (1991). The effects of induced mood on laboratory pain. *Pain, 46*(1), 105–111.

CHAPTER 2

The Neurobiology of Stress

Robert Murison
Department of Biological and Medical Psychology, University of Bergen, Bergen, Norway

THE STRESS CONCEPT

Attempts to define "stress" to everyone's satisfaction have remained elusive. In the vernacular, stress has become a negatively loaded term. Furthermore, the word is used to describe both a stimulus (more properly called a stressor) and a response, inevitably leading to circularity. If a stimulus produces a stress response, it must be a stressor. If it does not, it is not. The focus of this chapter is the neurobiology of the *stress response* and its ramifications, with some introductory remarks on what may constitute a *stressor*. The reader is referred to a number of historical discussions of the stress concept (Cannon, 1932; Lazarus, 1993; Selye, 1946, 1956). Others have argued that stress is no more or less than a general activation that becomes harmful only if sustained (e.g., Levine & Ursin, 1991). A more cognitively focused theory is provided by Ursin and Eriksen (2010), and more biologically/ethologically based approaches are provided by Koolhaas et al. (2011). For detailed coverage of the basic neuroendocrinology of stress, the reader is referred to Fink (2010).

For the purposes of this chapter, we take as our starting point the General Adaptation of Selye (1946) and the Fight–Flight Response of Cannon (1932). For Selye, the stress response is the nonspecific response of the body to any demand for change, thus explicitly linking stress to homeostasis. Although Selye's definition has been the subject of much discussion and criticism, it continues to serve as a useful starting point. It is important to note that Selye used the term "adaptation"; that is, the stress response has developed through evolution to be adaptive and to further the survival of the individual and the species. It is not a maladaptive response per se. See also Herman (2013).

Optimal functioning of the organism is dependent on the maintenance of a stable internal environment through homeostasis, which is ensured by the process of allostasis, the dynamic maintenance of stability through change (McEwen, 1998). The stress response contributes by allocating energy resources and initiating biological and behavioral processes that serve to reduce deviations from the optimal state. Homeostasis and allostasis come at a price, using energy resources, and the term allostatic load is

The Neuroscience of Pain, Stress, and Emotion
http://dx.doi.org/10.1016/B978-0-12-800538-5.00002-9

used to refer to the wear and tear imposed upon the body by allostatic processes. Sustained activation of the stress system or its inappropriate activation is both costly and deleterious at several levels, and appropriate termination of the response is essential to ensure that the catabolic, anti-reproductive, and immunosuppressive effects are limited. The optimal response to a stressor is rapid activation followed by rapid deactivation once the threat to homeostasis is no longer present. When the allostatic processes demand energy that is not immediately available, the body is under allostatic load (McEwen, 1998). Not dissimilar to the sustained activation theory of stress (Levine & Ursin, 1991), allostatic load is increased (1) when the organism fails to habituate to repeated presentations of homotypic stressors; (2) when it is exposed repeatedly to heterotypic stressors, without time to recover between; (3) when the response is inappropriately prolonged; and (4) when the response is inappropriately *not* activated, calling on other compensatory mechanisms (McEwen, 1998). Allostatic load of types 1, 2, and 3 are associated with chronically elevated levels of hypothalamopituitary–adrenocortical (HPA) activation and potential deleterious consequences.

The stress response occurs not only in response to what we typically interpret as negative stimuli and events (predation, threat, etc.), but also in response to what would typically be regarded as positive events but that require energy mobilization, for example, sexual behaviors (Koolhaas et al., 2011; Leuner, Glasper, & Gould, 2010).

THE STRESS STIMULUS

The environment (including both exogenous and endogenous milieux) presents the organism with several challenges—changes in temperature, the need to obtain food and water, the threat of attack by both conspecifics and predators, and the need to find a mate. To survive, flourish, and reproduce in the face of these and other challenges and the associated threat to homeostasis, the animal must mobilize energy. The stimulus may be internal or external, systemic (often not impinging on consciousness), or psychogenic (associated with anticipation of threat without an existing physiological insult). Herman and colleagues make the intuitively useful distinction between "reactive responses" primarily to internal stimuli (pain, homeostatic, and inflammatory signals) and "anticipatory responses" to external stimuli (predators, social challenges, etc.) as well as to memory programs (Herman et al., 2003).

For the purposes of pragmatism, any stimulus that elicits what is generally accepted as a biological stress response is regarded as a stressor. This must be so because it is impossible at the individual level to reliably predict which stimulus or set of stimuli will elicit the response. The stimulus must first be perceived and evaluated and processed at both subcortical and cortical levels before the stress response system(s) is activated or not. The elicitation (or not) of a stress response will depend on multiple factors, including stimulus intensity, valence, and other intrinsic properties, as well as learning processes, including habituation and sensitization, and early experience.

The process of identifying a stimulus as a threat or stressor will depend on both innate mechanisms and learning, and the interactions between these. Some stimuli are normally automatically interpreted by the brain as threatening and a stressor (e.g., the sight of a snake), while others will be perceived as nonthreatening (e.g., the sight of a flower) and these will be differentially susceptible to fear conditioning (Mineka & Ohman, 2002; Seligman, 1971). Superimposed on these "prepared" interpretations of stimuli will be conditioning and learning, which may lead the snake to be perceived as nonthreatening and the flower even as threatening. Perception and appraisal are therefore central to whether or not a stress response is mounted to any particular stimulus or set of stimuli.

Several psychological filtering mechanisms may modulate the interpretation of the stimulus, at least in humans. Distortions of stimulus expectancies—defense—involve denial of the threat content of the stimulus. Typically, individuals with high defense mechanisms show a low cortisol response to threat stimuli, but a high and prolonged sympathetic response (Eriksen, Olff, Murison, & Ursin, 1999).

Studies of the fear circuitry of the brain have contributed to our understanding of perception and interpretation of a stimulus as threatening or not. Based on studies of fear conditioning in animals (Phelps & LeDoux, 2005), it is accepted that stimuli (visual, auditory, somatic—including pain and gustatory) are analyzed at several neural levels in a hierarchical fashion. Visual and auditory psychogenic stimuli are first processed at the thalamic level (lateral geniculate and medial geniculate nuclei, respectively) before information is relayed through two pathways. Low-level analysis of the stimulus occurs in the amygdala, a central structure in the mediation of the stress response both for stimulus processing and for mounting the endocrine and autonomic motor responses from other brain areas. The thalamoamygdala pathway represents a shortcut, providing only undetailed information, without filtering by consciousness and higher cognitive functions, and represents an evolutionarily primitive pathway. A second, but slower, pathway involves reciprocal thalamocorticoamygdala projections, which provide higher level processing.

The lateral amygdala (LA) is regarded as the sensory input gateway, receiving information from both the thalamus and the cortical areas, including polysensory areas and the prefrontal cortex (PFC). By inhibiting the amygdala output, the infralimbic subregion of the PFC plays a role in extinction of fear. These influences on the LA allow for higher order cognitive processes such as emotion, imagination, and rumination to influence amygdala function and subsequent endocrine and autonomic output from the motor response systems. The LA and the basal nucleus of the amygdala (B) also receive projections from the hippocampus providing information about stimulus context. Stress responses and fear expression responses are thus modulated by the PFC via LA, B, and intercalated cells of the amygdala (Herman et al., 2003; Tsigos & Chrousos, 2002).

THE STRESS RESPONSE

The biological stress response has become well described although much remains to be discovered. Traditionally the stress responses system comprises two arms—the HPA axis and the sympathetic nervous system (SNS), including the sympathoadrenal–medullary (SAM) axis (see Figure 1). Both arms are influenced by the amygdala and the hypothalamus. The first and fastest acting part of the response is SNS activation, largely equivalent to the fight–flight response of Cannon and the initial stage of Selye's alarm response. The HPA axis is slower to respond in terms of endocrine output.

While the LA acts as the input station of the amygdala, the central nucleus (CE) acts as the main output station, mediating behavioral and autonomic expressions of fear, as well as autonomic and endocrine stress responses by downstream indirect connections to the hypothalamus, to the central gray area, and to the dorsal motor nucleus of the vagus (Rodrigues, LeDoux, & Sapolsky, 2009). There are few direct connections between the LA and the CE. Rather, the information is processed in the B and then projected to the CE. The B also projects to the striatum, mediating behavioral instrumental responses such as avoidance and escape, which are central to coping with the stressor.

MAJOR PATHWAYS OF THE TWO ARMS OF THE STRESS
RESPONSE

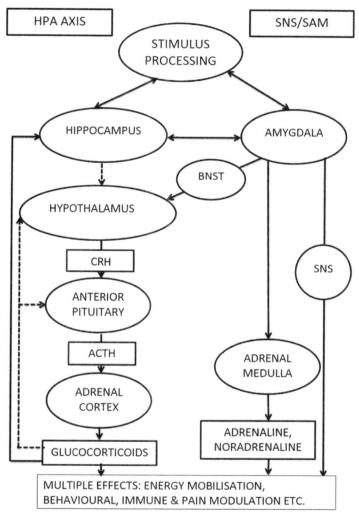

Figure 1 Schematic overview of the two major arms of the stress response system. ACTH, adrenocorticotropic hormone; BNST, bed nucleus of the stria terminalis; CRH, corticotropin-releasing hormone; HPA axis, hypothalamopituitary–adrenal axis; SAM, sympathoadrenal–medullary system; SNS, sympathetic nervous system. Inhibitory pathways are represented by dashed lines.

SNS and the SAM Axis

The SNS influences the cardiovascular system, the gastrointestinal (GI) tract, respiration, renal, endocrine, and other systems, while the parasympathetic nervous system contributes by "withdrawing" and inhibiting the SNS. The SNS response is mediated by the locus coeruleus (LC)/ noradrenergic system, comprising the noradrenergic cells of the medulla and pons. The CE projects to the brain stem to increase noradrenaline (NA) release from sympathetic nerve endings, sympathetic activation, and activation of the adrenal medulla, resulting in increased adrenaline and NA levels, arousal, and vigilance, that is, enhanced processing of external cues. The SAM system releases catecholamines (mostly adrenaline) into the bloodstream while the SNS with cholinergic preganglionic fibers releases NA from postganglionic axons. SNS innervation of peripheral organs is mediated by efferent preganglionic fibers, with cell bodies in the intermediolateral column of the spinal cord. These synapse in the sympathetic ganglia with postganglionic neurons, which innervate the vascular smooth muscle, heart, skeletal muscles, gut, kidney, fat, etc. Blood pressure and heart rate are elevated and energy resources are diverted to the musculature and away from vegetative functions.

At the same time, the hypothalamus is activated by the amygdala (largely indirectly; Herman et al., 2003) to release corticotropin-releasing hormone (CRH), and HPA activation ensues. Thus the two arms of the stress response system are both closely connected with amygdala and brain-stem function. Through its projections to the amygdala, the SNS enhances long-term storage of aversive emotional memories in the hippocampus and striatum. Noradrenergic responses to stressors may be modulated by higher centers such as the mesocortical/mesolimbic systems (influencing affect and anticipation); the amygdala and hippocampus, modulating the stress output (initiation, propagation, and termination of the response); and the arcuate nucleus, modulating pain.

The HPA Response

CRH is secreted from cells of the medial parvocellular division of the paraventricular nucleus (PVN) of the hypothalamus into the hypophyseal portal system and acts on CRH receptors in the anterior pituitary to release adrenocorticotropic hormone (ACTH) into the systemic circulation. CRH and its receptors are found also in extrahypothalamic structures, including limbic areas and the arousal systems of the LC and spinal cord, as well as in several peripheral tissues—adrenal medulla, heart, prostate, gut, liver, kidney, and testes. CRH receptors comprise two subtypes—CRH-R1, the most abundant in the anterior pituitary but also found throughout the brain, and CRH-R2, found in both peripheral tissues and subcortical brain areas.

ACTH is, together with α-MSH (melanocyte-stimulating hormone) and the endogenous opioids β-endorphin and encephalin, a product of cleavage of the proopiomelanocortin (POMC) molecule. Vasopressin (AVP) may synergistically interact with the CRH system to activate the anterior pituitary, although, by itself, AVP has little corticotropic action (Tsigos & Chrousos, 2002).

There are few direct projections between the amygdala and the PVN. Rather, amygdala influence over HPA activity is mediated by projections of the amygdala to the bed nucleus of the stria terminalis. Additionally, the PVN is influenced by input from the nucleus of the solitary tract, the Raphé nuclei, the subfornical organ, the thalamus, other hypothalamic areas (dorsomedial nucleus, medial preoptic area, lateral hypothalamic area, arcuate nucleus, etc.), the hippocampus, the PFC, and the lateral septum. Thus responses to both psychogenic and systemic stressors are mediated by brain-stem structures, allowing for an integrated response (Herman et al., 2003).

Circulating ACTH from the anterior pituitary leads to secretion from the adrenal cortex of glucocorticoid (GC) hormones, including cortisol and corticosterone. ACTH also stimulates release from the adrenal cortex of the neurosteroid dehydroepiandrosterone, a precursor for testosterone and dihydrotestosterone.

The HPA and SNS arms interact. NA and CRH stimulate each other, partly through α-1-NA receptors, and both systems are self-regulating through autoregulatory feedback loops. Both systems are regulated by the same central neurotransmitter systems and both are stimulated by serotonin and acetylcholine. Negative feedback systems involve GCs, *gamma*-aminobutyric acid (GABA), ACTH, and opioid peptides. NA-stimulated glycogenolysis is facilitated by GCs, being just one example of the interdependence of the HPA and SAM systems. In addition to facilitating energy mobilization, the HPA axis functions to inhibit the sympathetic and adrenomedullary systems and to terminate the immediate defense response, while promoting behavioral adaptation (de Kloet & Joëls, 2013; Munck, Guyre, & Holbrook, 1984).

GCs stimulate the release of stored energy (gluconeogenesis) by glycogenolysis, lipolysis, and proteolysis and act on several, if not most, organ systems, including the brain, the immune system, and the reproductive endocrine system. GC effects are exerted at cytoplasmic receptors but also have membrane effects via endocanniboid mobilization (de Kloet & Joëls, 2013). Activated cytoplasmic receptors migrate to the cell nucleus where they interact with DNA to activate specific hormone-response genes, also inhibiting other transcription factors including NF-κB, which are positive regulators of genes involved in the activation and growth of immune cells, among others (Tsigos & Chrousos, 2002).

GCs act on two nuclear receptors, high-affinity mineralocorticoid receptors (MRs) and low-affinity GC receptors (GRs). The levels of circulating GCs activate these receptors differentially, with resting levels stimulating primarily MRs and high levels stimulating GRs and MRs. This differential activation forms the basis of the inverted U-shaped curve relating GC levels to cognitive performance and organismic function (Herbert et al., 2006). Poor performance is associated with moderate activation of the MRs and no activation of GRs, as well as with high activations of both. Performance is enhanced when most of the MRs and some of the GRs are activated (de Kloet & Joëls, 2013).

Because the GCs are relatively accessible to measurement in blood, urine, saliva, hair, and feces and because they are relatively stable, they are commonly used indices of the stress response, particularly in field and clinical settings. Measurement of the sympathetic arm and SAM is less straightforward because of the rapidity of the response. Peak serum levels of cortisol are generally found at 15–20 min after the HPA system is activated, allowing a reasonable time for sampling, in contrast to ACTH and sympathetic activation, with rise times of seconds and less stability (Eriksen et al., 1999). GC levels in other tissues and body fluids have different rise times, which need to be taken into account in laboratory or field studies. The development of assays for GCs in hair is particularly useful for estimating long-term output of the axis (Stalder & Kirschbaum, 2012). Noninvasive measures in animal laboratory and field studies, primarily in feces, are increasingly used, avoiding the complications of handling and anesthesia (Lane, 2006; Rehbinder & Hau, 2006).

Interpretation of GC levels must take into account that much (c. 95%) of the GCs secreted from the adrenal cortex are bound to corticosteroid-binding globulin (CBG; transcortin) (Henley & Lightman, 2011). Thus only about 5% of secreted GCs are available for acting on tissue receptors. CBG levels may themselves be affected by stress. Some stressors in animals (e.g., inescapable shock and chronic social stress) downregulate levels of CBG, increasing free levels of GCs available to the tissues (e.g., Fleshner et al., 1995; Spencer et al., 1996). CBG also binds pro-gesterone, and women on oral contraceptives have elevated levels, lower salivary cortisol levels, and higher total cortisol levels following the Trier Social Stress Test (Kumsta, Entringer, Hellhammer, & Wüst, 2007). The choice of measurement (free, bound, or total GC) will depend on whether the experimenter is concerned with total output of the HPA axis or only the biologically active component.

In nonstressful situations, CRH and AVP are secreted in a pulsatile fashion with a circadian pattern generated by inputs from the suprachias-matic nucleus (Lightman et al., 2008; Walker, Terry, & Lightman, 2010). Pulsatile activity increases in the early hours of the active cycle, manifest in increased GC levels in the early morning in humans (the opposite in nocturnal species), and a fall through the day, reaching a nadir in the evening. The cycle is affected by factors such as light and feeding schedules, with light being the most potent zeitgeber, and by stressors.

The output of the HPA system is modulated by several factors, including AVP of magnocellular origin, cytokines, inflammatory mediators, and angiotensin II. Furthermore, although adrenocortical secretion of cortisol is primarily under the influence of ACTH, the adrenal cortex also receives innervation from the autonomic nervous system.

STRESS RESPONSE INTERACTIONS WITH OTHER SYSTEMS
Immune System

Cytokines and other humoral mediators of the immune system are potent activators of the stress response and the inflammatory cytokines tumor necrosis factor-α (TNF-α), interleukin (IL)-1β, and IL-6 stimulate the HPA axis. Because these are too large to cross the blood–brain barrier, several mechanisms have been suggested to explain how this is mediated. These include vagal stimulation, penetration of the brain at areas lacking a blood–brain barrier (the circumventricular organs, such as the median eminence, the organum vasculosum laminae terminalis, or the area postrema), selective active transport into the brain, stimulation of peripheral tissues whose products can penetrate the blood–brain barrier (e.g., endothelial cells), or infiltration of the brain by immune cells (Dunn, 2006).

In the opposite direction the HPA has primarily inhibitory effects on the immune system. However, the effects of stress on immune function depend on duration, intensity, and choice of measure. The well-known immu-nosuppressive effects of high levels of GCs are manifest in altered traffic and function of immune cells, reduced cytokine levels and mediators of inflammation, lower effects of these at target organs, and increased synthesis of anti-inflammatory agents (lipocortin 1, IL-10, IL-1 receptor antagonist; Mawdsley & Rampton, 2005). And chronic sustained stress, in for example depression or bereavement, is associated with impaired immune response as well as sustained high levels of GCs (Irwin, Daniels, & Weiner, 1987). At lower levels, however, GCs may have an immune-stimulatory effect, temporarily increasing production of the proinflammatory cytokines IL-6 and TNF-α (Mawdsley & Rampton, 2005). Acute and experimental stress is associated with immune enhancement, with increased levels of proinflammatory cytokines (Maes et al., 1998), similar to the effects of adrenal infusion (Sondergaard, Ostrowski, Ullum, & Pedersen, 2000).

Sympathetic innervation of the lymphoid tissues, particularly the spleen, impinges on the immune response (Jänig, 2014) and may have immunosuppressive, anti-inflammatory, or immune-potentiating effects. This will in turn feed back to the central nervous system, affecting cytokine levels in the brain and sickness behaviors (Dantzer, 2005). Lymphocytes also carry receptors for products of the HPA axis (CRH and GCs), and CRH secreted at post-ganglionic SNS neurons at inflammatory sites has proinflammatory properties.

Reproduction

The stress response is associated with inhibition of the hypothalamogonadal system and reproductive behavior. CRH inhibits the actions of gonadotropin-releasing hormone neurons at the hypothalamic level, and GCs have inhibitory effects at the pituitary level (gonadotrophs) and at the gonads, also reducing sensitivity of the target tissues to sex steroids (Tsigos & Chrousos, 2002). Inflammatory stress also inhibits the reproductive system via cytokine-induced secretion of CRH and POMC-derived peptides.

Growth Hormone

Chronic elevation of GCs is associated with suppression of growth hormone (GH) and somatomedin C, but acute elevation of GH may be seen at stress onset or after acute administration of GCs. This effect may be mediated by activation of GC-responsive elements in the promoter region of the GH gene. GCs stimulate somatostatin at the hypothalamus, decrease production of thyroid-stimulating hormone, and inhibit the conversion of the relatively inactive thyroxin to active tri-iodothyronine (Tsigos & Chrousos, 2002).

Pain

Because stress–pain interactions are covered by others in this volume, only a brief overview will be given here. Stress response systems impinge on nociception in at least two ways. The first is via the SNS. Descending projections arising from noradrenergic and serotonergic neurons in the brain stem provide tonic control of spinal afferent projections in the dorsal horn, providing a stress-induced suppression of pain. The second pathway involves secretion of endogenous opioids that bind to afferent neurons, "on" and "off" cells in the brain stem, and cortical and subcortical neurons (Schlereth & Birklein, 2008). Cortical structures involved include the PFC, anterior cingulate gyrus, insula, and amygdala. Brain-stem structures involved include the periaqueductal gray, dorsoreticular nucleus, nucleus tractus solitarii, and parabrachial nucleus.

Stress may modulate nociception by inducing opposite effects—analgesia or hyperalgesia. Both may be subject to conditioning and involve the amygdala and brain stem (Strobel, Hunt, Sullivan, Sun, & Sah, 2014). Stress-induced analgesia (SIA) is mediated by cortical mechanisms, the CE of the amygdala, distinct subregions of the hypothalamus, periaqueductal gray, rostroventral medulla (activating "off" cells), and spinal cord (Butler & Finn, 2009). SIA may be either opioid-mediated (naloxone sensitive) or non–opioid-mediated. Opioid-mediated analgesia is associated with brief stressors, while non–opioid-mediated analgesia is associated with intense longer-lasting stressors (McEwen & Kalia, 2010). Because the HPA system contributes to the release of endogenous opioids, it is implicated in opioid mechanisms of stress analgesia (see Butler & Finn, 2009). Immune cell products may also mediate local analgesia at inflammation sites.

Stress-induced hyperalgesia is associated with repeated or chronic stressors, either psychogenic or physical, and anxiety. In humans, SIA is associated with fear, while hyperalgesia is associated with anxiety (Rhudy & Meagher, 2000). Stress exacerbates pain associated with chronic disorders such as inflammatory bowel disease and fibromyalgia, and there is high comorbidity between affective disorders and pain. A number of experimental animal models of human stress-induced hyperalgesia have been employed, including forced swim, cold, and restraint, as well as psychogenic stressors such as social defeat, water avoidance, chronic mild stress, maternal deprivation, and models of posttraumatic stress disorder (PTSD). Neural substrates include the cortex (PFC, cingulate and insular cortex), amygdala, rostroventromedial medulla (activating "on" cells), periaqueductal gray, and spinal cord. As with SIA, both arms of the stress response system are implicated (Jennings, Okine, Roche, & Finn, 2014).

In summary, the stress response system is antireproductive, antigrowth, catabolic, and often immunosuppressive and antinociceptive—these being temporarily beneficial but deleterious in the long term.

TERMINATION OF THE STRESS RESPONSE

The stress response system must be terminated to conserve resources and to avoid potential deleterious side effects of the response. Sustained activation of the sympathetic system leads to chronic high heart rate and elevated blood pressure, placing the cardiovascular system at risk. Chronic inhibition of vegetative systems such as the GI tract may put those organs at risk of injury. Chronic inhibition of the GI system is associated with disturbances of motor and digestive function, and chronic immunosuppression leads to vulnerability to infections.

Chronic stress is associated with CRH hyperdrive, and downregulation of GRs in the hippocampus and PFC, thus removing a break from the system. As long ago as 1986, Sapolsky proposed the cascade theory of aging, whereby high levels of GCs impair the GR receptors in the hippocampus, which in turn results in increased levels of GCs (Sapolsky, Krey, & McEwen, 1986). Shutoff of the HPA axis is both rapid and delayed. Immediate shutoff, occurring within minutes, is mediated by membrane GR mechanisms and direct actions on the pituitary and the PVN, mediated by mobilization of endocannabinoids, while delayed shutoff is mediated by genomic actions.

Chronically high levels of GC place the brain at risk for neuronal dysfunction and damage, as well as deficits in cognitive performance, particularly on tasks involving the hippocampus (Herbert et al., 2006). Aging accompanied by high levels of GCs is associated with lower hippocampus volume as well as with impaired performance in spatial learning tasks and delayed recall (Lupien, McEwen, Gunnar, & Heim, 2009). Nontermination of the response due to dysfunction of feedback mechanisms is also associated with melancholic depression. In humans at least, the stress responses may be inappropriately and chronically activated by rumination and worry ("anticipatory stress"; Herman et al., 2003). Such activation of cognitive and noncognitive processes might be a particular aspect of the human condition that puts us at risk for affective disorders but may at the same time provide us with a unique problem-solving capacity.

The amygdala is positively regulated by chronic stress, a feed-forward rather than a feedback loop. Chronic stress leads to increased expression of CRH in the CE, and GC implants into the amygdala increase GC responses to acute stress. Chronic stress furthermore upregulates POMC mRNA expression and enhances the capacity for ACTH release at the pituitary. At the adrenal level, chronic stress results in hyperplasia and hypertrophy in the zona fasciculate and elevated responsiveness.

INDIVIDUAL VARIATION IN THE STRESS RESPONSE

Cortisol levels in humans are heavily under genetic influence (see Herbert et al., 2006). However, the response to a stressor is modulated by the expectations of the organism as to how it will be able to master the challenge (control). If the stimulus represents a situation with which the animal has coped in the past, the response will be modulated by response outcome expectancies (Ursin & Eriksen, 2010). Rats that have learned to avoid foot shocks by responding to a warning signal show attenuated corticosterone activation on reexposure to the warning signal (Coover, Ursin, & Levine, 1973). Similarly, parachute jumpers show an attenuated stress response after learning that they can survive the first training jumps (Ursin, Baade, & Levine, 1978). Negative response outcome expectancies and lack of control are associated with hopelessness and disturbances in homeostasis. These cognitive mechanisms of stimulus and response expectancies are mediated by the cortex and the limbic system.

In addition to stimulus properties (intrinsic and learned) and expectancies, other experiential factors will influence the amplitude of the stress response. In addition to the effects of prenatal stress (see Maccari, Krugers, Morley-Fletcher, Szyf, & Brunton, 2014, for a review), the effects of early life conditions in animals have attracted a renewal of interest. In summary, early-handled rats develop into stress-resistant adults in terms of HPA function and behavior (Levine, 2005). Rats separated from their mothers for significant periods (typically 3 h) over the first 14 days of life develop stress-sensitive phenotypes (e.g., Lippmann, Bress, Nemeroff, Plotsky, & Monteggia, 2007). Such studies have commonly used undisturbed non-handled animals as the control group for these two conditions. However, because the constant presence of the mother is an abnormal situation for the wild rat, such a control group is inappropriate (Levine, 2005). The three conditions (early handling, maternal separation, and nonhandling) should be considered as qualitatively different, and at best the nonhandled condition is a comparison rather than a control condition. An ecologically more valid approach is to study animals in an environment conducive to "natural" maternal behaviors, which would allow the mother to leave the pups several times during the day to forage.

A number of studies have carefully explored those perinatal factors that influence the adult stress responsiveness in rats, most importantly mother–pup interactions (see Zhang, Labonte, Wen, Turecki, & Meaney, 2013, for a review). Pups reared by mothers who naturally show high levels of licking and grooming and arched-back nursing are similar to early-handled animals in showing resistance to stressors in adulthood, while those of mothers showing low licking and grooming and low arched-back nursing resemble maternally separated animals. The effects of low maternal behaviors are mediated by methylation of the GR gene, downregulating the inhibitory influence of the hippocampus on the PVN and enhanced activation of the HPA system during a sensitive developmental period. There is evidence for a similar epigenetic phenomenon in humans, and in rats at least it appears to be transmittable across generations. A postmortem study of suicide victims has demonstrated higher levels of methylation of the GR gene in the hippocampi of those who had been exposed to abuse as children compared to those not so exposed and to nonvictims of suicide (McGowan et al., 2009). Although studies of methylation in human brain tissue are limited, studies of methylation of GRs on peripheral lymphocytes are used as proxies for brain effects. And results similar to those of McGowan et al. (2009) on brain tissue but from studies of GR methylation on lymphocytes suggest that GRs on lymphocytes are indeed valid proxies (Perroud et al., 2011).

Initially, the programming effects of early experience on stress responsiveness were interpreted in terms of a cumulative stress hypothesis and a triple-hit model (de Kloet & Joëls, 2013). Genetic vulnerability plus early adverse conditions plus a third "precipitatory" stressor in adolescence or adulthood increases the risk for somatic and behavioral disorders. But an alternative view to this is the "mismatch hypothesis," by which animals (or humans) exposed to adverse conditions during upbringing function better under stressful conditions in adulthood and less well under low-stress conditions. Similarly, those exposed to low-stress conditions during upbringing would be at a disadvantage when later exposed to stressful conditions. Experimentally, there is support for both the cumulative stress and the mismatch views and a number of attempts have been made to integrate the approaches (e.g., Homberg, 2012; Nederhof & Schmidt, 2012).

In animals, stress responsiveness is related to social status (Sakai & Tamashiro, 2005). Dominant baboons under stable social and environmental conditions in the wild exhibit lower levels of cortisol than subdominant animals (Sapolsky, 1989). And dominant rodents in a colony setting may have a more efficient HPA feedback, returning to control levels faster than subdominants after removal from a visual burrow housing system (McKittrick et al., 2000). In humans the relationship between social status and cortisol is more complex and will depend on the conditions under which the measurements are taken and an appropriate definition of social status. Rather, cortisol levels in humans may be more related to perceived status and self-esteem rather than to an arbitrary classification of social status and rank (Liu, Wrosch, Miller, & Pruessner, 2014).

The potential influence of the microbiome on stress responsiveness has been illustrated. Bacteria of the GI tract may directly affect levels of neurotransmitters in animals and humans (Lyte, 2011; Mayer, Knight, Mazmanian, Cryan, & Tillisch, 2014). And manipulations of the microbiome in young animals have significant effects on adult emotional behaviors and stress responses (e.g., Sudo et al., 2004).

THE STRESS RESPONSE AND AFFECTIVE DISORDERS

The relationship between psychiatry and stress relies on the diathesis–stress model (Monroe & Simons, 1991). While not necessarily being the *cause* of a psychiatric disorder, the stress response, in combination with other factors (genetic, developmental, etc.), contributes to several disorders, particularly depression. Melancholic depression is associated with hypersecretion of CRH, HPA activation, and immunosuppression. Predisposing factors include 5-HT transporter gene alleles and adversity. A role for stress systems in depression is also indicated by Cushing syndrome. These patients, with excessively high levels of cortisol, exhibit cognitive impairments and heightened risk for depression. And depression has for a long time been known to be associated with enhanced levels of cortisol and dysfunctional feedback mechanisms within the HPA system (Altemus & Gold, 1990; Stokes, 1995).

Learned helplessness (LH) in rats, an experimental model for depression, involves exposing animals to a number of uncontrollable and unpredictable aversive stimuli. Such animals later exhibit an inability to learn, increased turnover and reduced levels of NA in the nucleus coeruleus, as well as resistance to dexamethasone (Overmier & Seligman, 1967; Vollmayr &

Henn, 2003; Weiss, Simson, & Simson, 1989). Although there are parallels between LH and depression, there are important differences. LH is transient, lasting only 2 or 3 days, although it may be reinstated by cues associated with the inducing stimuli or context (Maier, 2001); but human depression is not context dependent. While LH in rats requires a certain minimum number and intensity of shocks (e.g., a minimum of 50 foot shocks at 1 mA), a far lower number of shocks at the same intensity induces a long-lasting increase in vigilance in the sudden silence test, an effect not seen after the LH induction procedures (van Dijken, Mos, van der Heyden, & Tilders, 1992; Murison & Overmier, 1998), reflecting an anxiety-like state rather than a depression-like state. Thus even stressors of the same modality but of different durations do not invariably produce the same effects, and the effects are qualitatively different. While the LH effect may be prevented by treatment with the opioid antagonist naltrexone, indicating opioid mediation, the effects of a shorter shock regimen are not, at least on some outcome measures (Overmier & Murison, 1994).

Hypocortisolemia has been associated with a number of symptoms, including PTSD, atypical seasonal depression, fibromyalgia, autoimmune disorders, and hypothyroidism. A number of studies, both human and animal, suggest that HPA dysfunction may be a risk factor for PTSD or PTSD-like symptoms rather than a consequence (Cohen et al., 2006; Milde, Sundberg, Roseth, & Murison, 2003; Yehuda & LeDoux, 2007). Like depression, PTSD is associated with lower hippocampal volume. Studies of Vietnam veterans and their twins suggest that low hippocampal volume represents a familial vulnerability rather than a consequence of trauma (Pitman et al., 2006). A 2013 review of human data suggests that vulnerability to PTSD is associated with lower GC responsiveness at the time of or shortly after the trauma, associated with a preexisting high sensitivity to GCs (van Zuiden, Kavelaars, Geuze, Olff, & Heijnen, 2013). An alternative is that the hypocortisolemia is a consequence of earlier trauma, excessive secretion of GCs, and a subsequent downregulation of the system or overshoot (Fries, Hesse, Hellhammer, & Hellhammer, 2005).

CONCLUSIONS

In summary, stimuli perceived as a threat to homeostasis trigger endocrine and autonomic responses with the purpose of increasing and appropriately channeling energy resources needed to cope with the threat while inappropriate bodily functions are inhibited. The responses are organized in a hierarchical and interdependent manner and are modified by cognitive functions. Termination of the responses is necessary to avoid persistent wear and tear on the body. The stress response impinges on multiple systems, including reproduction, growth, immune function, and pain. For most of these, the effects are not straightforward and depend subtly on the nature, intensity, and duration of the stress.

REFERENCES

Altemus, M., & Gold, P. W. (1990). Neuroendocrinology and psychiatric illness. *Frontiers in Neuroendocrinology, 11*(3), 238–265.

Butler, R. K., & Finn, D. P. (2009). Stress-induced analgesia. *Progress in Neurobiology, 88*(3), 184–202. http://dx.doi.org/10.1016/j.pneurobio.2009.04.003.

Cannon, W. B. (1932). *The wisdom of the body.* New York: W.W. Norton & Company, Inc.

Cohen, H., Zohar, J., Gidron, Y., Matar, M. A., Belkind, D., Loewenthal, U., et al. (2006). Blunted HPA axis response to stress influences susceptibility to posttraumatic stress response in rats. *Biological Psychiatry, 59*(12), 1208–1218. http://dx.doi.org/10.1016/j.biopsych.2005.12.003.

Coover, G. D., Ursin, H., & Levine, S. (1973). Plasma-corticosterone levels during active-avoidance learning in rats. *Journal of Comparative & Physiological Psychology, 82*(1), 170–174.

Dantzer, R. (2005). Somatization: a psychoneuroimmune perspective. *Psychoneuroendocrinology, 30*(10), 947–952. http://dx.doi.org/10.1016/j.psyneuen.2005.03.011.

van Dijken, H. H., Mos, J., van der Heyden, J. A., & Tilders, F. J. (1992). Characterization of stress-induced long-term behavioural changes in rats: evidence in favor of anxiety. *Physiology & Behavior, 52*(5), 945–951.

Dunn, A. J. (2006). Effects of cytokines and infections on brain neurochemistry. *Clinical Neuroscience Research, 6*(1–2), 52–68. http://dx.doi.org/10.1016/j.cnr.2006.04.002.

Eriksen, H. R., Olff, M., Murison, R., & Ursin, H. (1999). The time dimension in stress responses: relevance for survival and health. *Psychiatry Research, 85*(1), 39–50. http://dx.doi.org/10.1016/S0165-1781(98)00141-3.

Fink, G. (Ed.). (2010). *Stress science: Neuroendocrinology.* Amsterdam: Academic Press.

Fleshner, M., Deak, T., Spencer, R. L., Laudenslager, M. L., Watkins, L. R., & Maier, S. F. (1995). A long term increase in basal levels of corticosterone and a decrease in corticosteroid-binding globulin after acute stressor exposure. *Endocrinology, 136*, 1–7.

Fries, E., Hesse, J., Hellhammer, J., & Hellhammer, D. H. (2005). A new view on hypocortisolism. *Psychoneuroendocrinology, 30*(10), 1010–1016. http://dx.doi.org/10.1016/j.psyneuen.2005.04.006.

Henley, D. E., & Lightman, S. L. (2011). New insights into corticosteroid-binding globulin and glucocorticoid delivery. *Neuroscience, 180*, 1–8. http://dx.doi.org/10.1016/j.neuroscience.2011.02.053.

Herbert, J., Goodyer, I. M., Grossman, A. B., Hastings, M. H., de Kloet, E. R., Lightman, S., et al. (2006). Do corticosteroids damage the brain? *Journal of Neuroendocrinology, 18*(6), 393–411. http://dx.doi.org/10.1111/j.1365-2826.2006.01429.x.

Herman, J. P. (2013). Neural control of chronic stress adaptation. *Frontiers in Behavioral Neuroscience, 7,* 12. http://dx.doi.org/10.3389/fnbeh.2013.00061.

Herman, J. P., Figueiredo, H., Mueller, N. K., Ulrich-Lai, Y., Ostrander, M. M., Choi, D. C., & Cullinan, W. E. (2003). Central mechanisms of stress integration: hierarchical circuitry controlling hypothalamo–pituitary–adrenocortical responsiveness. *Frontiers in Neuroendocrinology, 24*(3), 151–180. http://dx.doi.org/10.1016/j.yfrne.2003.07.001.

Homberg, J. R. (2012). The stress-coping (mis)match hypothesis for nature × nurture interactions. *Brain Research, 1432*, 114–121. http://dx.doi.org/10.1016/j.brainres.2011.11.037.

Irwin, M., Daniels, M., & Weiner, H. (1987). Immune and neuroendocrine changes during bereavement. *Psychiatric Clinics of North America, 10*(3), 449–465.

Jänig, W. (2014). Sympathetic nervous system and inflammation: a conceptual view. *Autonomic Neuroscience, 182*(0), 4–14. http://dx.doi.org/10.1016/j.autneu.2014.01.004.

Jennings, E. M., Okine, B. N., Roche, M., & Finn, D. P. (2014). Stress-induced hyperalgesia. *Progress in Neurobiology, 121*, 1–18. http://dx.doi.org/10.1016/j.pneurobio.2014.06.003.

de Kloet, E. R., & Joëls, M. (2013). Stress research: past and present. In D. W. Pfaff (Ed.), *Neuroscience in the 21st century: From basic to clinical* (pp. 1979–2007). New York: Springer.

Koolhaas, J. M., Bartolomucci, A., Buwalda, B., de Boer, S. F., Flügge, G., Korte, S. M., et al. (2011). Stress revisited: a critical evaluation of the stress concept. *Neuroscience & Biobehavioral Reviews, 35*(5), 1291–1301. http://dx.doi.org/10.1016/j.neubiorev.2011.02.003.

Kumsta, R., Entringer, S., Hellhammer, D. H., & Wüst, S. (2007). Cortisol and ACTH responses to psychosocial stress are modulated by corticosteroid binding globulin levels. *Psychoneuroendocrinology, 32*, 1153.

Lane, J. (2006). Can non-invasive glucocorticoid measures be used as reliable indicators of stress in animals? *Animal Welfare, 15*(4), 331–342.

Lazarus, R. S. (1993). Coping theory and research: past, present, and future. *Psychosomatic Medicine, 55*(3), 234–247.

Leuner, B., Glasper, E. R., & Gould, E. (2010). Sexual experience promotes adult neurogenesis in the hippocampus despite an initial elevation in stress hormones. *PLoS One, 5*(7), e11597. doi:ARTN.

Levine, S. (2005). Developmental determinants of sensitivity and resistance to stress. *Psychoneuroendocrinology, 30*(10), 939–946. http://dx.doi.org/10.1016/j.psyneuen.2005.03.013.

Levine, S., & Ursin, H. (1991). What is stress? In M. R. Brown, G. F. Koob, & C. Rivier (Eds.), *Stress - neurobiology and neuroendocrinology* (pp. 3–21) New York: Marcel Dekker.

Lightman, S. L., Wiles, C. C., Atkinson, H. C., Henley, D. E., Russell, G. M., Leendertz, J. A., et al. (2008). The significance of glucocorticoid pulsatility. *European Journal of Pharmacology, 583*(2–3), 255–262. http://dx.doi.org/10.1016/j.ejphar.2007.11.073.

Lippmann, M., Bress, A., Nemeroff, C. B., Plotsky, P. M., & Monteggia, L. M. (2007). Long-term behavioural and molecular alterations associated with maternal separation in rats. *European Journal of Neuroscience, 25*(10), 3091–3098. http://dx.doi.org/10.1111/j.1460-9568.2007.05522.x.

Liu, S. Y., Wrosch, C., Miller, G. E., & Pruessner, J. C. (2014). Self-esteem change and diurnal cortisol secretion in older adulthood. *Psychoneuroendocrinology, 41*, 111–120. http://dx.doi.org/10.1016/j.psyneuen.2013.12.010.

Lupien, S. J., McEwen, B. S., Gunnar, M. R., & Heim, C. (2009). Effects of stress throughout the lifespan on the brain, behaviour and cognition. *Nature Reviews Neuroscience, 10*(6), 434–445. http://dx.doi.org/10.1038/nrn2639.

Lyte, M. (2011). Probiotics function mechanistically as delivery vehicles for neuroactive compounds: microbial endocrinology in the design and use of probiotics. *Bioessays, 33*(8), 574–581. http://dx.doi.org/10.1002/bies.201100024.

Maccari, S., Krugers, H. J., Morley-Fletcher, S., Szyf, M., & Brunton, P. J. (2014). The consequences of early-life adversity: neurobiological, behavioural and epigenetic adaptations. *Journal of Neuroendocrinology, 26*(10), 707–723. http://dx.doi.org/10.1111/jne.12175.

Maes, M., Song, C., Lin, A., De Jongh, R., Van Gastel, A., Kenis, G., et al. (1998). The effects of psychological stress on humans: increased production of pro-inflammatory cytokines and a Th1-like response in stress-induced anxiety. *Cytokine, 10*(4), 313–318.

Maier, S. F. (2001). Exposure to the stressor environment prevents the temporal dissipation of behavioural depression/learned helplessness. *Biological Psychiatry, 49*(9), 763–773.

Mawdsley, J. E., & Rampton, D. S. (2005). Psychological stress in IBD: new insights into pathogenic and therapeutic implications. *Gut, 54*(10), 1481–1491. http://dx.doi.org/10.1136/gut.2005.064261.

Mayer, E. A., Knight, R., Mazmanian, S. K., Cryan, J. F., & Tillisch, K. (2014). Gut microbes and the brain: paradigm shift in neuroscience. *Journal of Neuroscience, 34*(46), 15490–15496. http://dx.doi.org/10.1523/jneurosci.3299-14.2014.

McEwen, B. S. (1998). Stress, adaptation, and disease. Allostasis and allostatic load. *Annals of the New York Academy of Sciences, 840*, 33–44.

McEwen, B. S., & Kalia, M. (2010). The role of corticosteroids and stress in chronic pain conditions. *Metabolism, 59*(Suppl. 1), S9–S15. http://dx.doi.org/10.1016/j.metabol.2010.07.012.

McGowan, P. O., Sasaki, A., D'Alessio, A. C., Dymov, S., Labonte, B., Szyf, M., et al. (2009). Epigenetic regulation of the glucocorticoid receptor in human brain associates with childhood abuse. *Nature Neuroscience, 12*(3), 342–348. http://dx.doi.org/10.1038/nn.2270.

McKittrick, C. R., Magarinos, A. M., Blanchard, D. C., Blanchard, R. J., McEwen, B. S., & Sakai, R. R. (2000). Chronic social stress reduces dendritic arbors in CA3 of hippocampus and decreases binding to serotonin transporter sites. *Synapse, 36*(2), 85–94. http://dx.doi.org/10.1002/(SICI)1098-2396(200005)36:2<85::AID-SYN1>3.0.CO;2-Y.

Milde, A. M., Sundberg, H., Roseth, A. G., & Murison, R. (2003). Proactive sensitizing effects of acute stress on acoustic startle responses and experimentally induced colitis in rats: relationship to corticosterone. *Stress, 6*(1), 49–57. http://dx.doi.org/10.1080/1025389031000075808.

Mineka, S., & Ohman, A. (2002). Phobias and preparedness: the selective, automatic, and encapsulated nature of fear. *Biological Psychiatry, 52*(10), 927–937. http://dx.doi.org/10.1016/s0006-3223(02)01669-4.

Monroe, S. M., & Simons, A. D. (1991). Diathesis-stress theories in the context of life stress research: implications for the depressive disorders. *Psychological Bulletin, 110*, 406–425.

Munck, A., Guyre, P. M., & Holbrook, N. J. (1984). Physiological functions of glucocorticoids in stress and their relation to pharmacological actions. *Endocrine Reviews, 5*, 25–44.

Murison, R., & Overmier, J. B. (1998). Comparison of different animal models of stress reveals a non-monotonic effect. *Stress, 2*(3), 227–230.

Nederhof, E., & Schmidt, M. V. (2012). Mismatch or cumulative stress: toward an integrated hypothesis of programming effects. *Physiology & Behavior, 106*(5), 691–700. http://dx.doi.org/10.1016/j.physbeh.2011.12.008.

Overmier, J. B., & Murison, R. (1994). Differing mechanisms for proactive effects of intermittent and single shock on gastric ulceration. *Physiology & Behavior, 56*(5), 913–919.

Overmier, J. B., & Seligman, M. E. (1967). Effects of inescapable shock upon subsequent escape and avoidance responding. *Journal of Comparative & Physiological Psychology, 63*(1), 28–33.

Perroud, N., Paoloni-Giacobino, A., Prada, P., Olie, E., Salzmann, A., Nicastro, R., et al. (2011). Increased methylation of glucocorticoid receptor gene (NR3C1) in adults with a history of childhood maltreatment: a link with the severity and type of trauma. *Translational Psychiatry, 1*, e59. http://dx.doi.org/10.1038/tp.2011.60.

Phelps, E. A., & LeDoux, J. E. (2005). Contributions of the amygdala to emotion processing: from animal models to human behaviour. *Neuron, 48*(2), 175–187. http://dx.doi.org/10.1016/j.neuron.2005.09.025.

Pitman, R. K., Gilbertson, M. W., Gurvits, T. V., May, F. S., Lasko, N. B., Metzger, L. J., et al. (2006). Clarifying the origin of biological abnormalities in PTSD through the study of identical twins discordant for combat exposure. *Annals of the New York Academy of Sciences, 1071*, 242–254. http://dx.doi.org/10.1196/annals.1364.019.

Rehbinder, C., & Hau, J. (2006). Quantification of cortisol, cortisol immunoreactive me-
tabolites, and immunoglobulin A in serum, saliva, urine, and faeces for noninvasive
assessment of stress in reindeer. *Canadian Journal of Veterinary Research-Revue Canadienne
De Recherche Veterinaire, 70*(2), 151–154.

Rhudy, J. L., & Meagher, M. W. (2000). Fear and anxiety: divergent effects on human pain
thresholds. *Pain, 84*(1), 65–75.

Rodrigues, S. M., LeDoux, J. E., & Sapolsky, R. M. (2009). The influence of stress hormones on fear circuitry. *Annual Review of Neuroscience, 32*(1), 289–313. http://
dx.doi.org/10.1146/annurev.neuro.051508.135620.

Sakai, R. R., & Tamashiro, K. L. K. (2005). Social hierarchy and stress. In R. Steckler,
N. H. Kalin, & J. M. H. M. Reul (Eds.), *Handbook of stress and the brain* (Vol. 2, pp. 113–132).
Amsterdam: Elsevier.

Sapolsky, R. M. (1989). Hypercortisolism among socially subordinate wild baboons originates at the CNS level. *Archives of General Psychiatry, 46*(11), 1047–1051.

Sapolsky, R. M., Krey, L. C., & McEwen, B. S. (1986). The neuroendocrinology of stress
and aging: the glucocorticoid cascade hypothesis. *Endocrine Reviews, 7*(3), 284–301.
http://dx.doi.org/10.1210/edrv-7-3-284.

Schlereth, T., & Birklein, F. (2008). The sympathetic nervous system and pain. *Neuro-
molecular Medicine, 10*(3), 141–147. http://dx.doi.org/10.1007/s12017-007-8018-6.

Seligman, M. E. (1971). Phobias and preparedness. *Behavior Therapy, 2*(3), 307–320. http://
dx.doi.org/10.1016/s0005-7894(71)80064-3.

Selye, H. (1946). The general adaptation syndrome and the diseases of adaptation. *Journal of
Clinical Endocrinology, 6*, 117–196.

Selye, H. (1956). *The stress of life.* New York: McGraw-Hill.

Sondergaard, S. R., Ostrowski, K., Ullum, H., & Pedersen, B. K. (2000). Changes in plasma
concentrations of interleukin-6 and interleukin-1 receptor antagonists in response to
adrenaline infusion in humans. *European Journal of Applied Physiology, 83*(1), 95–98.
http://dx.doi.org/10.1007/s004210000257.

Spencer, R. L., Miller, A.-H., Moday, H., McEwen, B. S., Blanchard, R. J.,
Blanchard, D. C., et al. (1996). Chronic social stress produces reductions in available
splenic type II corticosteroid receptor binding and plasma corticosteroid binding
globulin levels. *Psychoneuroendocrinology, 21*, 95–109.

Stalder, T., & Kirschbaum, C. (2012). Analysis of cortisol in hair - state of the art and future
directions. *Brain Behavior and Immunity, 26*(7), 1019–1029. http://dx.doi.org/10.1016/
j.bbi.2012.02.002.

Stokes, P. E. (1995). The potential role of excessive cortisol induced by HPA hyperfunction
in the pathogenesis of depression. *European Neuropsychopharmacology, 5*, 77–82. http://
dx.doi.org/10.1016/0924-977x(95)00039-r.

Strobel, C., Hunt, S., Sullivan, R., Sun, J., & Sah, P. (2014). Emotional regulation of pain:
the role of noradrenaline in the amygdala. *Science China Life Sciences, 57*(4), 384–390.
http://dx.doi.org/10.1007/s11427-014-4638-x.

Sudo, N., Chida, Y., Aiba, Y., Sonoda, J., Oyama, N., Yu, X. N., et al. (2004). Postnatal
microbial colonization programs the hypothalamic-pituitary-adrenal system for stress
response in mice. *Journal of Physiology, 558*(Pt 1), 263–275. http://dx.doi.org/10.1113/
jphysiol.2004.063388.

Tsigos, C., & Chrousos, G. P. (2002). Hypothalamic-pituitary-adrenal axis, neuroendocrine
factors and stress. *Journal of Psychosomatic Research, 53*(4), 865–871.

Ursin, H., Baade, E., & Levine, S. (Eds.). (1978). *The psychobiology of stress: A study of coping
men.* New York: Academic Press.

Ursin, H., & Eriksen, H. R. (2010). Cognitive activation theory of stress (CATS). *Neuroscience and Biobehavioral Reviews, 34*(6), 877–881. http://dx.doi.org/10.1016/
j.neubiorev.2009.03.001.

Vollmayr, B., & Henn, F. A. (2003). Stress models of depression. *Clinical Neuroscience Research, 3*(4–5), 245–251. http://dx.doi.org/10.1016/s1566-2772(03)00086-0.

Walker, J. J., Terry, J. R., & Lightman, S. L. (2010). Origin of ultradian pulsatility in the hypothalamic-pituitary-adrenal axis. *Proceedings of the Royal Society B: Biological Sciences, 277*(1688), 1627–1633. http://dx.doi.org/10.1098/rspb.2009.2148.

Weiss, J. M., Simson, P. G., & Simson, P. E. (1989). Neurochemical basis of stress-induced depression. In H. Weiner, I. Florin, R. Murison, & D. H. Hellhammer (Eds.), *Frontiers of stress research* (pp. 37–50). Toronto: Hans Huber Publishers.

Yehuda, R., & LeDoux, J. (2007). Response variation following trauma: a translational neuroscience approach to understanding PTSD. *Neuron, 56*(1), 19–32. http://dx.doi.org/10.1016/j.neuron.2007.09.006.

Zhang, T. Y., Labonte, B., Wen, X. L., Turecki, G., & Meaney, M. J. (2013). Epigenetic mechanisms for the early environmental regulation of hippocampal glucocorticoid receptor gene expression in rodents and humans. *Neuropsychopharmacology: Official Publication of the American College of Neuropsychopharmacology, 38*(1), 111–123. http://dx.doi.org/10.1038/npp.2012.149.

van Zuiden, M., Kavelaars, A., Geuze, E., Olff, M., & Heijnen, C. J. (2013). Predicting PTSD: pre-existing vulnerabilities in glucocorticoid-signaling and implications for preventive interventions. *Brain Behavior and Immunity, 30*, 12–21. http://dx.doi.org/10.1016/j.bbi.2012.08.015.

CHAPTER 3

Emotional Modulation of Pain

Jamie L. Rhudy
Department of Psychology, The University of Tulsa, Tulsa, OK, USA

Pain is tremendously malleable. One of the first to document this was Beecher (1959), who found that soldiers wounded in battle requested fewer analgesics and reported less pain than civilians undergoing surgery with similar tissue damage. From these observations he hypothesized that the psychological state of the individual contributed to the pain experienced. Later, Melzack and Wall (1965) published the gate-control theory and provided the first mechanism by which emotions could influence pain. This theory suggested that inhibitory neurons in the spinal cord could regulate incoming nociceptive signals. Further, these neurons could be influenced by central controls, thus causing hypoalgesia (reduced pain) or even analgesia (elimination of pain). Much more is now known about the biological mechanisms of pain control and how emotions can engage them (Chapters 1 and 2). Indeed, publications on emotion and pain have increased exponentially since Melzack and Wall's paper (Figure 1), with a sharp increase in

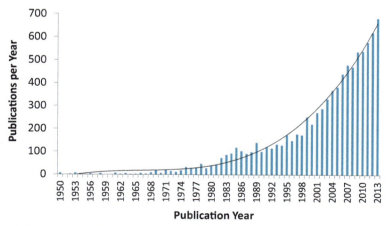

Figure 1 Number of publications by year that reference pain and emotion. As seen, the number of publications has grown exponentially since the early 1970s, with a particularly sharp increase in the mid-to-late 1990s. These data were obtained by conducting a combined search of Medline and PsycINFO using the search terms "pain" and "emotion or affective."

The Neuroscience of Pain, Stress, and Emotion
http://dx.doi.org/10.1016/B978-0-12-800538-5.00003-0

the mid-to-late 1990s (likely due to the birth of affective neuroscience). This chapter will examine what is currently known about emotional modulation of pain.

A BRIEF INTRODUCTION TO SOME TERMS

In this review, *nociception* refers to the neural signals promoted by intense, potentially harmful stimulation. *Pain* is the affective and sensory experience that can result from supraspinal processing of nociception. *Emotional/affective processing* refers to the neural signals associated with appetitive and defensive system activation (described below). *Emotions/affects* are state-like conscious experiences associated with these neural signals, whereas *affectivity* refers to stable, trait-like, emotional experiences. Although *stress* can refer to any organismic changes in response to disrupted homeostasis, here it will be used to mean the negative emotional state (distress) that results from disrupted homeostasis.

PAIN AND EMOTION WITHIN A MOTIVATIONAL CONTEXT

It is helpful to consider the emotion–pain relationship from within a broader motivational context. For organisms to survive, they must recognize and discriminate stimuli that are dangerous (e.g., predator) from those that are important for species survival (e.g., mate). As a result, neural systems have evolved to subserve these functions (Figure 2) (Lang & Davis, 2006). The *appetitive* system is activated by survival-promoting stimuli (e.g., sex, food) and results in appetitive behaviors (e.g., sustenance, procreation) and positive emotions. By contrast, the *defensive* system is activated by harmful or potentially harmful stimuli (e.g., predator, somatic threat) and results in defensive behaviors (e.g., withdrawal, attack) and negative emotions. Thus, emotions are the subjective experiences that result from activation of motivational systems and they imbue perception with a hedonic tone (like vs dislike).

Two orthogonal dimensions (valence and arousal) capture much of the variance in self-reported emotions (Figure 3) (Bradley, Codispoti, Cuthbert, &Lang, 2001), but see Tellegen, Watson, and Clark (1999) for another model. *Valence* refers to the pleasantness–unpleasantness of emotional experience and provides information about the motivation system activated (appetitive or defensive, respectively). *Arousal* refers to the intensity of the emotional experience and serves as an indirect readout of the degree of

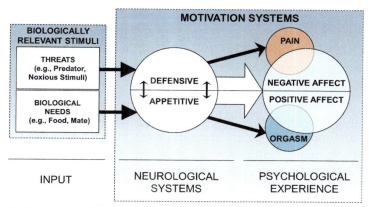

Figure 2 A hypothetical figure depicting the relationship between emotion and pain within a motivational context. Biologically relevant stimuli differentially activate the appetitive and defensive systems, which, in turn, results in emotion/affect, as well as other psychological states such as pain and orgasm. Stimuli that promote survival elicit positive affect via the appetitive system. Conversely, dangerous or threatening stimuli elicit negative affect via the defensive system. As can be seen, part of the variance in the experience of pain is shared with negative affect; however, unlike most emotional experiences (e.g., anxiety), pain also has a distinct sensory characteristic that provides information about location and intensity. An analogous experience emanating from activation of the appetitive system would be sexual orgasm, which has pleasant affective and sensory characteristics and promotes approach behaviors.

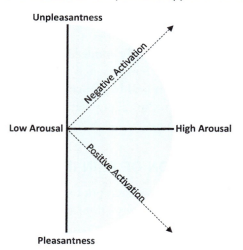

Figure 3 Valence (pleasantness vs unpleasantness) and arousal (low vs high) are two dimensions used to characterize variability in emotional experience. Pleasant emotions are associated with appetitive activation, whereas unpleasant emotions are associated with defensive activation. Yet, these experiences can vary in how arousing they are; more arousing emotions are psychologically more intense and promote greater motivation. Some researchers have characterized emotional experience from two orthogonal dimensions at a 45° rotation from valence and arousal. They refer to these dimensions as positive activation and negative activation (e.g., Tellegen et al., 1999).

motivation system activation. Thus, intense emotions are associated with greater arousal and motivation for appetitive/defensive behaviors.

Pain is a part of the defensive system and helps organisms detect and avoid somatic dangers. Pain system activation results in negative affect (pain and negative affect overlap in Figure 2) that promotes avoidance and learning so that danger can be circumvented in the present and future. Given this, pain and emotions are naturally linked. Nociceptive input triggers an unpleasant experience without which there would be no motivation to avoid harmful stimuli. However, activation of the pain system also results in sensory experiences that help determine the intensity and location of the threat (pain and negative affect nonoverlap in Figure 2).

Given the interconnectedness of emotion and pain systems, it is no surprise that they influence one another. As stated, pain system activation results in negative affect; therefore, pain inherently influences emotions. Interestingly, relief from pain not only reduces negative affect, but also increases positive affect via the dopaminergic reward system (Navratilova et al., 2012). Pain can also have long-term consequences on emotions. For example, chronic pain increases risk for affective disturbance (e.g., Kroenke et al., 2011) and impairs emotional awareness and decision-making (e.g., Ji et al., 2010). Although there are many relationships between emotion and pain (for a review, Lumley et al., 2011), this chapter will focus specifically on emotional modulation of pain.

The strongest causal evidence comes from studies in which both emotion and pain are experimentally induced; therefore, greater weight will be given to those studies. Further, it is important to first consider emotional modulation of pain in healthy humans because disruptions of the pain and/or emotion systems in clinical populations influence the emotion–pain connection.

EMOTIONAL MODULATION OF PAIN IN HEALTHY HUMANS

A number of models/theories have been put forth to explain the emotion–pain relationships: reciprocal inhibition (Smith & Wolpin, 1989), cognitive/memorial (Litt, 1996), attentional (e.g., Cornwall & Donderi, 1988), attribution (Nisbett & Schachter, 1966), parallel processing (schema modification) (Leventhal & Everhart, 1979), and perceptual–defensive–recuperative (Bolles & Fanselow, 1980). Although many of these explain certain aspects of the relationships, none provides a comprehensive explanation.

Motivational priming theory (MPT) was proposed by Lang and colleagues (Bradley et al., 2001; Lang, 1995) to explain the relationship between emotions and outputs/responses from appetitive and defensive systems. MPT argues that activation of a motivational system primes it, thus facilitating responses from the same system and inhibiting responses from the opposite system. For example, priming the defensive system with aversive stimuli leads to facilitation of startle (defensive reflex), whereas priming the appetitive system with pleasurable stimuli inhibits startle. Furthermore, the degree of motivation system activation plays a role: low levels of appetitive/defensive activation result in little inhibition/facilitation of motive system responses, whereas greater appetitive/defensive activation results in greater inhibition/facilitation.

Given that pain is part of the defensive system, some have used MPT to characterize the effects of emotion on pain (e.g., Kenntner-Mabiala & Pauli, 2005; Mini, Rau, Montoya, Palomba, & Birbaumer, 1995; Rhudy & Meagher, 2001c). Indeed, MPT explains much of the observed effects in healthy humans.

Observation 1: Positive Emotions Generally Inhibit Pain, Whereas Negative Emotions Generally Enhance Pain

Emotions evoked by painful stimuli (pain-related emotions) tend to direct attention toward pain, whereas emotions evoked by nonpainful stimuli (pain-unrelated emotions) tend to direct attention away from pain. Nonetheless, emotional modulation of pain does not appear to depend on the emotion source or on the specific emotion.

Pain-Related Emotions

In three innovative studies, Rainville, Bao, and Chretien (2005) used hypnotic suggestion to induce anger, fear, sadness, relief, and satisfaction about painfully hot water. They found that pain intensity and unpleasantness were increased by negative emotions and decreased by positive emotions (regardless of the emotion). In contrast to this study, most others have manipulated only pain-related *negative* emotions. For example, Cornwall and Donderi (1988) used a stressful interview or a warning about the pain test to induce anxiety and found that they enhanced pressure pain. Two studies used verbal threat of painful shock (never delivered) to induce anxiety and found it reduced heat pain thresholds (hyperalgesia) (Haslam, 1966; Rhudy & Meagher, 2000). Similarly, Weisenberg, Aviram, Wolf, and Raphaeli (1984) found that lights predicting the delivery of a painful shock generated anxiety and enhanced pain. Dougher, Goldstein, and Leight (1987) had participants read pain-related (e.g., slamming finger in car door) and pain-unrelated (e.g., walking down a dark alley) statements and found that only pain-related anxiety enhanced pain. Ploghaus et al. (2001) presented a neutral cue prior to a painful heat stimulus, but on some trials the cue was followed by more intense painful heat to cause anxiety. The cue ultimately led to hyperalgesia that was associated with activity in the entorhinal cortex of the hippocampal formation. Williams and Rhudy (2007b) paired mildly painful shocks with pictures of facial expressions. For some participants, shocks were paired with fearful expressions and for others they were paired with happy expressions. Later, the expressions were presented during pain testing in the absence of shocks. Fear expressions previously paired with shock produced hyperalgesia. Interestingly, happy facial expressions previously paired with shock did not modulate pain, suggesting some stimuli produce fear conditioning (negative affect) and hyperalgesia more readily.

What is more, pain-related negative emotions can activate brain-to-spinal cord mechanisms to enhance spinal nociception. Willer, Boureau, and Albe-Fessard (1979) assessed the nociceptive flexion reflex (NFR), a physiological marker of spinal nociception (Skljarevski & Ramadan, 2002), and found that pain and NFR were enhanced when participants anticipated a strong electric shock. Similarly, Hubbard et al. (2011) found NFRs were enhanced by a cue that signaled the possible delivery of a painful abdominal shock, relative to a cue that signaled no abdominal shock would occur.

Pain-Unrelated Emotions

Unlike pain-related emotions, numerous different emotion manipulations have been used to evoke pain-unrelated emotions. Worthington (1978) found that pleasant imagery, compared to neutral, had no effect on cold pressor pain; however, pain was reduced if the participants had choice over the imagery content, regardless of valence. Thus, imagery-evoked emotions may need to be personally relevant to have an effect. Indeed, personally relevant sad imagery was found to (a) decrease cold pressor pain tolerance (hyperalgesia) relative to personally relevant angry, pleasant, and neutral imagery (Smith & Wolpin, 1989) and (b) increase cold pressor pain ratings relative to recall of angry and joyful memories (Burns, Kubilus, & Bruehl, 2003). Further, Bruehl, Carlson, and McCubbin (1993) found personally relevant pleasant imagery increased happiness, reduced fear and anxiety, and reduced pain, relative to social-demand (told to reduce pain) and no-instruction controls.

Two studies found that reading sad statements enhanced pain relative to neutral statements (Berna et al., 2010; Willoughby, Hailey, Mulkana, & Rowe, 2002), an effect associated with activity in the supraspinal regions involved with mood and pain regulation (dorsolateral prefrontal cortex, inferior frontal gyrus) (Berna et al., 2010). Additionally, Zelman, Howland, Nichols, and Cleeland (1991) found elative statements produced higher cold pain tolerance (hypoalgesia) and depressive statements produced lower tolerance (hyperalgesia), whereas Carter et al. (2002) found that anxiety-related statements and depressive statements decreased pressure pain tolerance (hyperalgesia) relative to neutral statements, but that elative statements had no effect.

Cogan, Cogan, Waltz, and McCue (1987) had participants listen to humorous audiotapes and found that participants who laughed had increased ischemia thresholds (hypoalgesia) relative to those under conditions that controlled for attention and interest. Roy, Peretz, and Rainville (2008) found that heat pain intensity and unpleasantness were lowest during pleasant music, relative to neutral and unpleasant music. Stancak, Ward, and Fallon (2013) found that the presentation of short (4-s) unpleasant sounds (e.g., crying) enhanced laser-evoked pain relative to neutral (e.g., traffic) and pleasant (e.g., laughter) sounds, and their electroencephalogram data suggested that the hippocampal formation was involved, thus corroborating the findings of Ploghaus et al. (2001) discussed earlier.

Weisenberg, Tepper, and Schwarzwald (1995) found that a humorous (comedy) movie clip resulted in higher cold pressor pain tolerances (hypoalgesia) relative to a neutral (science) clip. In a follow-up study, this group measured cold pressor pain before, immediately after, and 30 min after emotional film clips (Weisenberg, Raz, & Hener, 1998). Humor (comedy) increased cold pressor tolerance relative to sad (holocaust) and neutral (nature) clips, but only at 30 min postassessment. Zillmann, de Wied, King-Jablonski, and Jenzowsky (1996) presented film clips that were supposed to be unpleasant/arousing (war scenes), unpleasant/unarousing (discussion of war experiences), pleasant/arousing (sex scene), pleasant/unarousing (dinner date), and neutral/unarousing (nature). However, manipulation checks found that pleasant clips were more arousing than unpleasant clips and the unpleasant clips did not differ in arousal. As a result, ischemia and cold pressor pain were inhibited during pleasant clips, but unpleasant clips did not enhance pain.

Villemure, Slotnick, and Bushnell (2003) examined the influence of computer-delivered pleasant and unpleasant odors on heat pain and also manipulated attention by having participants focus either on the pain or on the odors. Interestingly, valence and attention had independent effects: pain unpleasantness was lower during pleasant odors and higher during unpleasant odors (regardless of the attentional focus), whereas pain intensity was lower during odor focus and higher during pain focus (regardless of odor valence). Using the same paradigm, Villemure and Bushnell (2009) demonstrated that pleasant odors reduced pain-related activity in the anterior cingulate cortex, medial thalamus, and sensory cortices. Although Villemure and Bushnell did not include a neutral control, other laboratories found that, compared to neutral, sweet odors reduced cold pressor pain (Prescott & Wilkie, 2007), pleasant odors reduced heat pain (but only in women) (Marchand & Arsenault, 2002), and unpleasant odors enhanced cold pressor pain (Martin, 2006).

To promote standardization of emotion-induction procedures across studies and laboratories, Lang, Bradley, and Cuthbert (2001) created the International Affective Picture System (IAPS), a set of pictures that vary in content and include normative valence and arousal ratings (CSEA, 2006). The first known experiment to use IAPS to modulate pain was that of Mini et al. (1995). They presented randomized pictures for 6 s (with a random interpicture intervals), during which painful electric stimuli were delivered. Relative to neutral, pain was inhibited by pleasant pictures and enhanced by unpleasant pictures, and pain was strongly correlated with picture valence ratings ($r = -0.90$, $p < 0.0001$). A series of studies by Rhudy and colleagues used the same experimental design, but measured both pain and NFR (Palit et al., 2013; Rhudy & Bartley, 2010; Rhudy, Bartley, et al., 2013; Rhudy et al., 2010; Rhudy et al., 2012; Rhudy, Williams, McCabe, Nguyen, & Rambo, 2005; Rhudy, Williams, McCabe, Rambo, & Russell, 2006; Rhudy, Williams, McCabe, Russell, & Maynard, 2008). These studies found pain and NFR were enhanced during unpleasant pictures and reduced during pleasant pictures. Given that NFR was modulated, this indicates that positive and negative emotions engage brain-to-spinal cord circuits to modulate spinal nociception. Subsequent studies by this group found that emotional modulation of pain and NFR are mediated by independent mechanisms (Rhudy, Williams, et al., 2006) and do not vary across menstrual phases in women with or without premenstrual dysphoric disorder (Rhudy & Bartley, 2010; Rhudy et al., 2014), even though emotional modulation of pain/NFR is enhanced by natural increases in estrogen (Rhudy, Bartley, et al., 2013).

Other laboratories have shown that emotional pictures modulate markers of supraspinal nociception. Kenntner-Mabiala and Pauli (2005) found that pain and pain-evoked event-related potentials (ERPs; N150) were enhanced by unpleasant pictures and inhibited by pleasant pictures, although the unpleasant versus neutral comparison was nonsignificant. Further, Roy, Piche, Chen, Peretz, and Rainville (2009) used functional magnetic resonance imaging (fMRI) and confirmed the notion that emotional modulation of pain and NFR is mediated by different modulatory mechanisms. Emotional modulation of pain was associated with activity in the orbitofrontal cortex, subgenual anterior cingulate cortex, cuneus, and insula, whereas emotional modulation of NFR was associated with activity in the dorsolateral prefrontal cortex, parahippocampal gyrus, thalamus, amygdala, and brain-stem nuclei.

Importantly, emotional pictures modulate experimental pain evoked by a variety of stimuli. For example, emotional pictures modulate heat pain (Wunsch, Philippot, & Plaghki, 2003), cold pressor pain (Meagher, Arnau, & Rhudy, 2001; Rhudy, Dubbert, Parker, Burke, & Williams, 2006; de Wied & Verbaten, 2001), pressure pain (Kenntner-Mabiala, Weyers, & Pauli, 2007), laser-evoked pain (Stancak & Fallon, 2013), and jaw pain induced by saline injection (Horjales-Araujo et al., 2013). Interestingly, this last study found that emotional modulation of jaw pain was noted only in participants with a genetic polymorphism associated with high expression of the serotonin transporter gene (5-HTTLPR), suggesting that serotonin plays a role in emotional modulation of pain.

Observation 2: Degree of Motivation System Activation Affects the Degree of Pain Inhibition/Facilitation

As noted, valence reflects which motivational system is activated (pleasant = appetitive, unpleasant = defensive), whereas arousal provides an indirect readout of the degree of motivational system activation. Two studies independently manipulated valence and arousal (Rhudy et al., 2010; Rhudy et al., 2008) and found that pain and NFR are facilitated by unpleasant pictures and inhibited by pleasant pictures, but the degree of picture-evoked arousal was associated with the degree of facilitation/inhibition (Figure 4). Specifically, the most arousing unpleasant pictures (mutilation) led to the greatest facilitation and the most arousing pleasant pictures (erotica) led to the greatest inhibition. This valence-by-arousal interaction was later confirmed by an independent laboratory

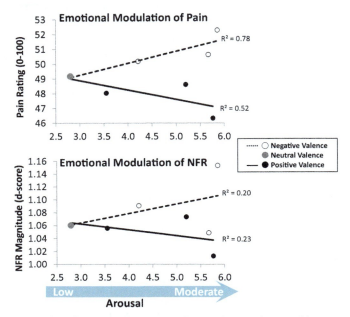

Figure 4 Empirical evidence demonstrating that, under conditions of low-to-moderate affective arousal induced by emotional picture viewing, negatively valenced emotions enhance pain and spinal nociception (nociceptive flexion reflex; NFR), whereas positively valenced emotions inhibit pain and spinal nociception *(adapted from Rhudy et al., 2010)*. Further, the greater the arousal (*x* axis values represent average arousal ratings of each picture content), the greater the degree of facilitation/inhibition. Dashed (unpleasant emotions) and solid (pleasant emotions) lines represent the lines of best fit for the relationship between arousal level and pain and NFR. As noted by the R^2 values for these lines, the arousal/intensity effect is stronger on pain perception than on NFR.

(Roy, Lebuis, Peretz, & Rainville, 2011) and is consistent with the Zillmann et al. study described earlier.

In a series of provocative studies, Whipple and Komisaruk examined self-applied vaginal stimulation on experimental pain in women (for a review, Komisaruk & Whipple, 2000). They found that pressure exerted against the anterior vaginal wall increased pain threshold by 53%, but did not affect tactile thresholds. This was not due to distraction, because several attentional controls were included. In a second study, *pleasurable* vaginal stimulation increased pain threshold by 84%, and in the subset of women who were able to achieve orgasm, pain threshold increased by 107% and pain tolerance by 75%. Therefore, highly arousing pleasure can profoundly inhibit pain. Unfortunately, analogous studies have not been conducted in men.

Given that low-intensity emotions should produce little (if any) inhibition/facilitation of pain, this could explain why some emotion manipulations failed to modulate pain (e.g., Burns et al., 2003; Smith & Wolpin, 1989; Weisenberg et al., 1998) and why personally relevant imagery modulates pain better than nonrelevant imagery (Worthington, 1978). Unfortunately, many studies fail to assess measures of valence and arousal to confirm these hypotheses.

One limitation of studies that manipulate arousal, however, is that arousal level is often confounded with the content of the manipulation (e.g., pictures of families elicit pleasant affect with low arousal, erotica elicits pleasant affect with moderate arousal). Indeed, one study found that pictures did not modulate pain if they did not contain human bodies, even though they elicited similar self-reported valence and arousal compared to pictures with bodies (Godinho, Magnin, Frot, Perchet, & Garcia-Larrea, 2006). These findings are intriguing and warrant further study; however, it is important to consider that subjective arousal is an *indirect* indicator of motivational activation, and pictures that include human bodies (e.g., erotica, mutilation) are more likely to activate motives (in humans) than the non-body pictures used in the Godinho et al. study (e.g., fashionable clothes, perfume, motorcycles). Future studies are needed to manipulate valence and arousal using all body-related pictures.

Observation 3: Emotional Stimuli that Elicit Simultaneous (and Equal) Defensive and Appetitive Activation Have No Net Effect on Pain

MPT states that pleasant stimuli activate the appetitive system to inhibit pain and unpleasant stimuli activate the defensive system to enhance pain, but it also implies that stimuli that elicit a mix of appetitive and defensive activation will have a zero net effect on pain, because simultaneous inhibition and facilitation cancel each other out. This issue has rarely been studied, but a few observations support it. For example, Meagher, Arnau, and Rhudy (2001) assessed cold pressor pain following the presentation of erotic pictures. Women reacted with sexual arousal (appetitive) and disgust (defensive), resulting in no modulation of their pain response. However, men reacted with only appetitive activation and pain was inhibited. In another study, Rhudy and Meagher (2003a) evoked negative emotion by presenting a painful shock. They found that heat pain thresholds were modulated when participants reacted with fear (defensive), but no pain modulation was observed when participants reacted with fear (defensive) and humor (appetitive).

Observation 4: Emotions Modulate All Pain-Related (Defensive) Outcomes in Parallel

If pain and pain-related responses emanate from defensive activation, then all should be inhibited by appetitive activation and facilitated by defensive activation. As previously noted, emotional modulation of the NFR (e.g., Rhudy et al., 2005; Rhudy et al., 2008; Willer et al., 1979) and pain-evoked ERPs (e.g., Kenntner-Mabiala & Pauli, 2005) parallel the modulation of pain. Similarly, studies have shown that emotional pictures modulate pain-evoked skin conductance response, pain-evoked heart rate acceleration, and pain-evoked blink magnitude (Rhudy, McCabe, & Williams, 2007; Rhudy et al., 2008; Williams & Rhudy, 2007a), as well as experimental head pain and the nociceptive blink reflex (a physiological marker of trigeminal nociception) (Williams & Rhudy, 2009).

INTENSE NEGATIVE EMOTIONS INHIBIT PAIN: A REVISION TO MPT

A number of studies have found that intense, highly arousing negative emotions inhibit pain. Willer (1980) repeatedly presented a cue that announced the possible delivery of an intense (70-mA) shock during NFR testing. The cues produced NFR inhibition (hypoalgesia) that was reversed by naloxone, suggesting the involvement of endogenous opioids. This was subsequently replicated (Willer & Albe-Fessard, 1980; Willer, Dehen, & Cambier, 1981) and extended to show the effect could be attenuated by anxiolytics (Willer & Ernst, 1986). In three studies, Rhudy and Meagher (2001a) used fear conditioning to pair a light with an intense, highly arousing shock (12.4 mA). Presentation of the light during heat pain produced hypoalgesia, but only in participants experiencing intense fear and arousal. This study emphasizes the importance of arousal level, because Williams and Rhudy (2007b) found that conditioned fear produced hyperalgesia when the shock (5 mA) elicited negative emotion with low-to-moderate arousal. Rhudy and Meagher (2000, 2003a, 2003b) and Rhudy, Grimes, and Meagher (2004) examined the effect that threat and delivery of a painful (12.4 mA) shock had on heat pain. When shock elicited intense, highly arousing negative emotions, hypoalgesia was always produced.

Even intense, highly arousing, *pain-unrelated*, negative emotions inhibit pain. Pitman, van der Kolk, Orr, and Greenberg (1990) presented a combat-related video (*Platoon*) to war veterans with post-traumatic stress disorder (PTSD) and healthy controls and then tested heat pain. The PTSD group experienced an opioid-mediated hypoalgesia, whereas controls experienced hyperalgesia. Importantly, the PTSD group reacted with greater negative affect (e.g., fear) and arousal than controls. Janssen and Arntz (1996) presented a live spider to spider phobics, which produced negative affect, high arousal (sympathetic activation), and an opioid-mediated hypoalgesia; however, it is unclear if phobic stimuli reliably elicit hypoalgesia (cf., Janssen & Arntz, 1997). Janssen and Arntz (2001) found that a first-time parachute jump produced anxiety (that correlated with β-endorphin levels) and opioid-mediated hypoalgesia on electric and pressure pain outcomes. Weisenberg et al. (1995) found that watching a horror movie clip resulted in higher cold pressor pain tolerances (hypoalgesia) relative to a neutral (science) clip. Rhudy and Meagher (2001b) assessed heat pain thresholds before and after negative emotion induction from startling noise bursts. Hypoalgesia was observed in women, whereas hyperalgesia was observed in men. Explaining this, manipulation checks found that women reacted to the noises with intense negative emotion and high arousal, whereas men reacted with negative emotion but low-to-moderate arousal. And finally, two studies paired a neutral cue with nonpainful unconditioned stimuli (noise bursts plus stressful mental arithmetic) and tested the effect of the cue on electric pain threshold and tolerance (Flor, Birbaumer, Schulz, Grusser, & Mucha, 2002; Flor & Grusser, 1999). The cue produced hypoalgesia that was partially mediated by opioids.

As a result of these findings, Rhudy and colleagues proposed a revision to MPT (Figure 5), arguing that MPT characterizes the effect of emotions on pain only when motivational systems are low-to-moderately activated (Rhudy & Meagher, 2001c; Rhudy & Williams, 2005). This explains why most studies find negative emotion-induced hyperalgesia, because the emotion-induction procedures (e.g., pictures, sounds, imagery) should not produce active defense (fight or flight) and intense, highly arousing, negative emotions in nonclinical samples. By contrast, when negative emotion induction involved a somatic threat (e.g., highly painful shocks), cues paired with severe somatic threat (e.g., light paired with highly painful shock), feared phobic stimuli (e.g., live spider), or life-threatening events (e.g., parachute jump), it evoked highly arousing negative emotions and hypoalgesia.

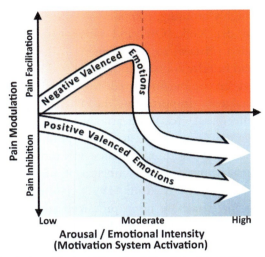

Figure 5 Hypothetical graph depicting the influence of emotion on pain modulatory processes. Available evidence suggests that the influence of emotion on pain is determined by a valence × arousal interaction. At low-to-moderate levels of arousal (emotional intensity), negative emotions enhance (facilitate) pain, whereas positive emotions reduce (inhibit) pain. Further, the degree of facilitation/inhibition is determined by the arousal level (i.e., there is greater facilitation/inhibition as arousal increases to moderate levels). However, under conditions of high arousal (very intense emotions, e.g., fear, panic, orgasmic pleasure) pain is inhibited, regardless of the emotional valence.

Therefore, the relationship between negative emotions and pain is nonmonotonic, such that low–to-moderately arousing negative emotions result in hyperalgesia, whereas highly arousing negative emotions result in hypoalgesia. Functionally, it would be adaptive to promote environmental scanning, vigilance, and sensory intake as a means to improve threat detection in situations associated with low-to-moderate threat (in which less intense negative emotion would predominate) (Meagher, Ferguson, et al., 2001; Walters, 1994). Thus, hyperalgesia would be adaptive because it promotes detection of somatic threats and recuperation from tissue damage that might have happened during a time of high threat. However, when threat is present and imminent (situations in which intense negative emotion would predominate), pain and pain-related behaviors could interfere with active defense (fight or flight), so they are inhibited (Bolles & Fanselow, 1980; Meagher, Ferguson, et al., 2001).

Importantly, pain modulation is not simply determined from arousal alone, because the relationship between positive emotions and pain is monotonic. Indeed, there is no known published study that found that positive emotions enhanced pain. Rather, positive emotions always inhibit pain as long as adequate appetitive activation was elicited. This probably explains why sexually arousing stimuli produce the most reliable pain inhibition, because sexual stimuli evoke reliable appetitive motivation even when the individual has not been deprived (Bradley et al., 2001). Indeed, when appetitive stimulation produces intense, highly arousing, positive emotions (orgasmic pleasure), profound hypoalgesia is elicited (Komisaruk & Whipple, 2000).

To summarize, a modified version of MPT that takes into account the degree of motivational activation can explain the emotion–pain relationships. This theory predicts that pain modulation is determined from a valence by arousal interaction, with arousal (emotional intensity) used as an indirect measure of motivation system activation.

EMOTIONAL MODULATION OF PAIN IN CLINICAL POPULATIONS

Disorders of emotion (e.g., depression) and pain are often comorbid (e.g., Bair, Robinson, Katon, & Kroenke, 2003), and there is evidence that affective disturbance might serve as a risk factor for chronic pain (e.g., Carroll, Cassidy, & Côté, 2004; Casey, Greenberg, Nicassio, Harpin, & Hubbard, 2008). Moreover, emerging evidence suggests that dysfunctions within emotion circuitry might promote disorders of both affect and pain (e.g., Lapate et al., 2012; Neugebauer, Galhardo, Maione, & Mackey, 2009). This could lead to higher thresholds to experience positive emotions, lower thresholds to experience negative emotions, prolongation of negative emotions, or augmented levels of negative emotions in patients. In addition, chronic pain patients may have a reduced capacity to engage pain-inhibitory mechanisms (e.g., Lautenbacher & Rollman, 1997). Thus, positive emotions and intense negative emotions may not be able to elicit hypoalgesia as they do in healthy individuals. For these reasons, it is important to examine emotional modulation of pain in chronic pain populations to determine whether the emotion–pain relationship is altered and/or contributes to pain persistence. Indeed, these studies generally find there is a link between enhanced negative emotions and pain and a failure of positive emotions to reduce pain.

Three studies manipulated emotion and pain in patients with irritable bowel syndrome (IBS). Posserud et al. (2004) evoked stress (Stroop test and mental arithmetic) in patients with IBS and controls and found patients had an abnormal stress response (e.g., higher reported stress, corticotropic releasing hormone) and experienced hyperalgesia in response to rectal distention. No controls experienced distention-related pain, so it is unclear whether hyperalgesia was specific to (or enhanced in) the IBS group. Similarly, Dickhaus et al. (2003) exposed patients with IBS and controls to noise stress (conflicting music) or relaxing sounds (ocean waves) and found that stress elicited greater negative emotions and enhanced pain in response to rectal distension in the patients. By contrast, Bach, Erdmann, Schmidtmann, and Monnikes (2006) evoked stress (anticipation of public speaking) in patients with IBS and controls and found that the patients reacted with greater stress reactivity (faster heart rate), but rectal distention discomfort was not altered by stress in either group.

de Tommaso et al. (2009) examined the effect of emotional pictures on laser-evoked pain in patients with migraine without aura and controls. Surprisingly, emotional modulation of pain was not observed in either group; however, they used low-arousal pictures, so modulatory effects may have been attenuated.

Three studies manipulated emotion and pain in patients with fibromyalgia (FM). Arnold et al. (2008) presented mutilation, unpleasant (nonmutilation), neutral, and pleasant pictures to participants with FM, back pain, or somatoform disorder and pain-free healthy controls. In general, unpleasant and mutilation pictures enhanced pain relative to neutral pictures (mutilation enhanced more). Unfortunately, the study may have been underpowered, because there was a marginal group difference in emotional modulation that was not explored further. Rhudy, DelVentura, et al. (2013) used mutilation, neutral, and erotic pictures to study emotional modulation of electric pain and NFR in patients with FM, patients with rheumatoid arthritis (RA), and controls. All three groups demonstrated emotional modulation of the NFR, suggesting that descending modulation of spinal nociception was intact. However, emotional modulation of pain was observed only in RA and controls, not FM. Similarly, Kamping, Bomba, Kanske, Diesch, and Flor (2013) used unpleasant (mutilation, attack), neutral, and pleasant (nudes, babies) pictures to study laser-evoked pain in FM and controls. They found controls had normal emotional modulation of pain intensity, but emotional modulation of pain was disrupted in FM (pain higher during pleasant and unpleasant). Further, while processing pain during pleasant pictures, patients with FM had less brain activation in the right ventral anterior cingulate cortex, bilateral insula, right secondary somatosensory cortex, and left orbitofrontal cortex, suggesting supraspinal mechanisms were disrupted.

Rhudy and colleagues also studied emotional modulation of pain/NFR in disorders known to increase risk for chronic pain: major depression (Terry, DelVentura, Bartley, Vincent, & Rhudy, 2013) and insomnia (DelVentura, Terry, Bartley, & Rhudy, 2014). As with FM, emotional modulation of pain, but not NFR, was disrupted in these groups. These data are consistent with the study noted earlier that found that individuals with a genetic risk for affective disturbance also fail to show emotional modulation of pain (Horjales-Araujo et al., 2013). As a result, Rhudy and colleagues argue that failure to emotionally modulate experimental pain could be a phenotype for risk of pain and affective disturbance, perhaps resulting from an inability to modulate pain signals once they reach the brain (even though spinal nociception is modulated).

A few studies have experimentally manipulated emotions and examined the effect on clinical (nonexperimental) pain. Gannon, Haynes, Cuevas, and Chavez (1987) asked controls and patients with frequent migraine or tension-type headache to engage in a stressful mental arithmetic task. Over 68% of headache patients developed a headache, compared to only 25% of controls. Davis, Zautra, and Reich (2001) exposed women with FM or osteoarthritis to either sad or neutral imagery followed by the recall of a stressful interpersonal conflict. Stress-induced increases in clinical pain were enhanced by the sad imagery, but only in the FM group. Furthermore, increased pain was associated with decreased positive affect in FM. Montoya et al. (2005) presented pleasant and unpleasant pictures to patients with FM or non-FM musculoskeletal pain. Unpleasant pictures enhanced FM pain relative to pleasant pictures and a no-picture control, whereas emotional modulation was not present in the non-FM group. Burns (2006) asked patients with chronic lower back pain (CLBP) and controls to recall personally relevant sad and angry events. Compared to sadness, anger elicited significantly greater back muscle tension, blood pressure, and pain in patients with CLBP. By contrast, controls showed similar physiological responses to sadness and anger. Unfortunately a neutral control condition was not included in many of these studies.

Consistent with experimental evidence, correlational studies generally find that day-to-day fluctuations in negative emotions exacerbate chronic pain and that there are deficits in the beneficial effects of positive emotions (e.g., Bruehl, Liu, Burns, Chont, & Jamison, 2012; Davis, Zautra, & Smith, 2004; Harrigan, Kues, Ricks, & Smith, 1984; Labus, Mayer, Chang, Bolus,

& Naliboff, 2007; van Middendorp et al., 2008; Staud, Price, Robinson, & Vierck, 2004).

SUMMARY AND IMPLICATIONS

Experimental evidence from healthy humans suggests that positive emotions generally inhibit pain/nociception, and negative emotions generally facilitate pain/nociception, with greater inhibition/facilitation occurring (to a degree) with greater emotional intensity. Preliminary evidence suggests a role for serotonin in these effects (Horjales-Araujo et al., 2013). Further, emotional modulation is more reliable when it is tested using within-subject designs, standardized emotional stimuli (e.g., IAPS pictures), and punctate pain stimuli (e.g., electric, laser). Greater variability is found with tonic measures of pain (e.g., cold pressor), perhaps resulting from difficulties manipulating and generating emotions that persist over the total duration of the pain test. Nonetheless, data supporting emotional modulation are surprisingly consistent across emotion-induction strategies and pain stimulus modalities.

However, when negative emotions are intense, are highly arousing, and promote active defense (fight or flight), they inhibit pain/nociception via opioid mechanisms. But, intense negative emotions that elicit active defense are relatively rare; therefore, negative emotions should enhance pain and nociception in most circumstances.

The emotion–pain relationship can be characterized by a modified version of MPT that takes into account emotional valence and the degree of motivation system activation. Further, it has several implications. First, pain regulation strategies should use positive emotions with at least moderate arousal, because positive emotions with low arousal may have no effect on pain. Second, individual differences in subjective and physiological emotional reactivity (valence, arousal) should be measured in emotional modulation research. And third, arousal/intensity level is particularly important for determining the effect of negative emotions. Indeed, if some individuals react with moderate arousal and others react with high arousal, the net effect of negative emotion may average to zero at the group level.

Clinical findings indicate that emotions can play an important role in some pain disorders (e.g., FM, IBS) and a disruption of supraspinal circuits that mediate emotional modulation of pain may be involved. However, there are currently too few studies that have examined these issues in clinical populations; thus, additional experimental and longitudinal research is needed. But, if the current findings hold up, it could mean that: (1) preexisting deficits in emotional modulation confer risk for chronic pain, (2) deficits in supra-spinal circuits may need to be reversed before affective strategies can be used to manage pain, and (3) new technologies may need to be developed to reverse emotional modulation deficits and improve pain management (e.g., real-time fMRI to improve emotional regulation).

ACKNOWLEDGMENTS

This work was partly supported by R03AR054571 and R01MD007807 awarded to Jamie L. Rhudy. The content is solely the responsibility of the author and does not necessarily represent the official views of NIAMS, NIMHD, or the NIH.

REFERENCES

Arnold, B. S., Alpers, G. W., Suss, H., Friedel, E., Kosmutzky, G., Geier, A., et al. (2008). Affective pain modulation in fibromyalgia, somatoform pain disorder, back pain, and healthy controls. *European Journal of Pain (London, England), 12*(3), 329–338.

Bach, D. R., Erdmann, G., Schmidtmann, M., & Monnikes, H. (2006). Emotional stress reactivity in irritable bowel syndrome. *European Journal of Gastroenterology & Hepatology, 18*(6), 629–636.

Bair, M. J., Robinson, R. L., Katon, W., & Kroenke, K. (2003). Depression and pain comorbidity: a literature review. *Archives of Internal Medicine, 163*(20), 2433–2445.

Beecher, H. K. (1959). *Measurement of subjective responses.* New York: Oxford University Press.

Berna, C., Leknes, S., Holmes, E. A., Edwards, R. R., Goodwin, G. M., & Tracey, I. (2010). Induction of depressed mood disrupts emotion regulation neurocircuitry and enhances pain unpleasantness. *Biological Psychiatry, 67*(11), 1083–1090. http://dx.doi.org/10.1016/j.biopsych.2010.01.014.

Bolles, R. C., & Fanselow, M. S. (1980). A perceptual-defensive-recuperative model of fear and pain. *Behavioral & Brain Sciences, 3*(2), 291–323.

Bradley, M. M., Codispoti, M., Cuthbert, B. N., & Lang, P. J. (2001). Emotion and motivation I: defensive and appetitive reactions in picture processing. *Emotion, 1*(3), 276–298.

Bruehl, S., Carlson, C. R., & McCubbin, J. A. (1993). Two brief interventions for acute pain. *Pain, 54*(1), 29–36.

Bruehl, S., Liu, X., Burns, J. W., Chont, M., & Jamison, R. N. (2012). Associations between daily chronic pain intensity, daily anger expression, and trait anger expressiveness: an ecological momentary assessment study. *Pain, 153*(12), 2352–2358. http://dx.doi.org/10.1016/j.pain.2012.08.001.

Burns, J. W. (2006). Arousal of negative emotions and symptom-specific reactivity in chronic low back pain patients. *Emotion, 6*(2), 309–319.

Burns, J. W., Kubilus, A., & Bruehl, S. (2003). Emotion induction moderates effects of anger management style on acute pain sensitivity. *Pain, 106*(1), 109–118.

Carroll, L. J., Cassidy, J. D., & Côté, P. (2004). Depression as a risk factor for onset of an episode of troublesome neck and low back pain. *Pain, 107*(1), 134–139.

Carter, L. E., McNeil, D. W., Vowles, K. E., Sorrell, J. T., Turk, C. L., Ries, B. J., et al. (2002). Effects of emotion on pain reports, tolerance and physiology. *Pain Research & Management, 7*(1), 21–30.

Casey, C. Y., Greenberg, M. A., Nicassio, P. M., Harpin, R. E., & Hubbard, D. (2008). Transition from acute to chronic pain and disability: a model including cognitive, affective, and trauma factors. *Pain, 134*(1–2), 69–79. http://dx.doi.org/10.1016/j.pain.2007.03.032.

Cogan, R., Cogan, D., Waltz, W., & McCue, M. (1987). Effects of laughter and relaxation on discomfort thresholds. *Journal of Behavioral Medicine, 10*(2), 139–144.

Cornwall, A., & Donderi, D. C. (1988). The effect of experimentally induced anxiety on the experience of pressure pain. *Pain, 35*, 105–113.

CSEA. (2006). *The international affective picture system: Digitized photographs.*

Davis, M. C., Zautra, A. J., & Reich, J. W. (2001). Vulnerability to stress among women in chronic pain from fibromyalgia and osteoarthritis. *Annals of Behavioral Medicine: A Publication of The Society of Behavioral Medicine, 23*(3), 215.

Davis, M. C., Zautra, A. J., & Smith, B. W. (2004). Chronic pain, stress, and the dynamics of affective differentiation. *Journal of Personality, 72*(6), 1133–1159. http://dx.doi.org/10.1111/j.1467-6494.2004.00293.x.

DelVentura, J. L., Terry, E. L., Bartley, E. J., & Rhudy, J. L. (2014). Emotional modulation of pain and spinal nociception in persons with severe insomnia symptoms. *Annals of Behavioral Medicine, 47*(3), 303–315.

Dickhaus, B., Mayer, E. A., Firooz, N., Stains, J., Conde, F., Olivas, T. I., et al. (2003). Irritable bowel syndrome patients show enhanced modulation of visceral perception by auditory stress. *The American Journal of Gastroenterology, 98*(1), 135–143.

Dougher, M. J., Goldstein, D., & Leight, K. A. (1987). Induced anxiety and pain. *Journal of Anxiety Disorders, 1*(3), 259–264.

Flor, H., Birbaumer, N., Schulz, R., Grusser, S. M., & Mucha, R. F. (2002). Pavlovian conditioning of opioid and nonopioid pain inhibitory mechanisms in humans. *European Journal of Pain, 6*(5), 395–402.

Flor, H., & Grusser, S. M. (1999). Conditioned stress-induced analgesia in humans. *European Journal of Pain, 3*, 317–324.

Gannon, L. R., Haynes, S. N., Cuevas, J., & Chavez, R. (1987). Psychophysiological correlates of induced headaches. *Journal of Behavioral Medicine, 10*(4), 411–423.

Godinho, F., Magnin, M., Frot, M., Perchet, C., & Garcia-Larrea, L. (2006). Emotional modulation of pain: is it the sensation or what we recall? *The Journal of Neuroscience, 26*(44), 11454–11461. http://dx.doi.org/10.1523/JNEUROSCI.2260-06.2006.

Harrigan, J. A., Kues, J. R., Ricks, D. F., & Smith, R. (1984). Moods that predict coming migraine headaches. *Pain, 20*(4), 385–396.

Haslam, D. R. (1966). The effect of threatened shock upon pain threshold. *Psychonomic Science, 6*, 309–310.

Horjales-Araujo, E., Demontis, D., Lund, E. K., Vase, L., Finnerup, N. B., Børglum, A. D., et al. (2013). Emotional modulation of muscle pain is associated with polymorphisms in the serotonin transporter gene. *Pain, 154*(8), 1469–1476. http://dx.doi.org/10.1016/j.pain.2013.05.011.

Hubbard, C. S., Ornitz, E. M., Gaspar, J. X., Smith, S., Amin, J., Labus, J. S., et al. (2011). Modulation of nociceptive and acoustic startle responses to an unpredictable threat in men and women. *Pain, 152*, 1632–1634. http://dx.doi.org/10.1016/j.pain.2011.03.001.

Janssen, S. A., & Arntz, A. (1996). Anxiety and pain: attentional and endorphinergic influences. *Pain, 66*(2–3), 145–150.

Janssen, S. A., & Arntz, A. (1997). No evidence for opioid-mediated analgesia induced by phobic fear. *Behaviour Research and Therapy, 35*(9), 823–830.

Janssen, S. A., & Arntz, A. (2001). Real-life stress and opioid-mediated analgesia in novice parachute jumpers. *Journal of Psychophysiology, 15*(2), 106–113.

Ji, G., Sun, H., Fu, Y., Li, Z., Pais-Vieira, M., Galhardo, V., et al. (2010). Cognitive impairment in pain through amygdala-driven prefrontal cortical deactivation. *The Journal of Neuroscience, 30*(15), 5451–5464. http://dx.doi.org/10.1523/JNEUROSCI.0225-10.2010.

Kamping, S., Bomba, I. C., Kanske, P., Diesch, E., & Flor, H. (2013). Deficient modulation of pain by a positive emotional context in fibromyalgia patients. *Pain, 154*(9), 1846–1855. http://dx.doi.org/10.1016/j.pain.2013.06.003.

Kenntner-Mabiala, R., & Pauli, P. (2005). Affective modulation of brain potentials to painful and nonpainful stimuli. *Psychophysiology, 42*(5), 559–567.

Kenntner-Mabiala, R., Weyers, P., & Pauli, P. (2007). Independent effects of emotion and attention on sensory and affective pain perception. *Cognition and Emotion, 21*(8), 1615–1629. http://dx.doi.org/10.1080/02699930701252249.

Komisaruk, B. R., & Whipple, B. (2000). How does vaginal stimulation produce pleasure, pain and analgesia?. In E. R. B. Fillingim (Ed.), *Sex, gender and pain, progress in pain research and management* (Vol. 17, pp. 109–134) IASP Press.

Kroenke, K., Wu, J., Bair, M. J., Krebs, E. E., Damush, T. M., & Tu, W. (2011). Reciprocal relationship between pain and depression: a 12-month longitudinal analysis in primary care. *Journal of Pain, 12*(9), 964–973.

Labus, J. S., Mayer, E. A., Chang, L., Bolus, R., & Naliboff, B. D. (2007). The central role of gastrointestinal-specific anxiety in irritable bowel syndrome: further validation of the visceral sensitivity index. *Psychosomatic Medicine, 69*(1), 89–98.

Lang, P. J. (1995). The emotion probe: studies of motivation and attention. *American Psychologist, 50*(5), 372–385.

Lang, P. J., Bradley, M. M., & Cuthbert, B. N. (2001). *International affective picture system (IAPS): Technical manual and affective ratings: NIMH center for the study of emotion and attention.*

Lang, P. J., & Davis, M. (2006). Emotion, motivation, and the brain: reflex foundations in animal and human research. *Progress In Brain Research, 156*, 3–29.

Lapate, R. C., Lee, H., Salomons, T. V., van Reekum, C. M., Greischar, L. L., & Davidson, R. J. (2012). Amygdalar function reflects common individual differences in emotion and pain regulation success. *Journal of Cognitive Neuroscience, 24*(1), 148–158. http://dx.doi.org/10.1162/jocn_a_00125.

Lautenbacher, S., & Rollman, G. B. (1997). Possible deficiencies of pain modulation in fibromyalgia. *The Clinical Journal of Pain, 13*(3), 189.

Leventhal, H., & Everhart, D. (1979). Emotion, pain, and physical illness. In C. Izard (Ed.), *Emotions in personality and psychopathology* (pp. 261–299). US: Springer.

Litt, M. D. (1996). A model of pain and anxiety associated with acute stressors: distress in dental procedures. *Behaviour Research and Therapy, 34*(5–6), 459–476.

Lumley, M. A., Cohen, J. L., Borszcz, G. S., Cano, A., Radcliffe, A. M., Porter, L. S., et al. (2011). Pain and emotion: a biopsychosocial review of recent research. *Journal of Clinical Psychology, 67*(9), 942–968. http://dx.doi.org/10.1002/jclp.20816.

Marchand, S., & Arsenault, P. (2002). Odors modulate pain perception: a gender-specific effect. *Physiology and Behavior, 76*(2), 251–256.

Martin, G. N. (2006). The effect of exposure to odor on the perception of pain. *Psychosomatic Medicine, 68*(4), 613–616.

Meagher, M. W., Arnau, R. C., & Rhudy, J. L. (2001). Pain and emotion: effects of affective picture modulation. *Psychosomatic Medicine, 63*(1), 79–90.

Meagher, M. W., Ferguson, A. R., Crown, E. D., McLemore, S., King, T. E., Sieve, A. N., et al. (2001). Shock-induced hyperalgesia: IV. generality. *Journal of Experimental Psychology: Animal Behavior Processes, 27*(3), 219–238.

Melzack, R., & Wall, P. D. (1965). Pain mechanisms: a new theory. *Science, 150.*

van Middendorp, H., Lumley, M. A., Jacobs, J. W. G., van Doornen, L. J. P., Bijlsma, J. W. J., & Geenen, R. (2008). Emotions and emotional approach and avoidance strategies in fibromyalgia. *Journal of Psychosomatic Research, 64*(2), 159–167.

Mini, A., Rau, H., Montoya, P., Palomba, D., & Birbaumer, N. (1995). Baroreceptor cortical effects, emotions and pain. *International Journal of Psychophysiology: Official Journal of the International Organization of Psychophysiology, 19*(1), 67.

Montoya, P., Sitges, C., Garcia-Herrera, M., Izquierdo, R., Truyols, M., Blay, N., et al. (2005). Abnormal affective modulation of somatosensory brain processing among patients with fibromyalgia. *Psychosomatic Medicine, 67*(6), 957.

Navratilova, E., Xie, J. Y., Okun, A., Qu, C., Eyde, N., Ci, S., et al. (2012). Pain relief produces negative reinforcement through activation of mesolimbic reward-valuation circuitry. *Proceedings of the National Academy of Sciences of the United States of America, 109*(50), 20709–20713. http://dx.doi.org/10.1073/pnas.1214605109.

Neugebauer, V., Galhardo, V., Maione, S., & Mackey, S. C. (2009). Forebrain pain mechanisms. *Brain Research Reviews, 60*(1), 226–242.

Nisbett, R. E., & Schachter, S. (1966). The cognitive manipulation of pain. *Journal of Experimental Social Psychology, 2*(3), 227–236.

Palit, S., Kerr, K. L., Kuhn, B. L., DelVentura, J. L., Terry, E. L., Bartley, E. J., et al. (2013). Examining emotional modulation of pain and spinal nociception in native Americans: a preliminary investigation. *International Journal of Psychophysiology, 90*(2), 272–281.

Pitman, R. K., van der Kolk, B. A., Orr, S. P., & Greenberg, M. S. (1990). Naloxone-reversible analgesic response to combat-related stimuli in posttraumatic stress disorder. A pilot study. *Archives of General Psychiatry, 47*(6), 541–544.

Ploghaus, A., Narain, C., Beckmann, C. F., Clare, S., Bantick, S., Wise, R., et al. (2001). Exacerbation of pain by anxiety is associated with activity in a hippocampal network. *The Journal of Neuroscience: The Official Journal of the Society for Neuroscience, 21*(24), 9896.

Posserud, I., Agerforz, P., Ekman, R., Björnsson, E. S., Abrahamsson, H., & Simrén, M. (2004). Altered visceral perceptual and neuroendocrine response in patients with irritable bowel syndrome during mental stress. *Gut, 53*(8), 1102–1108.

Prescott, J., & Wilkie, J. (2007). Pain tolerance selectively increased by a sweet-smelling odor. *Psychological Science, 18*(4), 308–311.

Rainville, P., Bao, Q. V. H., & Chretien, P. (2005). Pain-related emotions modulate experimental pain perception and autonomic responses. *Pain, 118*(3), 306.

Rhudy, J. L., & Bartley, E. J. (2010). The effect of the menstrual cycle on affective modulation of pain and nociception in healthy women. *Pain, 149*, 365–372.

Rhudy, J. L., Bartley, E. J., Palit, S., Kerr, K. L., Kuhn, B. L., Martin, S. L., et al. (2013). Do sex hormones influence emotional modulation of pain and nociception in healthy women? *Biological Psychology, 94*(3), 534–544.

Rhudy, J. L., Bartley, E. J., Palit, S., Kuhn, B. L., Kerr, K. L., Martin, S. L., et al. (2014). Affective disturbance associated with premenstrual dysphoric disorder (PMDD) does not disrupt emotional modulation of pain and spinal nociception. *Pain, 155*(10), 2144–2152. http://dx.doi.org/10.1016/j.pain.2014.08.011.

Rhudy, J. L., Bartley, E. J., Williams, A. E., McCabe, K. M., Chandler, M. C., Russell, J. L., et al. (2010). Are there sex differences in affective modulation of spinal nociception and pain? *The Journal of Pain, 11*, 1429–1441.

Rhudy, J. L., DelVentura, J. L., Terry, E. L., Bartley, E. J., Olech, E., Palit, S., et al. (2013). Emotional modulation of pain and spinal nociception in fibromyalgia. *Pain, 154*(7), 1045–1056.

Rhudy, J. L., Dubbert, P. M., Parker, J. D., Burke, R. S., & Williams, A. E. (2006). Affective modulation of pain in substance dependent veterans. *Pain Medicine, 7*, 483–500.

Rhudy, J. L., Grimes, J. S., & Meagher, M. W. (2004). Fear-induced hypoalgesia in humans: effects on low intensity thermal stimulation and finger temperature. *Journal of Pain, 5*(8), 458–468.

Rhudy, J. L., Martin, S. L., Terry, E. L., DelVentura, J. L., Kerr, K. L., & Palit, S. (2012). Using multilevel growth curve modeling to examine emotional modulation of temporal summation of pain (TS-pain) and the nociceptive flexion reflex (TS-NFR). *Pain, 153,* 2274–2282.

Rhudy, J. L., McCabe, K. M., & Williams, A. E. (2007). Affective modulation of autonomic reactions to noxious stimulation. *International Journal of Psychophysiology, 63,* 105–109.

Rhudy, J. L., & Meagher, M. W. (2000). Fear and anxiety: divergent effects on human pain thresholds. *Pain, 84*(1), 65–75.

Rhudy, J. L., & Meagher, M. W. (2001a). The effects of conditioned fear on human pain. *Society for Neuroscience Abstracts, 27,* 82.

Rhudy, J. L., & Meagher, M. W. (2001b). Noise stress and human pain thresholds: divergent effects in men and women. *Journal of Pain, 2*(1), 57–64.

Rhudy, J. L., & Meagher, M. W. (2001c). The role of emotion in pain modulation. *Current Opinion in Psychiatry, 14*(3), 241–245.

Rhudy, J. L., & Meagher, M. W. (2003a). Individual differences in the emotional reaction to shock determine whether hypoalgesia is observed. *Pain Medicine, 4*(3), 244–256.

Rhudy, J. L., & Meagher, M. W. (2003b). Negative affect: effects on an evaluative measure of human pain. *Pain, 104*(3), 617–626.

Rhudy, J. L., & Williams, A. E. (2005). Gender differences in pain: do emotions play a role? *Gender Medicine, 2*(4), 208–226.

Rhudy, J. L., Williams, A. E., McCabe, K., Nguyen, M. A., & Rambo, P. (2005). Affective modulation of nociception at spinal and supraspinal levels. *Psychophysiology, 42,* 579–587.

Rhudy, J. L., Williams, A. E., McCabe, K. M., Rambo, P. L., & Russell, J. L. (2006). Emotional modulation of spinal nociception and pain: the impact of predictable noxious stimulation. *Pain, 126,* 221–233.

Rhudy, J. L., Williams, A. E., McCabe, K. M., Russell, J. L., & Maynard, L. J. (2008). Emotional control of nociceptive reactions (ECON): do affective valence and arousal play a role? *Pain, 136*(3), 250–261.

Roy, M., Lebuis, A., Peretz, I., & Rainville, P. (2011). The modulation of pain by attention and emotion: a dissociation of perceptual and spinal nociceptive processes. *European Journal of Pain, 15*(6), e1–e10. http://dx.doi.org/10.1016/j.ejpain.2010.11.013.

Roy, M., Peretz, I., & Rainville, P. (2008). Emotional valence contributes to music-induced analgesia. *Pain, 134*(1–2), 140–147.

Roy, M., Piche, M., Chen, J.-I., Peretz, I., & Rainville, P. (2009). Cerebral and spinal modulation of pain by emotions. *PNAS Proceedings of the National Academy of Sciences of the United States of America, 106*(49), 20900–20905. http://dx.doi.org/10.1073/pnas.0904706106.

Skljarevski, V., & Ramadan, N. M. (2002). The nociceptive flexion reflex in humans—review article. *Pain, 96,* 3–8.

Smith, L. D., & Wolpin, M. (1989). Emotive imagery and pain tolerance. In J. E. Shorr, P. Robin, J. A. Connella, & M. Wolpin (Eds.), *Imagery: Current perspectives* (pp. 159–173). New York, NY: Plenum Press.

Stancak, A., & Fallon, N. (2013). Emotional modulation of experimental pain: a source imaging study of laser evoked potentials. *Frontiers in Human Neuroscience, 7.* http://dx.doi.org/10.3389/fnhum.2013.00552.

Stancak, A., Ward, H., & Fallon, N. (2013). Modulation of pain by emotional sounds: a laser-evoked potential study. *European Journal of Pain, 17*(3), 324–335. http://dx.doi.org/10.1002/j.1532-2149.2012.00206.x.

Staud, R., Price, D. D., Robinson, M. E., & Vierck, C. J., Jr. (2004). Body pain area and pain-related negative affect predict clinical pain intensity in patients with fibromyalgia. *The Journal of Pain: Official Journal of the American Pain Society, 5*(6), 338–343.

Tellegen, A., Watson, D., & Clark, L. A. (1999). On the dimensional and hierarchical structure of affect. *Psychological Science, 10*(4), 297–303. http://dx.doi.org/10.1111/1467-9280.00157.

Terry, E. L., DelVentura, J. L., Bartley, E. J., Vincent, A., & Rhudy, J. L. (2013). Emotional modulation of pain and spinal nociception in persons with major depressive disorder (MDD). *Pain, 154*(12), 2759–2768. http://dx.doi.org/10.1016/j.pain.2013.08.009.

de Tommaso, M., Calabrese, R., Vecchio, E., De Vito Francesco, V., Lancioni, G., & Livrea, P. (2009). Effects of affective pictures on pain sensitivity and cortical responses induced by laser stimuli in healthy subjects and migraine patients. *International Journal of Psychophysiology, 74*(2), 139–148. http://dx.doi.org/10.1016/j.ijpsycho.2009.08.004.

Villemure, C., & Bushnell, M. C. (2009). Mood influences supraspinal pain processing separately from attention. *The Journal of Neuroscience, 29*(3), 705–715. http://dx.doi.org/10.1523/JNEUROSCI.3822-08.2009.

Villemure, C., Slotnick, B. M., & Bushnell, M. C. (2003). Effects of odors on pain perception: deciphering the roles of emotion and attention. *Pain, 106*(1–2), 101–108.

Walters, E. T. (1994). Injury related behavior and neural plasticity: an evolutionary perspective on sensitization, hyperalgesia, and analgesia. *International Review of Neurobiology, 36*, 325–426.

Weisenberg, M., Aviram, O., Wolf, Y., & Raphaeli, N. (1984). Relevant and irrelevant anxiety in the reaction to pain. *Pain, 20*(4), 371–383.

Weisenberg, M., Raz, T., & Hener, T. (1998). The influence of film-induced mood on pain perception. *Pain, 76*(3), 365–375.

Weisenberg, M., Tepper, I., & Schwarzwald, J. (1995). Humor as a cognitive technique for increasing pain tolerance. *Pain, 63*(2), 207–212.

de Wied, M., & Verbaten, M. N. (2001). Affective pictures processing, attention, and pain tolerance. *Pain, 90*(1–2), 163–172.

Willer, J. C. (1980). Anticipation of pain-produced stress: electrophysiological study in man. *Physiology & Behavior, 25*(1), 49–51.

Willer, J. C., & Albe-Fessard, D. (1980). Electrophysiological evidence for a release of endogenous opiates in stress-induced 'analgesia' in man. *Brain Research, 198*(2), 419–426.

Willer, J. C., Boureau, F., & Albe-Fessard, D. (1979). Supraspinal influences on nociceptive flexion reflex and pain sensation in man. *Brain Research, 179*, 61–68.

Willer, J. C., Dehen, H., & Cambier, J. (1981). Stress-induced analgesia in humans: endogenous opioids and naloxone-reversible depression of pain reflexes. *Science, 212*(4495), 689–691.

Willer, J. C., & Ernst, M. (1986). Diazepam reduces stress-induced analgesia in humans. *Brain Research, 362*(2), 398–402.

Williams, A. E., & Rhudy, J. L. (2007a). Affective modulation of eyeblink reactions to noxious sural nerve stimulation: a supraspinal measure of nociceptive reactivity? *International Journal of Psychophysiology, 66*(3), 255–265.

Williams, A. E., & Rhudy, J. L. (2007b). The influence of conditioned fear on human pain thresholds: does preparedness play a role? *The Journal of Pain, 8*(7), 598–606.

Williams, A. E., & Rhudy, J. L. (2009). Supraspinal modulation of trigeminal nociception and pain. *Headache, 49*, 704–720.

Willoughby, S. G., Hailey, B. J., Mulkana, S., & Rowe, J. (2002). The effect of laboratory-induced depressed mood state on responses to pain. *Behavioral Medicine, 28*(1), 23–31.

Worthington, E. L. (1978). The effects of imagery content, choice of imagery content, and self-verbalization on the self-control of pain. *Cognitive Therapy & Research, 2*(3), 225–240.

Wunsch, A., Philippot, P., & Plaghki, L. (2003). Affective associative learning modifies the sensory perception of nociceptive stimuli without participant's awareness. *Pain, 102*(1), 27–38.

Zelman, D. C., Howland, E. W., Nichols, S. N., & Cleeland, C. S. (1991). The effects of induced mood on laboratory pain. *Pain, 46*(1), 105–111.

Zillmann, D., de Wied, M., King-Jablonski, C., & Jenzowsky, S. (1996). Drama-induced affect and pain sensitivity. *Psychosomatic Medicine, 58*(4), 333–341.

CHAPTER 4

Sex Differences in Pain and Stress

Emily J. Bartley, Roger B. Fillingim

University of Florida, Pain Research and Intervention Center of Excellence, Gainesville, FL, USA

INTRODUCTION

The prevalence and societal impact of chronic pain are staggering. Chronic pain affects 100 million U.S. adults and produces costs exceeding $600 billion annually; indeed, chronic pain affects more individuals and produces greater societal costs than cancer, AIDS, and heart disease combined (Gaskin & Richard, 2012; Institute of Medicine Committee on Advancing Pain Research & Education, 2011). While pain affects individuals from all population groups, abundant evidence suggests that many common chronic pain conditions are more prevalent among women than men (Fillingim, King, Ribeiro-Dasilva, Rahim-Williams, & Riley, 2009; Institute of Medicine Committee on Advancing Pain Research & Education, 2011; LeResche, 1999). Importantly, psychosocial stress represents a significant risk factor for development and increased clinical severity of chronic pain, and stress may contribute to sex differences in the experience of pain (Kulich, Mencher, Bertrand, & Maciewicz, 2000; McBeth, Morris, Benjamin, Silman, & Macfarlane, 2001; Schell, Theorell, Hasson, Arnetz, & Saraste, 2008). The purpose of this chapter is to review the evidence regarding sex differences in pain and to discuss the contributions of stress to these sex differences in pain. First, we will provide an overview of the literature regarding sex differences in both clinical pain and responses to laboratory-induced pain. Then, we will briefly discuss the contributions of stress to pain, including sex differences in stress responses and their potential contributions to sex differences in pain. Next, we will highlight the biopsychosocial mechanisms underlying sex differences in pain and the contributions of stress thereto. The chapter will conclude with a discussion of overall findings and important directions for future research.

The Neuroscience of Pain, Stress, and Emotion
http://dx.doi.org/10.1016/B978-0-12-800538-5.00004-2

SEX DIFFERENCES IN CLINICAL PAIN

Numerous epidemiologic studies have examined whether there are sex differences in the prevalence of chronic pain. For example, using a general case definition of chronic pain (e.g., pain on more days than not that has lasted for at least 3 months), women in the general population are significantly more likely to report chronic pain than men (Fillingim et al., 2009; Institute of Medicine Committee on Advancing Pain Research & Education, 2011). More recently, in the National Health and Nutrition Examination Survey (NHANES), the point prevalence of chronic pain (pain lasting more than 3 months) anywhere in the body was significantly higher in women (18.3%) than in men (12.9%) (Riskowski, 2014). Prevalence of acute pain (pain of <3 months duration) was also significantly greater in women (13%) than in men (11.4%), but less dramatically so. An Internet-based survey of more than 27,000 individuals in the United States found that significantly more women (34.3%) than men (26.7%) reported chronic pain (Johannes, Le, Zhou, Johnston, & Dworkin, 2010). Other studies have examined sex differences in specific pain conditions or pain in specific anatomical locations. For example, in another analysis of NHANES data, women showed higher prevalence of chronic pain in several, but not all, body regions as well as higher prevalence of widespread pain than men (Hardt, Jacobsen, Goldberg, Nickel, & Buchwald, 2008) (see Figure 1). Additional studies from multiple countries report similar results (Fernández-de-las-Peñas et al., 2011; Klijs, Nusselder, Looman, & Mackenbach, 2014), as summarized by Mogil (2012). Thus, the existing findings regarding sex differences in the prevalence of chronic pain reveal a highly consistent pattern of greater chronic pain prevalence among women; however, the magnitude of these sex differences varies across pain locations and across studies, and the observed sex differences are sometimes statistically significant and sometimes not.

The above findings generally derive from studies of adults and do not reflect any potential influence of age on sex differences in pain prevalence; however, it is important to acknowledge that sex differences in pain may vary across the life span. A meta-analysis of studies of pain prevalence in children and adolescents found that prevalence rates for most types of pain were greater for girls than for boys and prevalence increased with age (King et al., 2011). In particular, headache, abdominal pain, musculoskeletal pain, multiple pains, and general pain were more common in girls, while back pain showed less evidence of sex differences in prevalence, and lower limb

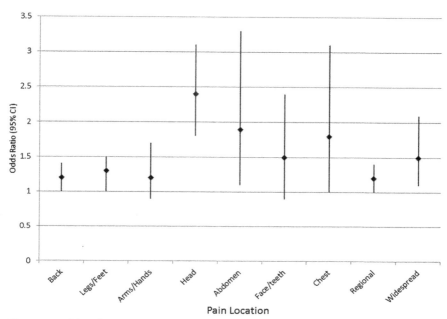

Figure 1 Odds of chronic pain conditions for women relative to men. The figure presents odds (and 95% confidence intervals) of each type of pain for women relative to men. Respondents were asked if they had a problem with pain that had lasted for at least 24 h and was not "fleeting or minor." If yes, then they were asked about the duration of pain, and chronic pain was defined as pain lasting at least 3 months. Widespread pain was defined as pain occurring above and below the waist, on both sides of the body, and in at least one axial location (spine, chest, upper or lower back). Regional pain was defined as any chronic pain that did not meet criteria for widespread pain. *(Data are from Hardt et al. (2008).)*

pain was more common in boys. At the other end of the life span, sex differences in pain prevalence in older adults have been examined in several studies. Data from the U.S. Health and Retirement Study, a nationally representative study of adults aged 60 and older, reported higher prevalence of chronic pain among women than men (Andrews, Cenzer, Yelin, & Covinsky, 2013). Similar results have been reported by others (Blyth et al., 2001; Tsang et al., 2008). However, age-related prevalence patterns for females and males can vary across pain conditions. For example, while joint pain is increasingly prevalent with age for both women and men, sex differences in prevalence of migraine, abdominal pain, and temporomandibular disorders generally peak in the reproductive years, with lower prevalence in females before adolescence and later in life (LeResche, 2000).

These findings highlight the importance of taking a life-span perspective when examining sex differences in pain.

SEX DIFFERENCES IN EXPERIMENTAL PAIN RESPONSES

Because clinical pain can be influenced by multiple uncontrolled factors, including severity of disease or tissue damage and the effects of treatment, many investigators have sought to examine sex differences in pain using carefully controlled laboratory-based pain induction methods. Common experimental pain stimuli include heat, cold, mechanical pressure, electrical, and chemical stimuli. The most commonly assessed measures are pain threshold (the lowest stimulus intensity required to induce pain) and pain tolerance (the highest stimulus intensity the participant is willing and able to tolerate). However, in recent years, there has been increased interest in using more dynamic stimulus configurations to assess pain-facilitatory and pain-inhibitory processes, including temporal summation of pain and CPM, respectively (Yarnitsky, Granot, & Granovsky, 2014). This literature has been thoroughly reviewed and summarized numerous times (Bartley & Fillingim, 2013; Fillingim et al., 2009; Hashmi & Davis, 2014; Mogil, 2012; Racine et al., 2012a). Despite varying interpretations of the findings, the pattern of results is quite clear and inarguable. In laboratory pain studies, women consistently report lower pain thresholds and tolerances and provide higher pain ratings in response to suprathreshold stimuli. This is true across all stimulus modalities that have been tested. However, the magnitude of these sex differences varies considerably across studies and even within studies across pain stimuli. With regard to the life-span perspective recommended above, a meta-analysis of sex differences in experimental pain responses among children and adolescents was published in 2014. This analysis revealed less consistent sex differences in children and adolescents compared to what has been observed in adults; however, in children over the age of 12, girls reported greater cold pressor pain intensity and lower heat pain threshold and tolerance compared to boys (Boerner, Birnie, Caes, Schinkel, & Chambers, 2014). Unfortunately, limited information is available regarding sex differences in laboratory pain responses among older adults, although a previous study showed that older women using hormone replacement were more sensitive to heat pain compared to both older women not using hormones and older men, who did not differ from each other (Fillingim & Edwards, 2001).

The above studies refer to traditional measures of pain perception, such as pain threshold and tolerance, which are relatively static and unidimensional, while more recent research has witnessed increased interest in more dynamic measures of pain-facilitatory and pain-inhibitory functions. Several studies have examined sex differences in temporal summation of pain, a measure of pain facilitation, which refers to the increase in pain that occurs when a fixed painful stimulus is repeatedly administered in rapid succession. Most of the studies have revealed significantly greater temporal summation of pain among women than men, in response to both heat and mechanical stimuli (Fillingim et al., 2009; Racine et al., 2012a), suggesting greater pain facilitation among women. Regarding pain-inhibitory function, the most common experimental method for assessment involves testing whether the ability of a painful stimulus applied to one body site is able to reduce the painfulness of a second stimulus applied at a remote body site, which is known as conditioned pain modulation (CPM) (Yarnitsky et al., 2010). A meta-analysis of studies examining CPM showed that males exhibit significantly greater CPM than females, suggesting enhanced pain-inhibitory responses among males (Popescu, LeResche, Truelove, & Drangsholt, 2010). However, studies of a different pain-inhibitory process have revealed that women show greater habituation to sustained heat stimuli compared to men (Hashmi & Davis, 2010, 2014). Also, as further discussed below, stress-induced analgesia (SIA) may produce greater pain inhibition in females than in males (Fillingim et al., 2009). Thus, while there is considerable variability across studies in the magnitude of the effects, the literature on sex differences in response to laboratory-induced pain consistently demonstrates greater sensitivity to pain and increased pain facilitation among women. While studies of CPM show more robust pain-inhibitory responses among men, other forms of pain inhibition may be greater for women.

STRESS AND PAIN: AN INTRODUCTION

Considerable evidence indicates bidirectional interactions between stress and pain. An acute injury serves as a prime example of this relationship. As is well known, pain is vital to the survival of the organism. It serves as a warning signal—signifying the presence of threat and enhancing motivation toward elimination of the threat or dampening its effects to prevent further injury. In the case of injury, and accompanying pain, the stress response is automatically activated, triggering a series of physiological events intended to help the organism adapt to the stressor and reach a level of homeostatic balance. Although this response system is adaptive, as it enables the body to acclimate to various environmental and internal challenges—a process known as allostasis (Logan & Barksdale, 2008), the continuous activation of the stress response may increase health-related burden and facilitate progression of chronic disease, including persistent pain (McEwen, 1998). While a discussion of the stress response system is beyond the scope of this chapter (see Chapter 2 for a more comprehensive review), the following sections are directed toward discussing the dynamic relationship between stress and pain.

RELATIONSHIP BETWEEN STRESS AND PAIN

It is not surprising that stress and pain are related, especially given that multiple neuroendocrine, immune, and autonomic mediators play a role in stress responsivity as well as neuromodulatory responses that regulate pain (McEwen & Kalia, 2010). Chapman and colleagues postulate that chronic pain may develop from dysregulation in endocrine, nervous, and immune subsystems, a consequence that can lead to supersystem dysfunction. Given the interactive nature of these systems, dysregulation in one subsystem would give rise to deficits in another. Hence, the authors posit that transition from acute pain to chronic pain probably arises from maladaptive changes within the supersystem, which can lead to systemic pathology and dysregulation in facilitatory and inhibitory systems responsible for nociceptive processing (Chapman, Tuckett, & Song, 2008).

Numerous animal and human studies have reported on the effects of stress on both pain inhibition and suppression. If an organism is under threat from a predator and becomes wounded, the peripheral and central nervous system pathways that modulate pain expression are activated and facilitate a set of responses to suppress the perception of pain. This is advantageous in that it allows the organism to redirect its resources and mobilize energy toward either escape or approach behavior. Conversely, energy directed toward focus on the pain would not be beneficial as this would diminish attention toward protection from the threat. This phenomenon, termed SIA, is a reduced pain response believed to be mediated by descending pain-inhibitory circuits and engaged by intense and highly arousing stressors (Butler & Finn, 2009; Rhudy & Meagher, 2000; Wagner et al., 2013).

In contrast, stress can also enhance pain, which is commonly observed in cases of mild and prolonged stressors (i.e., stress-induced hyperalgesia). For example, in preclinical studies the same stressor that acutely invokes SIA produces hyperalgesia with repeated exposure (Jennings, Okine, Roche, & Finn, 2014). If we consider the systems perspective proposed by Chapman and colleagues, persistent activation of the stress response will probably lead to dysregulation in both pain-facilitatory and -inhibitory processes and enhance vulnerability to chronic pain. Ample evidence implicates persistent stress in pain and functioning in multiple chronic pain conditions including fibromyalgia (FM), irritable bowel syndrome (IBS), and temporomandibular disorder. Indeed, healthy individuals with higher levels of overall perceived distress (as measured by psychological distress and somatization) have been found to be two to nine times more likely to develop widespread pain after a follow-up of 12 months (McBeth, Macfarlane, Benjamin, & Silman, 2001). Cathcart and Pritchard observed that daily stress was a significant predictor of increased muscle tenderness and reduced pressure pain thresholds in individuals with chronic tension-type headache over a 2-week period (Cathcart & Pritchard, 2008). Further, among patients with rheumatoid arthritis, Fifield and colleagues found that on workdays with a higher degree of stressors, patients reported greater midday pain (Fifield et al., 2004).

Pain is also typically conceived as a potent stressor. The stress associated with chronic pain can lead to lower quality of life, increased disability, occupational and economic hardship, and decrements in social well-being. A number of studies have also reported on the presence of affective distress in patients with chronic pain, with evidence suggesting that approximately 35% of individuals with chronic pain are affected by various psychiatric disorders such as depression (Miller & Cano, 2009). Further, the risk of depression is reported to increase when pain is of a diffuse nature (Lépine & Briley, 2004). Because women tend to have a higher risk for chronic pain, as well as stress-related disorders such as depression and anxiety, it has been suggested that alterations in noradrenergic and hypothalamic–pituitary–adrenal (HPA) axis activity may give rise to aberrations in opioidergic functioning and serve as a mechanism underlying sex differences in pain and stress.

SEX DIFFERENCES IN NEUROENDOCRINE RESPONSES TO STRESS

Sexually dimorphic responses in stress regulatory systems have been implicated in the etiology of sex differences in pain. Although this chapter primarily focuses on human models, research in animals has demonstrated a relatively consistent pattern of responses, with female rodents exhibiting higher basal levels of glucocorticoids and corticosterone, higher peak amplitudes of corticosterone, and greater levels of adrenocorticotropic hormone (ACTH) and corticosterone release in response to a stressor (Bangasser & Valentino, 2012; Kudielka & Kirschbaum, 2005). The picture appears to be more complex among humans, an effect probably influenced by numerous factors including variability in the type of stressor or experimental methodology, hormone status, psychiatric comorbidity, demographic factors, and outcomes measured. While some studies have reported no differences among males and females in both basal levels (Allen, Lu, Tsao, Worthman, & Zeltzer, 2009) and reactivity (Kelly, Tyrka, Anderson, Price, & Carpenter, 2008; Paris et al., 2010; van Stegeren, Wolf, & Kindt, 2008) of stress-related hormones such as ACTH or corticosteroids, others have established clear sex differences, with larger cortisol and ACTH responses in men. For instance, men had higher cortisol reactivity to a harassment stressor (Earle, Linden, & Weinberg, 1999), while the same was observed in another study examining responsivity to a mental stressor (i.e., reaction time test and mental arithmetic) (Lovallo, Farag, Vincent, Thomas, & Wilson, 2006). Interestingly, the latter study found that women had greater cortisol responses after a standardized postexercise meal, suggesting differences in metabolic functioning among men and women. In response to a cold pain induction, Zimmer, Basler, Vedder, & Lautenbacher (2003) found greater cortisol responses in men compared to women; however, these effects differed according to the type of stressor. In a study by Stroud, Salovey, & Epel (2002), men had higher cortisol reactivity in response to an achievement-oriented task, while women had greater cortisol responses to a social rejection task. The authors hypothesized that women's greater adrenocortical responses to interpersonal rejection may be a potential mechanism underlying higher rates of affective distress in this group.

Age also appears to be an important determinant of sex differences in HPA response patterns. Allen and colleagues (Allen et al., 2009) found no sex differences in cortisol reactivity to a cold pressor test in children aged 8–18. However, when the groups were compared separately, higher cortisol levels were associated with increased pressure tolerance among boys, while greater cortisol reactivity was related to higher pain intensity and unpleasantness in girls. Further, in a meta-analysis of sex and age effects on HPA reactivity, Otte and colleagues noted that older adults exhibited large cortisol responses to psychosocial stressors, and these effects were stronger in women (Otte, Hart, Neylan, & Marmar, 2005). In addition to age influences, menstrual cycle and hormone status have been found to play a role in HPA axis and adrenocortical reactivity. For example, Kirschbaum, Kudielka, Gaab, Schommer, & Hellhammer (1999) assessed responsivity to a psychosocial speech challenge in 81 healthy adults including women in the luteal and follicular phases, women using oral contraceptives, and men. While no sex differences emerged for total plasma cortisol, ACTH responses were elevated in men compared to women in all groups. However, women in the luteal phase and men had relatively comparable salivary cortisol responses, whereas the other two groups had lower free cortisol responses. Taken together, results from these studies suggest that HPA axis response patterns appear to differ across males and females, but multiple unmeasured factors have an impact on these responses, thus contributing to the complexity of findings across studies.

THE RELATIONSHIP OF STRESS TO CHRONIC PAIN PREVALENCE IN WOMEN

There is ample evidence reflecting the reciprocal relationship between stress and pain. Stress can certainly worsen pain-related symptomatology and individuals with chronic pain are at greater risk for increased sensitivity to interpersonal and environmental stressors. As mentioned previously, women have a higher predisposition for development of a number of chronic pain conditions, including temporomandibular disorder, FM, IBS, tension-type headache, interstitial cystitis, and chronic fatigue syndrome (CFS), and stress is reported to be a major contributor to the onset and maintenance of these conditions.

Because of the link between stress and pain, several studies have investigated alterations in HPA axis and sympathetic nervous system functioning as a potential etiological factor in chronic pain. While higher basal levels of cortisol (Chang et al., 2009) and noradrenaline (Posserud et al., 2004) have been observed in IBS, others have found blunted levels of cortisol (Böhmelt, Nater, Franke, Hellhammer, & Ehlert, 2005) and ACTH (Chang et al., 2009) in this group. Upon the induction of a psychosocial stressor, patients with IBS have demonstrated higher levels of ACTH (Posserud et al., 2004) and cortisol (Chang et al., 2009) or no differences in norepinephrine, cortisol, or ACTH (Dickhaus et al., 2003).

Findings in patients with FM have been just as inconsistent, as there is evidence of both hyper- and hypocortisolism in this group. In a meta-analysis of 85 studies examining neuroendocrine activity in FM, IBS, and CFS, the authors found that while hypocortisolism was significantly observed in CFS, there were no consistent abnormalities in functioning in IBS or FM (Tak et al., 2011). However, it is important to note that multiple factors may hinder consistency among studies. For example, in a sample of patients with FM, Crofford and colleagues observed that approximately half demonstrated heightened levels of cortisol in the evening hours, compared with healthy subjects (Crofford et al., 2004). Further, in a study comparing morning wakening cortisol responses in patients with FM and patients with shoulder and neck pain (SNP), Riva and colleagues observed that women with SNP had hypercortisolism, whereas patients with FM had hypo-cortisolism, upon waking. The authors speculated that the hypercortisolism observed in regional pain syndrome may be a preliminary step toward development of hypocortisolism and subsequent widespread pain (Riva, Mork, Westgaard, & Lundberg, 2012). Overall, results suggest that dysre-gulation in HPA axis and sympathetic-adrenal-medullary axis activity may play an important role in the development and/or persistence of chronic pain, but a number of factors such as the salience of the stressor and the timing of biomarker collection could influence results.

SEX DIFFERENCES IN SIA

Depending on the nature of the stimulus, stress can induce a hypoalgesic effect and dampen the perception of pain. A number of preclinical studies have reported on sex differences in SIA, with several noting greater SIA in males than in females (Butler & Finn, 2009; Craft, 2003). Moreover, qualitative sex differences in SIA have been reported, as analgesia induced by forced swim stress was reversed by either opioid or N-methyl-D-aspartate blockade in male but not female animals (Mogil, Sternberg, Kest, Marek, & Liebeskind, 1993). Results from human studies vary, with some finding no sex differences, whereas others note greater SIA in females. For example, no sex differences in SIA were observed in response to a speech induction (al'Absi & Petersen, 2003) or an argument stressor (Bragdon et al., 2002). In contrast, Rhudy and

Meagher found that when using radiant heat as a test stimulus and acoustic startle as the stressor, women exhibited greater SIA (as evidenced by greater heat pain thresholds), while the opposite effect was observed in men (Rhudy & Meagher, 2001). Sternberg et al. found that after a period of treadmill running, women demonstrated greater SIA during a cold pressor test; however, in the same study, men showed greater analgesia after a video game competition (Sternberg, Boka, Kas, Alboyadjia, & Gracely, 2001). Interestingly, there were no sex differences across these two stress conditions using radiant heat as the pain stimulus. Overall, the characteristics of the stressor and the nature of the pain being assessed likely dictate the presence of sex differences in SIA.

MECHANISMS UNDERLYING SEX DIFFERENCES IN PAIN

Multiple biological and psychosocial variables contribute to sex differences in pain. In addition to differences in stress regulatory systems, male–female differences in central nervous system processing of pain-related information could contribute to the observed sex differences in clinical and experimental pain responses. Several studies of brain imaging have examined sex differences in pain-induced cerebral activation. Overall, these studies show some sex differences in pain-related brain activation, but there is also substantial overlap in pain-evoked brain activity between females and males (Fillingim et al., 2009). More recently, sex differences in functional and structural connectivity in pain-related networks have been reported, with women showing greater connectivity of descending pain modulatory systems, while men showed greater connectivity in salience and attention networks (Wang, Erpelding, & Davis, 2014). Also, studies in females and males with migraine and abdominal pain have revealed sex differences in functional and structural connectivity (Hong et al., 2014; Jiang et al., 2013; Maleki et al., 2012). Overall, these studies suggest that differences in brain structure and function between females and males may contribute to differences in the experience of pain; however, additional studies are needed to further characterize the influence of pain-related brain activity on sex differences in pain.

Reproductive hormones represent another potentially important factor contributing to sex differences in pain. For example, menstrual cycle influences on clinical and experimental pain responses have been demonstrated (Fillingim et al., 2009; Hassan, Muere, & Einstein, 2014). Considerable evidence indicates that estrogens affect pain responses in a complex fashion, as both pain-facilitatory and pain-inhibitory effects of estrogens have been reported. For example, use of hormone replacement among postmenopausal women has been associated with increased risk for clinical pain and enhanced experimental pain sensitivity. In contrast, exogenous administration of estrogen reduced muscle pain sensitivity and enhanced pain-related brain μ-opioid receptor binding in healthy women, suggesting that estrogen enhances endogenous opioid-mediated pain inhibition. Also, testosterone has been associated with reduced pain sensitivity (Bartley et al., 2015; Cairns & Gazerani, 2009). Thus, while gonadal hormones influence pain responses, the magnitude and direction of these effects remain unclear, and the precise biological mechanisms whereby sex hormones influence pain responses remain unknown.

Genetic factors may also contribute to sex differences in pain. The catechol-O-methyl-transferase gene (*COMT*), which represents the most widely studied gene in the pain field, has been associated with pain in a sex-dependent fashion (Belfer et al., 2013). Specifically, a haplotype coding for low *COMT* activity was associated with increased capsaicin-induced pain among women but not men. Another commonly studied pain gene is the μ-opioid receptor gene (*OPRM1*). The *OPRM1* A118G single-nucleotide polymorphism (SNP) has been associated with pain in several studies, such that the minor (G) allele is associated with reduced pain sensitivity (Fillingim, Wallace, Herbstman, Ribeiro-Dasilva, & Staud, 2008). The minor (G) allele of this SNP was associated with pressure pain sensitivity, marginally more strongly in males than in females, and a gene-by-sex interaction emerged for thermal pain sensitivity, such that the minor allele predicted lower thermal pain sensitivity in males but higher thermal pain sensitivity in females (Fillingim et al., 2005). A similar pattern of results emerged in a clinical study, in which the G allele predicted lower pain and disability scores 12 months after lumbar disc herniation in males, while females with the G allele showed greater pain and disability at follow-up (Olsen et al., 2012).

A translational study demonstrated that both sex and genotype can interact with stress to influence pain responses. Mogil et al. (2011) examined the association of the vasopressin receptor (*AVPR1A*) with capsaicin-induced pain. An SNP of *AVPR1A* was associated with capsaicin pain, but only among males who reported high levels of stress at the time of testing, which corroborated the findings observed in mice (Mogil et al., 2011). These results were further supported by findings that high stress predicted poorer desmopressin (a synthetic AVPR1A agonist) analgesia only among men with this *AVPR1A* genotype. These findings suggest that vasopressin activates endogenous analgesic mechanisms, except when they have already been activated by stress, as in males with high functioning of the AVPR1A receptor. This genotype-by-sex-by-stress interaction indicates the complexity of biopsychosocial influences on pain.

In addition to biological processes, multiple psychosocial factors contribute to sex differences in pain. For example, stereotypic gender roles appear to be associated with experimental pain responses, as women are more willing to report pain, which has been associated with sex differences in experimental pain responses. Pain coping may also play a role in sex differences in pain. Women report higher levels of pain catastrophizing, which can contribute to sex differences in clinical and experimental pain responses. Additional pain-related psychosocial processes that may contribute to sex differences in pain include negative mood, including depression and anxiety; more detailed discussions of psychosocial contributions to sex differences in pain can be found elsewhere (Fillingim et al., 2009; Racine et al., 2012b).

CONCLUSIONS

In laboratory settings, mounting evidence supports differences between men and women with respect to responsivity to painful experimental stimuli, with women reporting lower pain thresholds and tolerances, higher ratings of pain, greater pain facilitation, and lower pain inhibition, compared to men. Similarly, chronic pain prevalence is higher among women. However, the magnitude of these differences varies by pain location, age, and study.

Multiple biopsychosocial mechanisms are likely to contribute to sex differences in pain, including variation in brain structure and function, sex hormones, genetic factors, gender roles, and pain-related coping. Stress has been identified as a potential precipitant of chronic pain, and several investigations support the role that stress-related triggers have on the onset and maintenance of persistent pain. When stressors are prolonged, this may confer risk for chronic pain by enhancing dysregulation in peripheral and central nervous system processing and reducing the capacity for recovery and adaptation. We propose a model that aligns with the systems perspective paradigm proposed by Chapman et al. (2008), but considers the role of sex differences on various levels of this system. We postulate that upon the induction of a stressor (e.g., physical, psychological, social), supersystem dysregulation may be facilitated by sexually dimorphic differences in coping, as well as male–female differences in neural, endocrine, and immune system functioning. Through persistent activation of the stress response, allostatic load is initiated, which may prompt vulnerability to chronic pain among women (see Figure 2). Hence, given the prevalence of chronic pain in women, the extent to which stress has meaningful implications for susceptibility to pain may be an important consideration for understanding and eliminating sex-related disparities in chronic pain. Ultimately, treatment for chronic pain may benefit from taking a systems-based approach and considering the multiple interactive factors (both psychosocial and biological) that influence health and human functioning and the dynamic role that stress plays in these functions.

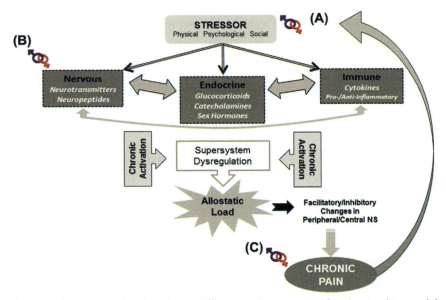

Figure 2 Hypothetical role of sex differences in stress and pain. In this model, physical, psychological, and social stressors activate stress regulatory systems at the nervous, endocrine, and immune system levels. Persistent activation of stressors leads to supersystem dysregulation and generates an allostatic load response. This facilitates aberrations in facilitatory and inhibitory functions in peripheral and central nervous system processing, an effect that may reduce recovery capacity and enhance risk for development and maintenance of chronic pain. In turn, persistent pain serves as a powerful stressor, which could ultimately perpetuate a pain–stress cycle. It is proposed that sex differences exist at multiple levels of this model. Sex differences in stress-related coping (A) may give rise to supersystem dysfunction and enhance sex differences in stress regulatory systems (B). As a result, dysregulation among nervous, endocrine, and immune systems prompts allostatic load and increases risk for chronic pain among women (C).

REFERENCES

al'Absi, M., & Petersen, K. L. (2003). Blood pressure but not cortisol mediates stress effects on subsequent pain perception in healthy men and women. *Pain, 106*(3), 285–295. http://dx.doi.org/10.1016/S0304-3959(03)00300-2.

Allen, L. B., Lu, Q., Tsao, J. C. I., Worthman, C. M., & Zeltzer, L. K. (2009). Sex differences in the association between cortisol concentrations and laboratory pain responses in healthy children. *Gender Medicine, 6*(Part 2), 193–207. http://dx.doi.org/10.1016/j.genm.2009.03.001.

Andrews, J. S., Cenzer, I. S., Yelin, E., & Covinsky, K. E. (2013). Pain as a risk factor for disability or death. *Journal of the American Geriatrics Society, 61*(4), 583–589. http://dx.doi.org/10.1111/jgs.12172.

Bangasser, D. A., & Valentino, R. J. (2012). Sex differences in molecular and cellular substrates of stress. *Cellular and Molecular Neurobiology, 32*(5), 709–723. http://dx.doi.org/10.1007/s10571-012-9824-4.

Bartley, E. J., & Fillingim, R. B. (2013). Sex differences in pain: a brief review of clinical and experimental findings. *British Journal of Anaesthesia, 111*(1), 52–58. http://dx.doi.org/10.1093/bja/aet127.

Bartley, E. J., Palit, S., Kuhn, B. L., Kerr, K. L., Terry, E. L., DelVentura, J. L., et al. (2015). Natural variation in testosterone is associated with hypoalgesia in healthy women. *The Clinical Journal of Pain, 31*(8), 730–739. http://dx.doi.org/10.1097/AJP.0000000000000153.

Belfer, I., Segall, S. K., Lariviere, W. R., Smith, S. B., Dai, F., Slade, G. D., & Diatchenko, L. (2013). Pain modality- and sex-specific effects of COMT genetic functional variants. *Pain, 154*(8), 1368–1376. http://dx.doi.org/10.1016/j.pain.2013.04.028.

Blyth, F. M., March, L. M., Brnabic, A. J. M., Jorm, L. R., Williamson, M., & Cousins, M. J. (2001). Chronic pain in Australia: a prevalence study. *Pain, 89*(2), 127–134. http://dx.doi.org/10.1016/S0304-3959(00)00355-9.

Boerner, K. E., Birnie, K. A., Caes, L., Schinkel, M., & Chambers, C. T. (2014). Sex differences in experimental pain among healthy children: a systematic review and meta-analysis. *Pain, 155*(5), 983–993. http://dx.doi.org/10.1016/j.pain.2014.01.031.

Böhmelt, A. H., Nater, U. M., Franke, S., Hellhammer, D. H., & Ehlert, U. (2005). Basal and stimulated hypothalamic-pituitary-adrenal axis activity in patients with functional gastrointestinal disorders and healthy controls. *Psychosomatic Medicine, 67*(2), 288–294. http://dx.doi.org/10.1097/01.psy.0000157064.72831.ba.

Bragdon, E. E., Light, K. C., Costello, N. L., Sigurdsson, A., Bunting, S., Bhalang, K., et al. (2002). Group differences in pain modulation: pain-free women compared to pain-free men and to women with TMD. *Pain, 96*(3), 227–237. http://dx.doi.org/10.1016/S0304-3959(01)00451-1.

Butler, R. K., & Finn, D. P. (2009). Stress-induced analgesia. *Progress in Neurobiology, 88*(3), 184–202. http://dx.doi.org/10.1016/j.pneurobio.2009.04.003.

Cairns, B. E., & Gazerani, P. (2009). Sex-related differences in pain. *Maturitas, 63*(4), 292–296. http://dx.doi.org/10.1016/j.maturitas.2009.06.004.

Cathcart, S., & Pritchard, D. (2008). Daily stress and pain sensitivity in chronic tension-type headache sufferers. *Stress and Health, 24*(2), 123–127. http://dx.doi.org/10.1002/smi.1167.

Chang, L., Sundaresh, S., Elliott, J., Anton, P. A., Baldi, P., Licudine, A., et al. (2009). Dysregulation of the hypothalamic-pituitary-adrenal (HPA) axis in irritable bowel syndrome. *Neurogastroenterology and Motility, 21*(2), 149–159. http://dx.doi.org/10.1605/01.301-0004412476.2009.

Chapman, C. R., Tuckett, R. P., & Song, C. W. (2008). Pain and stress in a systems perspective: reciprocal neural, endocrine, and immune interactions. *The Journal of Pain, 9*(2), 122–145. http://dx.doi.org/10.1016/j.jpain.2007.09.006.

Craft, R. M. (2003). Sex differences in drug- and non-drug-induced analgesia. *Life Sciences*, 72(24), 2675–2688. http://dx.doi.org/10.1016/S0024-3205(03)00178-4.

Crofford, L. J., Young, E. A., Engleberg, N. C., Korszun, A., Brucksch, C. B., McClure, L. A., et al. (2004). Basal circadian and pulsatile ACTH and cortisol secretion in patients with fibromyalgia and/or chronic fatigue syndrome. *Brain, Behavior, and Immunity*, 18(4), 314–325. http://dx.doi.org/10.1016/j.bbi.2003.12.011.

Dickhaus, B., Mayer, E. A., Firooz, N., Stains, J., Conde, F., Olivas, T. I., et al. (2003). Irritable bowel syndrome patients show enhanced modulation of visceral perception by auditory stress. *American Journal of Gastroenterology*, 98(1), 135–143.

Earle, T. L., Linden, W., & Weinberg, J. (1999). Differential effects of harassment on cardiovascular and salivary cortisol stress reactivity and recovery in women and men. *Journal of Psychosomatic Research*, 46(2), 125–141. http://dx.doi.org/10.1016/S0022-3999(98)00075-0.

Fernández-de-las-Peñas, C., Hernández-Barrera, V., Alonso-Blanco, C., Palacios-Ceña, D., Carrasco-Garrido, P., Jiménez-Sánchez, S., et al. (2011). Prevalence of neck and low back pain in community-dwelling adults in Spain: a population-based national study. *Spine*, 36(3), E213–E219. http://dx.doi.org/10.1097/BRS.0b013e3181d952c2.

Fifield, J., McQuillan, J., Armeli, S., Tennen, H., Reisine, S., & Affleck, G. (2004). Chronic strain, daily work stress and pain among workers with rheumatoid arthritis: does job stress make a bad day worse? *Work and Stress*, 18(4), 275–291. http://dx.doi.org/10.1080/02678370412331324996.

Fillingim, R. B., & Edwards, R. R. (2001). The association of hormone replacement therapy with experimental pain responses in postmenopausal women. *Pain*, 92(1–2), 229–234.

Fillingim, R. B., Kaplan, L., Staud, R., Ness, T. J., Glover, T. L., Campbell, C. M., et al. (2005). The A118G single nucleotide polymorphism of the μ-opioid receptor gene (OPRM1) is associated with pressure pain sensitivity in humans. *The Journal of Pain*, 6(3), 159–167. http://dx.doi.org/10.1016/j.jpain.2004.11.008.

Fillingim, R. B., King, C. D., Ribeiro-Dasilva, M. C., Rahim-Williams, B., & Riley, J. L., III (2009). Sex, gender, and pain: a review of recent clinical and experimental findings. *The Journal of Pain*, 10(5), 447–485. http://dx.doi.org/10.1016/j.jpain.2008.12.001.

Fillingim, R. B., Wallace, M. R., Herbstman, D. M., Ribeiro-Dasilva, M., & Staud, R. (2008). Genetic contributions to pain: a review of findings in humans. *Oral Diseases*, 14, 673–682.

Gaskin, D. J., & Richard, P. (2012). The economic costs of pain in the United States. *The Journal of Pain*, 13(8), 715–724. http://dx.doi.org/10.1016/j.jpain.2012.03.009.

Hardt, J., Jacobsen, C., Goldberg, J., Nickel, R., & Buchwald, D. (2008). Prevalence of chronic pain in a representative sample in the United States. *Pain Medicine*, 9(7), 803–812. http://dx.doi.org/10.1111/j.1526-4637.2008.00425.x.

Hashmi, J. A., & Davis, K. D. (2010). Effects of temperature on heat pain adaptation and habituation in men and women. *Pain*, 151(3), 737–743. http://dx.doi.org/10.1016/j.pain.2010.08.046.

Hashmi, J. A., & Davis, K. D. (2014). Deconstructing sex differences in pain sensitivity. *Pain*, 155(1), 10–13. http://dx.doi.org/10.1016/j.pain.2013.07.039.

Hassan, S., Muere, A., & Einstein, G. (2014). Ovarian hormones and chronic pain: a comprehensive review. *Pain*, 155(12), 2448–2460. http://dx.doi.org/10.1016/j.pain.2014.08.027.

Hong, J.-Y., Kilpatrick, L. A., Labus, J. S., Gupta, A., Katibian, D., Ashe-McNalley, C., et al. (2014). Sex and disease-related alterations of anterior insula functional connectivity in chronic abdominal pain. *The Journal of Neuroscience*, 34(43), 14252–14259. http://dx.doi.org/10.1523/JNEUROSCI.1683-14.2014.

Institute of Medicine Committee on Advancing Pain Research, Care, & Education. (2011). *Relieving pain in America a blueprint for transforming prevention, care, education, and research.* Washington, DC: National Academies Press.

Jennings, E. M., Okine, B. N., Roche, M., & Finn, D. P. (2014). Stress-induced hyperalgesia. *Progress in Neurobiology, 121,* 1–18. http://dx.doi.org/10.1016/j.pneurobio. 2014.06.003.

Jiang, Z., Dinov, I. D., Labus, J. S., Shi, Y., Zamanyan, A., Gupta, A., et al. (2013). Sexrelated differences of cortical thickness in patients with chronic abdominal pain. *PLoS One, 8*(9), e73932. http://dx.doi.org/10.1371/journal.pone.0073932.

Johannes, C. B., Le, T. K., Zhou, X. L., Johnston, J. A., & Dworkin, R. H. (2010). The prevalence of chronic pain in United States adults: results of an Internet-based survey. *Journal of Pain, 11*(11), 1230–1239. http://dx.doi.org/10.1016/j.jpain.2010.08.002.

Kelly, M. M., Tyrka, A. R., Anderson, G. M., Price, L. H., & Carpenter, L. L. (2008). Sex differences in emotional and physiological responses to the Trier Social Stress Test. *Journal of Behavior Therapy and Experimental Psychiatry, 39*(1), 87–98. http://dx.doi.org/ 10.1016/j.jbtep.2007.02.003.

King, S., Chambers, C. T., Huguet, A., MacNevin, R. C., McGrath, P. J., Parker, L., et al. (2011). The epidemiology of chronic pain in children and adolescents revisited: a systematic review. *Pain, 152*(12), 2729–2738. http://dx.doi.org/10.1016/ j.pain.2011.07.016.

Kirschbaum, C., Kudielka, B. M., Gaab, J., Schommer, N. C., & Hellhammer, D. H. (1999). Impact of gender, menstrual cycle phase, and oral contraceptives on the activity of the hypothalamus-pituitary-adrenal axis. *Psychosomatic Medicine, 61*(2), 154–162. http://dx.doi.org/10.1097/00006842-199903000-00006.

Klijs, B., Nusselder, W. J., Looman, C. W., & Mackenbach, J. P. (2014). Educational disparities in the burden of disability: contributions of disease prevalence and disabling impact. *American Journal of Public Health, 104*(8), e141–E148. http://dx.doi.org/ 10.2105/AJPH.2014.301924.

Kudielka, B. M., & Kirschbaum, C. (2005). Sex differences in HPA axis responses to stress: a review. *Biological Psychology, 69*(1), 113–132. http://dx.doi.org/10.1016/ j.biopsycho.2004.11.009.

Kulich, R. J., Mencher, P., Bertrand, C., & Maciewicz, R. (2000). Comorbidity of post-traumatic stress disorder and chronic pain: implications for clinical and forensic assessment. *Current Review of Pain, 4*(1), 36–48. http://dx.doi.org/10.1007/s11916-000-0008-4.

Lépine, J.-P., & Briley, M. (2004). The epidemiology of pain in depression. *Human Psychopharmacology, 19*(S1), S3–S7. http://dx.doi.org/10.1002/hup.618.

LeResche, L. (1999). Gender considerations in the epidemiology of chronic pain. In I. K. Crombie (Ed.), *Epidemiology of pain* (pp. 43–52). Seattle, WA: IASP Press.

LeResche, L. (2000). Epidemiological perspectives on sex differences in pain. In R. B. Fillingim (Ed.), *Sex, gender, and pain* (pp. 233–249). Seattle, WA: IASP Press.

Logan, J. G., & Barksdale, D. J. (2008). Allostasis and allostatic load: expanding the discourse on stress and cardiovascular disease. *Journal of Clinical Nursing, 17*(7b), 201–208. http:// dx.doi.org/10.1111/j.1365-2702.2008.02347.x.

Lovallo, W. R., Farag, N. H., Vincent, A. S., Thomas, T. L., & Wilson, M. F. (2006). Cortisol responses to mental stress, exercise, and meals following caffeine intake in men and women. *Pharmacology Biochemistry and Behavior, 83*(3), 441–447. http://dx.doi.org/ 10.1016/j.pbb.2006.03.005.

Maleki, N., Linnman, C., Brawn, J., Burstein, R., Becerra, L., & Borsook, D. (2012). Her versus his migraine: multiple sex differences in brain function and structure. *Brain, 135*(Pt 8), 2546–2559. http://dx.doi.org/10.1093/brain/aws175.

McBeth, J., Macfarlane, G. J., Benjamin, S., & Silman, A. J. (2001). Features of somatization predict the onset of chronic widespread pain: results of a large population-based study. *Arthritis & Rheumatism, 44*(4), 940–946. http://dx.doi.org/10.1002/1529-0131(200104) 44:4<940.

McBeth, J., Morris, S., Benjamin, S., Silman, A. J., & Macfarlane, G. J. (2001). Associations between adverse events in childhood and chronic widespread pain in adulthood: are they explained by differential recall? *The Journal of Rheumatology, 28*(10), 2305–2309.

McEwen, B. S. (1998). Stress, adaptation, and disease. Allostasis and allostatic load. *Annals of the New York Academy of Sciences, 840,* 33–44.

McEwen, B. S., & Kalia, M. (2010). The role of corticosteroids and stress in chronic pain conditions. *Metabolism, 59*(Suppl. 1), S9–S15. http://dx.doi.org/10.1016/j.metabol.2010.07.012.

Miller, L. R., & Cano, A. (2009). Comorbid chronic pain and depression: who is at risk? *The Journal of Pain, 10*(6), 619–627. http://dx.doi.org/10.1016/j.jpain.2008.12.007.

Mogil, J. S. (2012). Sex differences in pain and pain inhibition: multiple explanations of a controversial phenomenon. *Nature Reviews Neuroscience, 13*(12), 859–866. http://dx.doi.org/10.1038/nrn3360.

Mogil, J. S., Sorge, R. E., LaCroix-Fralish, M. L., Smith, S. B., Fortin, A., Sotocinal, S. G., et al. (2011). Pain sensitivity and vasopressin analgesia are mediated by a gene-sex-environment interaction. *Nature Neuroscience, 14*(12), 1569–1573. http://dx.doi.org/10.1038/nn.2941.

Mogil, J. S., Sternberg, W. F., Kest, B., Marek, P., & Liebeskind, J. C. (1993). Sex differences in the antagonism of swim stress-induced analgesia: effects of gonadectomy and estrogen replacement. *Pain, 53*(1), 17–25.

Olsen, M. B., Jacobsen, L. M., Schistad, E. I., Pedersen, L. M., Rygh, L. J., Røe, C., et al. (2012). Pain intensity the first year after lumbar disc herniation is associated with the A118G polymorphism in the opioid receptor mu 1 gene: evidence of a sex and genotype interaction. *The Journal of Neuroscience, 32*(29), 9831–9834. http://dx.doi.org/10.1523/JNEUROSCI.1742-12.2012.

Otte, C., Hart, S., Neylan, T., & Marmar, C. (2005). A meta-analysis of cortisol response to challenge in human aging: importance of gender. *Pharmacopsychiatry, 38*(5), 268.

Paris, J. J., Franco, C., Sodano, R., Freidenberg, B., Gordis, E., Anderson, D. A., et al. (2010). Sex differences in salivary cortisol in response to acute stressors among healthy participants, in recreational or pathological gamblers, and in those with posttraumatic stress disorder. *Hormones and Behavior, 57*(1), 35–45. http://dx.doi.org/10.1016/j.yhbeh.2009.06.003.

Popescu, A., LeResche, L., Truelove, E. L., & Drangsholt, M. T. (2010). Gender differences in pain modulation by diffuse noxious inhibitory controls: a systematic review. *Pain, 150*(2), 309–318. http://dx.doi.org/10.1016/j.pain.2010.05.013.

Posserud, I., Agerforz, P., Ekman, R., Bjornsson, E. S., Abrahamsson, H., Simren, M., & Institute of Clinical Neurosciences. (2004). Altered visceral perceptual and neuroendocrine response in patients with irritable bowel syndrome during mental stress. *Gut, 53*(8), 1102–1108. http://dx.doi.org/10.1136/gut.2003.017962.

Racine, M., Tousignant-Laflamme, Y., Kloda, L. A., Dion, D., Dupuis, G., & Choinière, M. (2012a). A systematic literature review of 10 years of research on sex/gender and experimental pain perception - part 1: are there really differences between women and men? *Pain, 153*(3), 602–618. http://dx.doi.org/10.1016/j.pain.2011.11.025.

Racine, M., Tousignant-Laflamme, Y., Kloda, L. A., Dion, D., Dupuis, G., & Choinière, M. (2012b). A systematic literature review of 10 years of research on sex/gender and pain perception - part 2: do biopsychosocial factors alter pain sensitivity differently in women and men? *Pain, 153*(3), 619–635. http://dx.doi.org/10.1016/j.pain.2011.11.026.

Rhudy, J. L., & Meagher, M. W. (2000). Fear and anxiety: divergent effects on human pain thresholds. *Pain, 84*(1), 65–75.

Rhudy, J. L., & Meagher, M. W. (2001). Noise stress and human pain thresholds: divergent effects in men and women. *The Journal of Pain, 2*(1), 57–64. http://dx.doi.org/10.1054/jpai.2000.19947.

Riskowski, J. L. (2014). Associations of socioeconomic position and pain prevalence in the United States: findings from the National Health and Nutrition Examination Survey. *Pain Medicine, 15*(9), 1508–1521. http://dx.doi.org/10.1111/pme.12528.

Riva, R., Mork, P. J., Westgaard, R. H., & Lundberg, U. (2012). Comparison of the cortisol awakening response in women with shoulder and neck pain and women with fibromyalgia. *Psychoneuroendocrinology, 37*(2), 299–306. http://dx.doi.org/10.1016/j.psyneuen.2011.06.014.

Schell, E., Theorell, T., Hasson, D., Arnetz, B., & Saraste, H. (2008). Stress biomarkers' associations to pain in the neck, shoulder and back in healthy media workers: 12-month prospective follow-up. *European Spine Journal, 17*(3), 393–405. http://dx.doi.org/10.1007/s00586-007-0554-0.

van Stegeren, A. H., Wolf, O. T., & Kindt, M. (2008). Salivary alpha amylase and cortisol responses to different stress tasks: impact of sex. *International Journal of Psychophysiology, 69*(1), 33–40. http://dx.doi.org/10.1605/01.301-0003274082.2008.

Sternberg, W. F., Boka, C., Kas, L., Alboyadjia, A., & Gracely, R. H. (2001). Sex-dependent components of the analgesia produced by athletic competition. *The Journal of Pain, 2*(1), 65–74. http://dx.doi.org/10.1054/jpai.2001.18236.

Stroud, L. R., Salovey, P., & Epel, E. S. (2002). Sex differences in stress responses: social rejection versus achievement stress. *Biological Psychiatry, 52*(4), 318–327. http://dx.doi.org/10.1016/S0006-3223(02)01333-1.

Tak, L. M., Cleare, A. J., Ormel, J., Manoharan, A., Kok, I. C., Wessely, S., et al. (2011). Meta-analysis and meta-regression of hypothalamic-pituitary-adrenal axis activity in functional somatic disorders. *Biological Psychology, 87*(2), 183–194. http://dx.doi.org/10.1016/j.biopsycho.2011.02.002.

Tsang, A., Von Korff, M., Lee, S., Alonso, J., Karam, E., Angermeyer, M. C., et al. (2008). Common chronic pain conditions in developed and developing countries: gender and age differences and comorbidity with depression-anxiety disorders. *The Journal of Pain, 9*(10), 883–891. http://dx.doi.org/10.1016/j.jpain.2008.05.005.

Wagner, K. M., Roeder, Z., DesRochers, K., Buhler, A. V., Heinricher, M. M., & Cleary, D. R. (2013). The dorsomedial hypothalamus mediates stress-induced hyperalgesia and is the source of the pronociceptive peptide cholecystokinin in the rostral ventromedial medulla. *Neuroscience, 238*(0), 29–38. http://dx.doi.org/10.1016/j.neuroscience.2013.02.009.

Wang, G., Erpelding, N., & Davis, K. D. (2014). Sex differences in connectivity of the subgenual anterior cingulate cortex. *Pain, 155*(4), 755–763. http://dx.doi.org/10.1016/j.pain.2014.01.005.

Yarnitsky, D., Arendt-Nielsen, L., Bouhassira, D., Edwards, R. R., Fillingim, R. B., Granot, M., et al. (2010). Recommendations on terminology and practice of psychophysical DNIC testing. *European Journal of Pain, 14*(4), 339. http://dx.doi.org/10.1016/j.ejpain.2010.02.004.

Yarnitsky, D., Granot, M., & Granovsky, Y. (2014). Pain modulation profile and pain therapy: between pro- and antinociception. *Pain, 155*(4), 663–665. http://dx.doi.org/10.1016/j.pain.2013.11.005.

Zimmer, C., Basler, H.-D., Vedder, H., & Lautenbacher, S. (2003). Sex differences in cortisol response to noxious stress. *The Clinical Journal of Pain, 19*(4), 233–239. http://dx.doi.org/10.1097/00002508-200307000-00006.

PART 2

Psychological Processes Related to Pain and Stress

CHAPTER 5

Pain and the Placebo Effect

Magne Arve Flaten[1], Mustafa al'Absi[2]
[1]Department of Psychology, Norwegian University of Science and Technology, Trondheim, Norway;
[2]University of Minnesota Medical School, Minneapolis, Duluth, MN, USA

INTRODUCTION

Beyond the biological and physiological processes there are many other psychological, behavioral, and sociodemographic factors that directly and indirectly contribute to maintaining health or causing dysregulation leading to disease states. Indeed, the biopsychosocial model of health and disease states that the causes of disease, and its treatment, can be found among biological, psychological, and environmental factors, not just the biological factors. Such conceptual framework provides explanation to account for processes that impact health and are beyond what can be explained using the traditional biomedical model. For example, an essential distinction of the biopsychosocial model is its accommodation of the hypothesis that the state of the brain or mind has consequences on a person's physical health. This may sound obvious to many, as the public media and the alternative medicine industry occasionally make this claim. However, generating scientific evidence that the brain can reduce or increase physical symptoms with consequences for health has only recently gained momentum. In this article the evidence that the state of the brain can reduce or increase pain and pain-related biological responses will be reviewed. This will be undertaken in the context of discussing placebo, its nature, and its impact on pain and related symptoms.

Pain is often variable across time, and to ascertain that alleviation of pain is due to the actual treatment, at least three elements must be considered. First, it is the cure itself, the drug or other treatments, that reduces the symptom. Additionally, many diseases or symptoms vary in intensity or severity across time, termed the natural history of the disease. So, second, periods of intense pain may be followed by periods without or with less pain. The third factor, which is the topic of this chapter, is that the expectations the patient has about the treatment may reduce, or under some circumstances increase, pain or other symptoms (Colloca, Flaten, & Meissner, 2013).

The Neuroscience of Pain, Stress, and Emotion
http://dx.doi.org/10.1016/B978-0-12-800538-5.00005-4

EXPECTATIONS

After the ingestion of a painkiller one expects that pain will be reduced. This expectation of improvement is of course the reason people seek treatment. Whether this expectation has consequences for the symptom is the question dealt with in this chapter. Expectations are beliefs that some event will occur in the future, and response expectations (Kirsch, 1999) are expectations of how one automatically will react to certain events, for example, the intake of a painkiller. It is hypothesized that response expectations can generate autonomic reactions. Expectations are difficult to study, and we know more about the effects of expectations than about them, but there are at least two important dimensions of expectations that should be described here: one is the confidence that the response will occur, that is, how sure the patient is that the painkiller will reduce pain. The other dimension is the magnitude of the response, that is, how much the painkiller will reduce the pain (Bjørkedal & Flaten, 2011; Flaten, 2014).

Expectations are often conceptualized as controlling a top-down system, in which cognitions and emotions modulate sensory input to the brain or may modulate the representation of sensory input in the brain. Expectations thus partly control how we react to events. Stress is one way of reacting to situations perceived as emotionally negative and uncontrollable, and stress has been linked to a number of symptoms. Consequently, cognitions and emotions may affect our health by changing our perceptions and, thereby, decrease or even increase stress.

PLACEBO ANALGESIA

Since the late twentieth century, studies have attempted to examine experimentally the nature of the placebo effect and to identify its psychological, cognitive, and neurobiological mechanisms. One example is a study by Levine and Gordon (1984) that examined how expectations can reduce pain, termed placebo analgesia. Postoperative pain was studied in dental patients who had their third molars extracted under local anesthesia. Without subsequent treatment, postoperative pain will increase for at least 4 h after the operation (Levine, Gordon, & Fields, 1978). Levine and Gordon (1984), however, used a natural history control group that, instead of an analgesic drug, received intravenous infusions of saline, controlled by a pump that gave no cues to the patient that the infusion was being performed. The procedure was performed so that the natural history group received the same amount of saline as an "open infusion" group. In that group, saline was administered by a person sitting at the patient's bedside; the patient was told that a powerful painkiller was being administered. The only difference between the natural history group and the open infusion group was that the latter group was told it was getting an infusion that could reduce the pain, whereas the natural history group did not receive this information. The result was a decrease in reported pain in the open infusion group compared to the natural history group of about 1.5 cm on a 10 cm scale. As the only difference between the groups was the information they had received about the pain treatment, the reduced pain report in the open infusion group must have been due to the expectation of reduced pain in this group, and the reduced pain was then a placebo analgesic response. Another group received an open infusion of naloxone, that is, they were led to believe that they received a painkiller but actually received an opioid antagonist. This group displayed a smaller reduction in pain than the first open infusion group, indicating that the placebo analgesic response was mediated by endogenous opioid activity.

THE NEUROBIOLOGICAL BASIS OF PLACEBO ANALGESIA

One of the findings that has been replicated in multiple studies is that placebo-induced analgesia is mediated by the endogenous opioid pathway. This has been demonstrated, for example, by the finding in multiple studies that naloxone reduces placebo analgesic responses (reviewed in Carlino, Pollo, & Benedetti, 2011; Meissner et al., 2011). Administration of naloxone is indirect evidence that endorphins are involved in placebo analgesia. Lipman et al. (1990) showed increased β-endorphin sampled from cerebrospinal fluid in chronic pain patients after intrathecal saline, but only in the patients showing a placebo analgesic response. In patients not showing a placebo response, no change in β-endorphin was observed.

It should be noted that while the observation that naloxone reverses, at least partially, the placebo response was found in multiple studies (Grevert, Albert, & Goldstein, 1983), some studies did not provide such evidence, suggesting a different pathway mediating placebo analgesia. Vase, Robinson, Verne, and Price (2005) showed large placebo analgesic responses in patients with irritable bowel syndrome, but naloxone did not reduce the placebo response. Amanzio and Benedetti (1999) showed that the way in which expectations were induced determined whether the placebo response was naloxone-reversible or not. They found placebo analgesia induced by verbal information to be completely antagonized by naloxone. However, placebo analgesia induced via classical conditioning was naloxone-reversible only if the subjects had experienced that morphine reduced pain. If the subjects had been exposed to a nonopioid painkiller, on the other hand, subsequent placebo analgesic response was not reduced by naloxone. These observations clearly suggest some heterogeneity in the effect of placebo, possibly due to individual differences, conditions, and methodological applications of the placebo manipulation. This issue is further illustrated next.

One central issue has been the role of endorphins and their antagonism by naloxone in experimental and clinical pain. As reviewed in ter Riet, de Craen, de Boer, and Kessels (1998) most studies on experimental pain have shown that naloxone does not increase pain ratings, indicating that painful stimulation does not elicit endorphin release. This is a critical point when interpreting the finding that naloxone reverses placebo analgesia: if naloxone increased pain, then this would indicate that what seemed like antagonism of a placebo analgesic response would be due to antagonism of pain-elicited (and not placebo-elicited) endorphin release. Thus, it is crucial that naloxone can be shown to not affect pain in this type of experiment.

Studies on clinical pain, on the other hand, have shown that naloxone administration can increase pain levels. This complicates the interpretation of naloxone-induced reduction in placebo analgesia. Therefore, other methods have also been employed to investigate the neurobiological mechanisms underlying placebo analgesia. Benedetti et al. (1998) recorded respiration under the influence of a placebo, as one effect of opioids is respiratory depression. It was hypothesized that a placebo respiratory depressant response should be correlated with a placebo analgesic response, and a placebo depressant response was indeed observed, which is indirect evidence that placebo analgesia is mediated by endorphin release.

One objective way of assessing whether placebo analgesia is a psychobiological process is by recordings of electroencephalographic responses to painful stimuli. Experimentally induced pain stimuli with abrupt onset generate event-related or evoked potentials that can be detected in the electroencephalogram (Apkarian, Bushnell, Treede, & Zubieta, 2005; Granovsky, Granot, Nir, & Yarnitsky, 2008). The event-related potentials (ERPs) reflect cortical activity in response to pain stimulation. The potentials are highly correlated with pain report (Granovsky et al., 2008). Since placebo analgesic responses are hypothesized to reflect reduced pain experience, not just pain report, placebo analgesia should be associated with reduced evoked potentials in response to pain stimuli. Such findings would support the idea that placebo analgesia is mediated by endogenous opioid descending inhibition leading to attenuated pain signal to the brain.

The role of the descending inhibition of pain transmission has been demonstrated in other studies. Watson, El-Deredy, Vogt, and Jones (2007) found that experimentally induced pain to the arm elicited cortical activity that was reduced by application of placebo cream. A placebo analgesic response was also seen in pain report. Wager, Matre, and Casey (2006) found smaller pain-elicited potentials in a placebo condition compared to a natural history condition, but only for the first half of the stimulations. In the second half of the experiment, no difference was found between the conditions, possibly owing to habituation to the painful stimulation. Aslaksen, Bystad, Vambheim, and Flaten (2011) as well found reduced ERPs in response to painful stimulation under the influence of a placebo. Together, these studies support the hypothesis that placebo analgesia is due to reduced pain signals to the brain.

Another illustration of this central modulation has been demonstrated by information manipulation. Goffaux, Redmond, Rainville, and Marchand (2007) told one group of subjects that the application of the second stimulus would decrease their pain, while another group was told that the second painful stimulus would increase pain. Pain ratings were reduced or increased according to the direction of the information, and pain-elicited reflexes, measured by electromyographic responses from the stimulated leg, were also changed according to the information. Moreover, ERPs recorded at about 200 ms and later showed large differences between the groups, with smaller potentials in the group that expected the second painful stimulus to reduce the pain. This study has been replicated (Bjørkedal & Flaten, 2012) and provides evidence that expectations can reduce pain signals to the brain, since both the pain-reflex and the ERPs were reduced by information that a second noxious stimulus would reduce pain.

In addition to data collected using surface and peripheral measures, there is also evidence from brain imaging studies that the placebo analgesic effect is partly due to activation of a descending pain modulatory pathway. Eippert, Finsterbusch, Bingel, and Buchel (2009) showed that pain-elicited activity in the spinal cord, in the segment in which the relevant pain pathway synapses with second-order neurons transmitting the pain signal to the brain, was reduced under the influence of a placebo. This fits well with another finding by Eippert et al. (2009), in which administration of naloxone reduced reported placebo analgesia and reduced neural responses in pain-related areas of the brain, including the thalamus, the insula, and the rostral anterior cingulate cortex. Naloxone was also found to modulate placebo-induced responses in important structures of a descending pain control system that involves the periaqueductal gray and the rostral ventromedial medulla. This descending system can inhibit, or under some circumstances increase, pain. Furthermore, naloxone abolished placebo-induced coupling between the rostral anterior cingulate cortex and the periaqueductal gray, which predicted neural and behavioral placebo effects, and activation of the rostral ventral medulla, a key part of the descending system that mediates pain modulation. Wager et al. (2004) reported that the prefrontal cortex was activated after administration of the placebo, but before administration of the painful stimulus. This activation fits well with the idea that expectations associated with cortical activity controlled activity in the pain-modulatory network that involved the periaqueductal gray. Exactly how expectations can control the descending system is still unknown, however.

In summary, reported studies, including those using brain imaging, support the hypothesis that placebo analgesia is due to activation of a top-down system, involving prefrontal cortical areas that control a pain-modulatory system that involves opioid mechanisms. However, other mechanisms are probably involved and an interactive influence may also produce different patterns of placebo effects in different populations. Indeed, some studies have shown that placebo analgesia may be opioid-independent, while other studies indicate that these effects are found in certain groups and are influenced by the nature of the placebo manipulation. Defining these different patterns of placebo-related activation and outcome should enhance our understanding of this process and how it could influence pain perception.

SOCIAL FACTORS AND PLACEBO MODULATION OF PAIN

It has been long recognized that social factors influence pain perception. Aslaksen, Myrbakk, Høifødt, and Flaten (2007) had male and female experimenters induce pain in and record pain from male and female students. They showed that male participants reported lower pain to female experimenters, compared to male participants who reported pain to male experimenters.

Pain Intensity

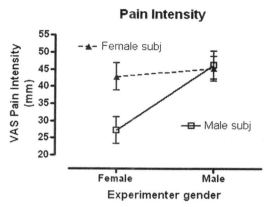

Figure 1 Pain intensity reported by male and female subjects tested by male and female experimenters. Pain intensity is reported on 100 mm visual analogue scales. Vertical bars are 1 standard error of the mean. *(Reprinted from Aslaksen et al. (2007) with kind permission of the publisher.)*

The pain reported to the female experimenters was almost 50% lower than the pain reported to the male experimenters (Figure 1). Interestingly, the autonomic response to painful stimulation, indexed by heart rate variability, which assesses the balance between sympathetic and parasympathetic activity, was similar in both sexes. Hence, the female experimenter seems to have induced a bias in the male participants to report less pain, whereas the experience of pain, indexed by the physiological reaction, may have been the same for both sexes. Such a response bias constitutes a serious threat to pain measurement reliability. It could also play a role in placebo analgesia.

The issue of reporting has been identified as a possible reason for the placebo effect. This issue can be addressed using methods of assessment that are informed by a more robust theoretical frame of reference. In the context of placebo, Allan and Siegel 2002 suggested that placebo responses can be explained by signal detection theory. Thus, pain report can be modulated by the consequences of reporting that pain was reduced or not. After pain medication has been administered, there will be an expectation in the patient and the health personnel that pain should be lower. Furthermore, saying that pain is not alleviated could have undesired consequences for the patient: it may seem like the patient is questioning the physician's credibility, or the patient may be classified as difficult. Thus, administration of pain medication may induce a bias toward reporting lower pain, which can lead to reports of lower pain in the absence of the actual experience of lower pain.

This response bias can be mitigated by using more objective measures, including physiological correlates of pain. ERPs refer to components that can be extracted from the electroencephalogram recorded at the time of painful stimulation (Granovsky et al., 2008). The painful stimulations give rise to components that are correlated with reported pain. To that end, some studies (Aslaksen et al., 2011; Wager et al., 2006; Watson et al., 2007) have shown that these components are reduced under placebo analgesia. These observations are important for at least two reasons: the smaller ERPs are an indication that the cortical response to the painful stimuli is reduced and that placebo analgesia is due to neurobiological processes that reduce transmission of the pain signal before it reaches the brain. Hence, reduced ERPs are evidence that placebo analgesia is not entirely due to response bias, although response bias probably explains a part of the placebo effect.

Other studies that have used functional magnetic resonance imaging and positron emission tomography have as well found reduced activity in brain areas involved in pain processing, further supporting that placebo analgesia is caused by processes that reduce pain in the brain (Wager et al., 2004, Wager, Scott, Zubieta, 2007).

The roles of social factors have been illustrated in various studies both clinically and experimentally, and several studies in humans and rodents suggest that the social environment can modulate pain (e.g., Aslaksen et al., 2007; Loggia, Mogil, & Bushnell, 2008; Langford et al., 2006). The concept of empathy is of central importance, as empathy means that you can take the viewpoint of another person and, by doing this, experience some of the same sensations as the observed person. In an experimental study, Loggia et al. (2008) made participants first like or dislike another person, before that person and the participant were exposed to painful stimuli. Participants who watched a person they liked receive painful stimuli reported more pain themselves, compared to participants who watched a person they did not like receive painful stimulation. These findings were extended by positive correlations between empathy and pain ratings, suggesting that higher pain scores were related to empathy.

Animal studies using rodents have obtained comparable results. Langford et al. (2006) observed a similar phenomenon in rodents, as they reported that mice exposed to cage mates displayed higher pain sensitivity compared to the same mice exposed to other mice they had never met before. When mice observed a cage mate in pain, pain sensitivity in a different modality was increased, indicating that nociceptive mechanisms in general were sensitized.

In summary, while pain does have physiological and biological signatures peripherally and centrally, it can be directly modulated by descending inhibitory and excitatory inputs. These findings show that the social environment can modulate pain and pain report. Thus, the studies show that the social environment can modulate physiological processes. This in turn suggests that the social environment can affect physical health.

ONE OR MULTIPLE PLACEBO EFFECTS?

The placebo effect is due to the expectation that one has received active and effective treatment for a symptom or disease. Expectations are thus a common factor for all types of treatment, whether it be treatment against pain, Parkinson disease, heart failure, or other diseases. The question is whether different expectations generate different reactions in different diseases. Expectations of analgesia are different from expectations that treatment should reduce the symptoms in Parkinson disease. Do these two expectations generate different physiological reactions?

There are varying views on the placebo response. One is the view that the mind controls the body in specific ways and that specific expectations have specific effects. Thus, an expectation that a pain-relieving cream is applied to one hand should have an effect on that hand and not at other extremities. This indeed was what Benedetti, Arduino, and Amanzio (1999) and Montgomery and Kirsch (1997) found in separate studies. A placebo analgesic response that was specific to one part of the body and not to other parts could be viewed as supporting the hypothesis that expectations have specific effects on some organs or response systems, and not others.

Watson, El-Deredy, Bentley, Vogt, and Jones (2006) used a procedure similar to Benedetti et al. (1999), with placebo cream applied to one arm and not the other, and with pain stimulation to both arms. The results were that one-third of the participants responded with a specific placebo response, that is, placebo analgesia was observed in the arm on which the placebo cream was applied, but not in the arm without the placebo cream. However, one-third of the participants displayed placebo responses in both arms. These findings are consistent with the conclusion that placebo response is a general psychophysiological reaction that affects multiple response systems. However, the results could also indicate that the descending pain-modulatory system is more specific in some individuals, which should be evident in more specific placebo responses in those participants.

The view presented here is that a general psychophysiological mechanism involved in stress and homeostatic regulation participates in shaping, directly and indirectly, the placebo response. Indeed the placebo response is seen as a regulation of psychophysiological processes, including pain. This view is supported by the outcome (both physiological and behavioral) observed in response to various types of treatments. As indicated by several authors (Aslaksen & Flaten, 2008, Aslaksen et al., 2011; Flaten et al., 1997; Petersen et al., 2012; Scott et al., 2007), receiving information that a painkiller has been administered reduces stress and negative emotions, which can improve several symptoms. Pain, for example, is often increased by negative emotions such as anxiety and tension, and a reduction in anxiety reduces pain. Thus, changes in general psychophysiological processes such as stress and anxiety may produce the results termed placebo effect. Several studies have shown that placebos can change the level of general arousal, supporting the idea that at least part of the placebo effect is a general process related to arousal and possibly homeostatic mechanisms (Flaten, 1998; Flaten, 2010; Flaten & Blumenthal, 1999; Flaten, Åsli, & Blumenthal, 2003) that can be recorded by psychophysiological methods (Flaten, 1993).

EMOTIONAL VALENCE AND AROUSAL MODULATE PAIN

Emotional valence refers to the content of the emotion, that is, basically whether the emotion is positive or negative. The context in which pain is experienced can modulate the unpleasantness of pain. Situations that induce negative emotions often increase pain, whereas situations that generate positive emotions often reduce pain. Thus, one way in which placebos may act is by reducing negative emotions or increasing positive emotions and thereby reducing pain via emotional modulation.

Several experiments have shown that negative emotional valence increases pain, and positive emotions decrease pain (Rhudy et al., 2008). In such studies, emotions were manipulated using photos from the International Affective Picture System, and pain was induced after offset of the pictures to control for the confounding effect of attention to the pictures. Rhudy et al. (2008) found that pain report, as well as the nociceptive flexion reflex and skin conductance responses, decreased as positive emotional valence increased. The effect is not large, but is reliable.

The relationship between pain and emotional valence suggests that emotional arousal could be important for pain modulation, since highly positive and highly negative emotions are associated with larger arousal. When arousal and valence are both at high levels, as in severe stress, pain is reduced, termed stress-induced analgesia. Flor and colleagues have shown that conditioned stress, induced by presenting a conditioned stimulus that had been paired with a difficult task and a distracter, reduced pain, and this was mediated via opioid mechanisms (Flor & Grusser, 1999). Thus, the relationship between emotional valence and/or arousal to pain seems to hold for positive emotions and moderately intense negative emotions, but not for intense negative emotions.

THE ROLE OF EMOTIONS IN PLACEBO RESPONDING

Administration of treatment for pain alleviates negative emotions, which reduces pain and initiates a negative feedback loop (Flaten, Aslaksen, Finset, Simonsen, & Johansen, 2006; Price et al., 1999). Aslaksen and Flaten (2008) (Figure 2) administered experimental painful heat stimuli before and after administration of capsules containing corn starch, that is, placebos, with information that the capsules contained a powerful painkiller. In the natural history control condition, the participants received the painful stimulation but no capsules and no information. Placebo analgesia was observed in the lower pain report when participants received information that a painkiller had been administered. Reported stress correlated with the placebo analgesic response, so stress reduction due to the placebo effect was associated with reduction in pain. Heart rate variability is a commonly used index of

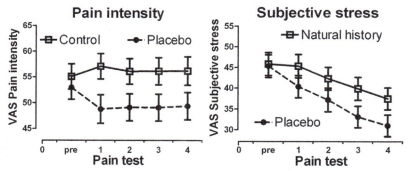

Figure 2 Left panel: Reported pain intensity before and after administration of a placebo in the placebo condition. In the control condition, pain was administered five times to control for the natural history of pain, but no information and no capsules were administered. The placebo analgesic response is the difference between the conditions in pain tests 1–4. Right panel: Reported stress levels before and after administration of a placebo in the placebo condition. In the natural history control condition, pain was applied without any treatment or suggestion of treatment. *(Reprinted from Aslaksen and Flaten (2008) with kind permission from the publisher.)*

sympathetic and parasympathetic influences on heart rate, and this measure provided more objective stress data, and there was lower sympathetic activation to painful stimulation after administration of a placebo. The same result has also been reported by Pollo, Vighetti, Rainero, and Benedetti (2003). Thus, placebo analgesia was correlated with reduced stress and negative emotions, suggesting the possibility that stress-reduction properties may mediate placebo effects.

The study by Aslaksen and Flaten (2008) could not establish the direction of causality between stress and pain. It could not be determined whether the reduced stress led to reduction in pain, or vice versa. To investigate the causal relation between perceived stress and placebo effects, stress should be recorded in the absence of pain. Aslaksen et al. (2011) did just this, and recorded stress in the absence of pain, to observe whether information that a painkiller was administered reduced stress. Experimental heat pain was presented before and after administration of a placebo with information that it was a powerful painkiller. The placebo reduced stress in two measurements after placebo, about 10 and 25 min after placebo administration, and the reduced stress explained 17% and 26% of the variance in the placebo analgesic response at these two time points. Nevertheless, the hypothesized stress-reduction properties of placebo and its mediating effect on pain warrant further research.

Scott et al. (2007) found that administration of a placebo reduced pain as well as negative affect. The lower negative affect was observed after placebo administration, but prior to pain administration, so the reduced negative emotions were not confounded with the reduction in pain. Thus, placebo reduced negative emotions prior to and independent of the subsequent reduction in pain, which indicates a causal link from reduced negative affect to lower pain. Another result in Scott et al. (2007) was that positive emotions increased after administration of placebo. These findings are in agreement with Vase et al. (2005), who recorded emotions in the absence of pain, as Scott et al. (2007) and Aslaksen et al. (2011) did. Vase et al. (2005) first presented phasic painful stimuli for an extended period of 20 min, and after this phase of the study expectations of pain levels and anxiety were recorded in the absence of painful stimuli. Subsequently, a second phase in which painful stimulation was presented for 20 min was carried out. It was shown that expected pain levels, desire for pain relief, and anxiety together accounted for 58% of the placebo effect in the second phase of the experiment. However, the reduction in expected pain was the only unique predictor of placebo analgesic response. These findings were replicated clinically by Petersen et al. (2012), who exposed patients with postoperative pain to a placebo such that the patients with postoperative pain received open or hidden administrations of lidocaine, a topical analgesic. The placebo reduced the area of hyperalgesia, and the placebo effect was correlated with reduced negative affect.

A definitive test of the hypothesis that placebo analgesia is reduced by high negative emotions can be performed by inducing negative emotions to investigate whether these emotions reduce placebo analgesia. Lyby, Åsli, Forsberg, and Flaten (2012) did exactly this. They induced negative emotions by instructing healthy subjects that an electric shock would be administered to the fingers during a period of about 10 min. Startle eyeblink reflexes were elicited as a physiological measure of negative emotions, as the startle reflex is increased by negative emotions. The results showed that the placebo effect was abolished by the induced fear and was most pronounced in subjects who were highest in measures of fear of pain. Fear of painful stimulation is high in some individuals, and these individuals show more signs of stress and negative emotions when pain is impending. Administration of the placebo resulted in a reduction in startle eyeblink reflex amplitude. However, this effect was abolished by the negative emotions induced by telling subjects they would get an electric shock, and the reduction in placebo analgesia was strongest among subjects high in fear of pain. Thus, the fear completely abolished the placebo analgesia, especially in subjects who had high scores on measures of fear (Figure 3).

Taken together, these findings suggest that a placebo reduces stress and negative emotions. These reductions possibly mediate the pain-attenuating effects of placebo, that is, placebo analgesia. Conversely, increased stress reduces or abolishes placebo analgesia.

INDIVIDUAL DIFFERENCES IN PLACEBO ANALGESIC RESPONSES

As discussed above, it has been shown that emotions modulate pain, and this observation is important in understanding why there are individual differences in placebo responses. Individual differences in personality traits or other stable characteristics of individuals are problematic for methodological reasons. Causal inference cannot be made from findings of correlations between placebo analgesic responding and personality measures. However, the observation that a particular trait may be associated with an increase or decrease in placebo analgesia can be translated into an experimental test

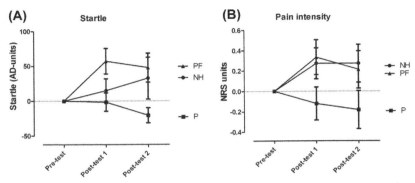

Figure 3 Condition-by-test interactions in the startle reflex (A) and in reported pain intensity (B). Vertical bars denote ±1 standard error of the mean. Negative numbers indicate a reduction in pain or startle reflex compared to the pretest, whereas positive numbers indicate an increase in response compared to the pretest. NH, natural history; P, placebo; PF, placebo + fear. Startle reflex data show fear potentiated startle in the PF condition, in which the participants expected a shock to the fingers. The pain intensity data show that the induced fear abolished the placebo analgesia. *(Reprinted from Lyby et al. (2012) with kind permission from the publisher.)*

of this hypothesis (e.g., Lyby et al., 2012). To examine individual differences in placebo effects, all subjects are usually exposed to both the placebo and the natural history conditions in order to compute a placebo response for each individual that can be correlated with measures of individual differences, such as a personality test. Within-subject designs must therefore be employed. Such designs may induce variability due to the order of the conditions, as the subjects often are more nervous at the beginning of the first session, and pain may be higher in that session. This may reduce the placebo response. Thus, the placebo response can be underestimated in subjects when the placebo session is run before the natural history session.

A few studies have examined the extent to which a trait measure of emotions can affect placebo analgesia. Lyby, Aslaksen, and Flaten (2010, 2011) showed that high fear of pain, a trait measure of how fearful individuals are of painful stimulation, reduced placebo analgesia. Furthermore, individuals high in fear of pain reacted with increased stress when anticipating painful stimulation and they reported increased pain. In sum, these findings suggest that increased levels of stress or negative emotions reduce placebo analgesic responding. This is most pronounced in subjects high in fear of pain, as they react with increased fear and nervousness in the anticipation of pain.

IMPLICATIONS FOR TREATMENT OF PAIN

The studies presented in this chapter show that information that effective treatment has been administered can reduce stress and other negative emotions. This may in turn contribute to reduction of pain perception. The extent to which induction of positive emotion is also involved in the placebo effect has been investigated less, however. Thus, modulation of emotions is one mechanism that mediates the placebo response.

This has implications for treatment of pain and possibly other symptoms. When the health personnel providing treatment manages to reduce stress and other negative emotions, the treatment has more of an effect. This is shown by, for example, Petersen et al. (2012): when pharmacological treatment against pain is administered without the patient's knowledge, the treatment has less of an effect compared to when the same amount of drug is administered with the patient's knowledge. The psychosocial context in which treatment is administered can explain part of the total effect of the treatment. Expectations are part of the psychosocial context, and when the patient is reassured that the treatment is effective, stress and negative feelings wane, and pain and possibly other distressing symptoms are reduced.

CONCLUSIONS

Research on the effect of expectations of treatment outcomes demonstrates that the benefit of treatment is increased when drug therapy (or other treatment) is paired with positive expectations about the therapy. These effects seem to occur across populations and conditions. Psychosocial factors, among other factors, influence pain and may be influenced by placebo effects. Processes involved in the placebo effects are well explained by an integrative approach of medicine guided by the biopsychosocial model, that health, disease, and treatment are dependent on multifaceted factors that include social, psychological, cultural, and biological factors.

REFERENCES

Allan, L. G., & Siegel, S. A. (2002). Signal detection theory analysis of the placebo effect. *Evaluation & the Health Professions, 25*(4), 410–420.

Amanzio, M., & Benedetti, F. (1999). Neuropharmacological dissection of placebo analgesia expectation-activated opioid systems versus conditioning-activated specific subsystems. *Journal of Neuroscience, 19*, 484–494.

Apkarian, A. V., Bushnell, M. C., Treede, R.-D., & Zubieta, J.-K. (2005). Human brain mechanisms of pain perception and regulation in health and disease. *European Journal of Pain, 9*, 463–484.

Aslaksen, P. M., Bystad, M., Vambheim, S. M., & Flaten, M. A. (2011). Gender differences in placebo analgesia: event-related potentials and emotional modulation. *Psychosomatic Medicine, 73*, 193–199.

Aslaksen, P. M., & Flaten, M. A. (2008). The roles of subjective and physiological stress in the effect of a placebo on experimentally induced pain. *Psychosomatic Medicine, 70*, 811–818.

Aslaksen, P. M., Myrbakk, I. N., Høifødt, R. S., & Flaten, M. A. (2007). The effect of experimenter gender on autonomic and subjective responses to pain stimuli. *Pain, 129*, 260–268.

Benedetti, F., Arduino, C., & Amanzio, M. (1999). Somatotopic activation of opioid systems by target-directed expectations of analgesia. *Journal of Neuroscience, 19*, 3639–3648.

Benedetti, F., et al. (1998). The specific effects of prior opioid exposure on placebo analgesia and placebo respiratory depression. *Pain, 75*, 313–319.

Bjørkedal, E., & Flaten, M. A. (2011). Interaction between expectancies and drug effects: an experimental investigation of placebo analgesia with caffeine as an active placebo. *Psychopharmacology, 215*, 537–548.

Bjørkedal, E., & Flaten, M. A. (2012). Expectations of increased or decreased pain explain the effect of conditioned pain modulation in females. *Journal of Pain Research, 5*, 289–300.

Carlino, E., Pollo, A., & Benedetti, F. (2011). Placebo analgesia and beyond: a melting pot of concepts and ideas for neuroscience. *Current Opinion in Anesthesiology, 24*(5), 540–544.

Colloca, L., Flaten, M. A., & Meissner, K. (2013). *Placebo and pain.* New York: Elsevier.

Eippert, F., et al. (2009). Activation of the opioidergic descending pain control system underlies placebo analgesia. *Neuron, 63*, 533–543.

Eippert, F., Finsterbusch, J., Bingel, U., & Buchel, C. (2009). Direct evidence for spinal cord involvement in placebo analgesia. *Science, 326*(5951), 404.

Flaten, M. A. (1993). A comparison of electromyographic and photoelectric techniques in the study of classical eyeblink conditioning and startle reflex modification. *Journal of Psychophysiology, 7*, 230–237.

Flaten, M. A. (1998). Information about drug effects modify arousal. An investigation of the placebo response. *Nordic Journal of Psychiatry, 52*, 147–151.

Flaten, M. A. (2010). Expectations of pharmacological treatment and their role for adjustment. In D. A. Powell (Ed.), *CNS mechanisms involved in learned autonomic adjustments* (pp. 115–131). Kerala, India: Research Signpost.

Flaten, M. A. (2014). Pain related negative emotions and placebo analgesia. In *Handbook of experimental pharmacology.* New York: Springer.

Flaten, M. A., Aslaksen, P. M., Finset, A., Simonsen, T., & Johansen, O. (2006). Cognitive and emotional factors in placebo analgesia. *Journal of Psychosomatic Research, 61*(1), 81–89.

Flaten, M. A., Åsli, O., & Blumenthal, T. D. (2003). Expectancy and placebo responses to caffeine-associated stimuli. *Psychopharmacology, 169*, 198–204.

Flaten, M. A., & Blumenthal, T. D. (1999). Caffeine-associated stimuli generate conditioned responses: an experimental investigation of the placebo effect. *Psychopharmacology, 145*, 105–112.

Flaten, M. A., Simonsen, T., Waterloo, K. K., & Olsen, H. (1997). Pharmacological classical conditioning in humans. Human Psychopharmacology. *Clinical and Experimental, 12*, 369–377.

Flor, H., & Grusser, S. M. (1999). Conditioned stress-induced analgesia in humans. *European Journal of Pain, 3*(4), 317–324.

Goffaux, P., Redmond, W. J., Rainville, P., & Marchand, S. (2007). Descending analgesia— when the spine echoes what the brain expects. *Pain, 130,* 137–143.

Granovsky, Y., Granot, M., Nir, R.-R., & Yarnitsky, D. (2008). Objective correlate of subjective pain perception by contact heat-evoked potentials. *Journal of Pain, 9,* 53–63.

Grevert, P., Albert, L. H., & Goldstein, A. (1983). Partial antagonism of placebo analgesia by naloxone. *Pain, 16,* 129–143.

Kirsch, I. (1999). Response expectancy: an introduction. In I. Kirsch (Ed.), *How expectancies shape experience* (pp. 3–13). Washington, DC: American Psychological Association.

Langford, D. J., Crager, S. E., Shehzad, Z., Smith, S. B., Sotocinal, S. G., Levenstadt, J. S., et al. (2006). Social modulation of pain as evidence for empathy in mice. *Science, 312*(5782), 1967–1970.

Levine, J. D., & Gordon, N. C. (1984). Influence of the method of drug administration on analgesic response. *Nature, 312*(5996), 755–756.

Levine, J. D., Gordon, N. C., & Fields, H. L. (1978). The mechanism of placebo analgesia. *The Lancet,* 654–657. September 23.

Lipman, J. J., et al. (1990). Peak B endorphin concentration in cerebrospinal fluid: reduced in chronic pain patients and increased during the placebo response. *Psychopharmacology, 102,* 112–116.

Loggia, M. L., Mogil, J. S., & Bushnell, M. C. (2008). Empathy hurts: compassion for another increases both sensory and affective components of pain perception. *Pain, 136,* 168–176.

Lyby, P. S., Aslaksen, P. M., & Flaten, M. A. (2010). Is fear of pain related to placebo analgesia? *Journal of Psychosomatic Research, 68*(4), 369–377.

Lyby, P. S., Aslaksen, P. M., & Flaten, M. A. (2011). Variability in placebo analgesia and the role of fear of pain—an ERP study. *Pain, 152*(10), 2405–2412.

Lyby, P. S., Åsli, O., Forsberg, J. T., & Flaten, M. A. (2012). Induced fear reduces the effectiveness of a placebo intervention on pain. *Pain, 153*(5), 1114–1121.

Meissner, K., et al. (2011). The placebo effect: advances from different methodological approaches. *Journal of Neuroscience, 31*(45), 16117–16124.

Montgomery, G. H., & Kirsch, I. (1997). Classical conditioning and the placebo effect. *Pain, 72,* 107–113.

Petersen, G. L., et al. (2012). Placebo manipulations reduce hyperalgesia in neuropathic pain. *Pain, 153*(6), 1292–1300.

Pollo, A., Vighetti, S., Rainero, I., & Benedetti, F. (2003). Placebo analgesia and the heart. *Pain, 102*(1–2), 125–133.

Price, D. D., et al. (1999). An analysis of factors that contribute to the magnitude of placebo analgesia in an experimental paradigm. *Pain, 83,* 147–156.

Rhudy, J. L., et al. (2008). Emotional control of nociceptive reactions (ECON): do affective valence and arousal play a role? *Pain, 136*(3), 250–261.

ter Riet, G., de Craen, A. J. M., de Boer, A., & Kessels, A. G. H. (1998). Is placebo analgesia mediated by endogenous opioids? A systematic review. *Pain, 76,* 273–275.

Scott, D. J., et al. (2007). Individual differences in reward responding explain placebo-induced expectations and effects. *Neuron, 55,* 325–336.

Vase, L., Robinson, M. E., Verne, G. N., & Price, D. D. (2005). Increased placebo analgesia over time in irritable bowel syndrome (IBS) patients is associated with desire and expectation but not endogenous opioid mechanisms. *Pain, 115,* 338–347.

Wager, T. D., et al. (2004). Placebo induced changes in fMRI in the anticipation and experience of pain. *Science, 303*(5661), 1162–1167.

Wager, T. D., Matre, D., & Casey, K. L. (2006). Placebo-effects in laser-evoked pain potentials. *Brain, Behavior and Immunity, 20,* 219–230.

Wager, T. D., Scott, D. J., & Zubieta, J.-K. (2007). Placebo effects on human mu-opioid activity during pain. *Proceedings of the National Academy of Sciences, 104,* 11056–11061.

Watson, A., El-Deredy, W., Bentley, D. E., Vogt, B. A., & Jones, A. K. P. (2006). Categories of placebo response in the absence of site-specific expectation of analgesia. *Pain, 126,* 115–122.

Watson, A., El-Deredy, W., Vogt, B. A., & Jones, A. K. P. (2007). Placebo analgesia is not due to compliance or habituation: EEG and behavioural evidence. *Neuroreport, 18,* 771–775.

CHAPTER 6

Nocebo and Pain

Martina Amanzio[1], Sara Palermo[2], Fabrizio Benedetti[2]
[1]Department of Psychology, University of Turin, Turin, Piedmont, Italy; [2]Department of Neuroscience, University of Turin Medical School, Turin, Piedmont, Italy

INTRODUCTION

A placebo effect is the effect that follows the administration of a placebo, that is, of an inert pharmacological or physical treatment. It is important to point out that the inert treatment is given along with contextual stimuli, for example, verbal suggestions of clinical improvement that make the patient believe that the treatment is real and effective. Therefore, a placebo would be better defined as an inert treatment plus the context that tells the patient a therapeutic act is being performed. The nocebo effect is a phenomenon that is opposite to the placebo effect. To induce a nocebo effect, the inert substance is given along with a negative context, for example, verbal suggestions of clinical worsening, so as to induce negative expectations about the outcome. The term nocebo ("I shall harm") was introduced in contrast to the term placebo ("I shall please") by some authors to distinguish the pleasing from the noxious effects of placebos (Kennedy, 1961; Pogge, 1963; Kissel & Barrucand, 1964; Hahn, 1985, 1997). Therefore, if the positive psychosocial context, which is typical of the placebo effect, is reversed, the nocebo effect can be studied. To differentiate nocebo effects and placebo effects from spontaneous remission and other confounding factors, they are calculated as the symptom difference between a nocebo-treated or placebo-treated group and a no-treatment group (Fields & Levine, 1984).

From an ethical point of view, the investigation of the nocebo effect is difficult to carry out. In fact, whereas the induction of placebo responses is certainly ethical in many circumstances (Benedetti & Colloca, 2004), the induction of nocebo responses represents a stressful and anxiogenic procedure, because verbally induced negative expectations of symptom worsening may lead to a real worsening. Certainly, a nocebo procedure is

The Neuroscience of Pain, Stress, and Emotion
http://dx.doi.org/10.1016/B978-0-12-800538-5.00006-6

unethical in patients, and this is one of the main reasons much less is known about nocebo phenomena.

NEGATIVE EXPECTATIONS MAY LEAD TO CLINICAL WORSENING

Many nocebo and nocebo-like effects are present in daily life and in routine clinical practice (Benedetti, Lanotte, Lopiano, & Colloca, 2007; Colloca & Benedetti, 2007). For example, negative diagnoses and prognoses can lead to an amplification of pain intensity and, more in general, negative communication within the healing context may have important effects on patients' emotions (Wells & Kaptchuk, 2012; Holloway, Gramling, & Kelly, 2013). Likewise, nocebo and nocebo-related effects may occur when distrust toward medical personnel and therapies is present. In this case, unwanted effects and side effects may occur as the result of negative expectations (Flaten, Simonsen, & Olsen, 1999; Barsky, Saintfort, Rogers, & Borus, 2002), and these may reduce, or even conceal, the efficacy of some treatments. For example, it has been found that verbal suggestions can change the direction of nitrous oxide action from analgesia to hyperalgesia (Dworkin, Chen, LeResche, & Clark, 1983). Another example is the health reports that are commonly issued in Western societies; negative warnings sent out by the mass media may have an important impact on the perceived symptoms of many people. In a study on headaches caused by mobile phone use, no evidence of radio-frequency-induced headache and pain was found, so the authors concluded that the pain increase was likely to be due to a nocebo effect (Oftedal, Straume, Johnsson, & Stovner, 2007). Diseases with an important psychological component, like irritable bowel syndrome, are also affected by nocebo effects; sedatives and opioids in postoperative pain management have been found to be influenced by nocebo effects as well (Manchikanti, Pampati, & Damron, 2005; Svedman, Ingvar, & Gordh, 2005). Similarly, some negative expectation-inducing procedures, like voodoo magic, may lead to symptom worsening. Finally, the fear-avoidance model of pain can be seen as a sort of nocebo-like effect, whereby the fear of pain may lead to pain worsening (Vlaeyen & Linton, 2000; Leeuw et al. 2007).

A 2014 meta-analysis investigated nocebo effects in pain (Petersen et al. 2014). Only studies that investigated nocebo effects as the effects that followed the administration of an inert treatment along with verbal suggestions of symptom worsening and that included a no-treatment control condition were eligible. The authors found that the overall magnitude of the nocebo effect was moderate to large and highly variable. Moreover, in studies in which nocebo effects were induced by a combination of verbal suggestions and conditioning, the effect size was larger than in studies in which nocebo effects were induced by verbal suggestions alone. Importantly, as the magnitude of the nocebo effect is variable and sometimes large, this meta-analysis demonstrates the importance of minimizing nocebo effects in clinical practice (Petersen et al. 2014).

In the clinical trials setting, patients who receive a placebo often report a high frequency of adverse events (see Figure 1(A)). Amanzio, Corazzini, Vase, and Benedetti (2009) compared the rates of adverse events reported in the placebo arms of clinical trials for three classes of antimigraine drugs: nonsteroidal anti-inflammatory drugs, triptans, and anticonvulsants. It was found that the rate of adverse events in the placebo arms of trials with antimigraine drugs was high. In addition, and most interestingly, the adverse events in the placebo arms corresponded to those of the anti-migraine medication against which the placebo was compared. For example, anorexia and memory difficulties, which are typical adverse events of anticonvulsants, were present only in the placebo arm of these trials. These results suggest that the adverse events in placebo arms of clinical trials of antimigraine medications depend on the adverse events of the active medication against which the placebo is compared. These findings are certainly in keeping with the expectation theory of placebo and nocebo effects, even if a role for learning in the form of conditioning

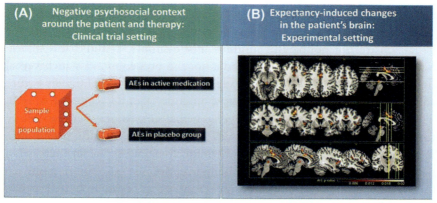

Figure 1 Two ways to analyze nocebo as a whole: the clinical trial setting (A) and the experimental setting (B).

with active treatments cannot be ruled out (Amanzio, 2011). Similar findings were obtained by Mitsikostas, Mantonakis, and Chalarakis (2011) for headache, Mitsikostas, Chalarakis, Mantonakis, Delicha, and Sfikakis (2012) for fibromyalgia, Häuser, Bartram, Bartram-Wunn, and Tölle (2012) for diabetic peripheral neuropathy, and Papadopoulos and Mitsikostas (2012) for neuropathic pain. These authors emphasized how dropouts due to nocebo effects may confound the interpretation of many clinical trials.

In both experimental and clinical settings, as also pointed out in the meta-analysis by Petersen et al. (2014), it has long been known that the perceived intensity of a painful stimulus following negative expectation of pain increase is higher than in the absence of negative expectations. For example, expectation of painful stimulation amplifies perceived unpleasantness of innocuous thermal stimulation (Sawamoto et al. 2000), and the level of expected pain intensity alters perceived pain intensity. In fact, by using two visual cues, each conditioned to one of two noxious thermal stimuli (high and low), Keltner et al. (2006) showed that subjects reported higher pain when the noxious stimulus was preceded by the high-intensity visual cue. In another study, Benedetti, Amanzio, Casadio, Oliaro, and Maggi (1997), Benedetti, Amanzio, Vighetti, and Asteggiano (2006) showed expectation-induced hyperalgesia in both the clinical and the experimental settings. In the clinical setting, the situation was a post-operative manipulation that induced expectations of pain increase, so that the patients were given an inert treatment that they expected to be painful (Benedetti et al., 1997). A straightforward increase in pain was found, and this also occurred in the experimental setting using the tourniquet technique, whereby ischemic pain was induced in one arm (Benedetti et al., 2006). These effects can be quite powerful, and sometimes pain can be generated from a nonpainful stimulus. For example, a study by Colloca, Sigaudo, and Benedetti (2008a) used a nocebo procedure, in which verbal suggestions of painful stimulation were given to healthy volunteers before administration of either tactile or low-intensity painful electrical stimuli. This study showed that these anxiogenic verbal suggestions were capable of turning tactile stimuli into pain, as well as low-intensity painful stimuli into high-intensity pain. Therefore, by defining hyperalgesia as an increase in pain sensitivity and allodynia as the perception of pain in response to innocuous stimulation, nocebo suggestions of a negative outcome can produce both hyperalgesic and allodynic effects. In general, several studies have shown that negative expectations have a dramatic effect on pain perception. Indeed, many works have shown that nocebo effects occur in different painful conditions, ranging from experimental to clinical pain (e.g., Varelmann, Pancaro, Cappiello, & Camann, 2010; Elsenbruch et al. 2012; Sanderson, Hardy, Spruyt, & Currow, 2013; van den Broeke, Geene, van Rijn, Wilder-Smith, & Oosterman, 2013).

The open–hidden (expected–unexpected) approach has also proven to be useful in understanding the importance of expectations in nocebo-related phenomena. In this case, open and hidden interruptions of treatments have been studied. An "open" interruption is performed by a doctor, who tells the patient that the treatment has been discontinued. A "hidden" interruption is carried out by a computer and the patient does not know about the interruption: he or she believes that the therapy is still being administered. Benedetti and collaborators (Benedetti et al. 2003; Colloca, Lopiano, Lanotte, & Benedetti, 2004) studied the effects of open (expected) versus hidden (unexpected) interruptions of morphine in postoperative patients. These patients, after having received morphine for 48 h, underwent either open or hidden interruption. In the open condition, they were told that morphine had been stopped; in the hidden condition, morphine was stopped without telling them anything. After interruption of morphine, the pain increase was larger in the open group than in the hidden group. At 10 h after morphine interruption, more patients of the open group requested further painkillers than in the hidden group. Therefore, the hidden interruption of morphine prolonged the postinterruption analgesia. This suggests that the open–hidden difference relates to the fact that in the open condition fear and negative expectations of pain relapse (because analgesics are no longer provided) play an important role.

Nocebo effects can also be learned through observation, which indicates that social learning plays an important role. Vögtle, Barke, and Kröner-Herwig (2013) and Swider and Bąbel (2013) studied simultaneously but independently subjects observing a model who simulated more pain in association with either a red light (Swider & Bąbel, 2013) or the application of an ointment on the skin (Vögtle et al. 2013). After the observation phase, the experimental subjects showed robust nocebo responses, that is, hyperalgesic responses, following the presentation of the red light, and this was correlated to empathy scores (Swider & Bąbel, 2013). Likewise, substantial nocebo responses were found after the observation of the ointment application, and this was correlated to pain catastrophizing (Vögtle et al. 2013). In addition, Swider and Bąbel (2013) found a gender effect, whereby nocebo hyperalgesia was greater after a male model was observed compared to a female model, regardless of the sex of the experimental subject.

Negative expectations and nocebo effects can spread across individuals very quickly through the propagation of negative information and communication, and this may produce biochemical changes that have a negative impact on health. Within this context, high-altitude headache has been studied as a model for the investigation of the products of cyclo-oxygenase, that is, prostaglandins and thromboxane (Benedetti, Durando, & Vighetti, 2014). In this experimental model, a subject (the trigger) receives negative information about the risk of headache at high altitude and disseminates this negative information across a number of other subjects. In one week, this negative information propagated across 36 subjects. This nocebo group showed a significant increase in headache and salivary prostaglandins and thromboxane when at high altitude compared to the control group. In this novel experimental model (Benedetti et al. 2014), negative information propagated across 36 subjects in one week. Hundreds or thousands of subjects might get "socially infected" in longer periods of time, thus emphasizing the possible important role of negative social communication in the dissemination of symptoms and illness across a population.

Therefore, observation and social interaction are important in the nocebo phenomenon, and some personality traits may play a key role, because a correlation was found between the magnitude of the nocebo hyperalgesic responses and empathy and catastrophizing (Vögtle et al. 2013). These findings may have implications both in the clinical trial setting and in medical practice. In the first case, observation of others must be taken into consideration whenever a clinical trial is performed. Patients participating in a clinical trial may be influenced by observing other patients in the same trial. For example, communication among patients enrolled in the same clinical trial is common, and this may influence either positively or negatively the therapeutic outcome. In the second case, doctors and psychologists must consider the possible negative impact that the observation of unsuccessful treatments may have on their patients. This holds true not only in routine medical practice but also in daily life as well, whenever others' suffering and negative outcomes are observed, for example, through the media. Social observational learning can lead to a negative emotional contagion across individuals, with the consequent activation of nocebo mechanisms.

CHOLECYSTOKININ IS A MEDIATOR
OF NOCEBO HYPERALGESIA

In 1997, a trial in postoperative patients was run with the nonspecific cholecystokinin CCK-A/CCK-B (or CCK-1 and -2) receptor antagonist proglumide (Benedetti et al. 1997). The situation was a postoperative manipulation that induced expectations of pain worsening. It was found that proglumide prevented nocebo hyperalgesia in a dose-dependent manner, even though it is not specifically a painkiller, thus suggesting that the nocebo hyperalgesic effect is mediated by CCK. In fact, a dose as low as 0.05 mg was totally ineffective, while a dose increase to 0.5 and 5 mg proved to be effective. As CCK is also involved in anxiety mechanisms, it was hypothesized that proglumide affects anticipatory anxiety (Benedetti et al. 1997; Benedetti & Amanzio, 1997). Importantly, this effect was not antagonized by naloxone. However, owing to ethical constraints, these effects were not investigated further in these patients.

To better understand the mechanisms underlying nocebo hyperalgesia and to overcome the ethical constraints inherent to the clinical approach, a similar procedure was used in healthy volunteers in whom experimental pain was induced (Benedetti et al., 2006). It was found that the oral administration of an inert substance, along with verbal suggestions of hyperalgesia, induced both hyperalgesia and hyperactivity of the hypothalamic–pituitary–adrenal (HPA) axis, as assessed by means of adrenocorticotropic hormone and cortisol plasma concentrations. Both nocebo-induced hyperalgesia and HPA hyperactivity were blocked by the benzodiazepine diazepam, which suggests the involvement of anxiety mechanisms. By contrast, the administration of the mixed CCK-A/CCK-B receptor antagonist, proglumide, blocked nocebo hyperalgesia completely, but had no effect on HPA hyperactivity, suggesting a specific involvement of CCK in the hyperalgesic but not in the anxiety component of the nocebo effect. Interestingly, neither diazepam nor proglumide showed analgesic properties on baseline pain, as they acted on the nocebo-induced pain increase only. These data suggest that a close relationship between anxiety and nocebo hyperalgesia exists, but also that proglumide does not act by blocking anticipatory anxiety, as previously hypothesized (Benedetti et al., 1997; Benedetti & Amanzio, 1997); rather it interrupts a CCK-ergic link between anxiety and pain. Therefore, in contrast to the anxiolytic action of diazepam, proglumide blocks a CCK-ergic pronociceptive system, which is activated by anxiety and is responsible for anxiety-induced hyperalgesia. Support for this view comes from a social-defeat model of anxiety in rats, in which CI-988, a selective CCK-B receptor antagonist, prevents anxiety-induced hyperalgesia (Andre et al. 2005).

Nocebo hyperalgesia is thus an interesting model to better understand when and how the endogenous pronociceptive systems are activated. The pronociceptive and antiopioid action of CCK has been documented in many brain regions (Benedetti, 1997; Hebb, Poulin, Roach, Zacharko, & Drolet, 2005; Benedetti et al., 2007). It has been shown that CCK reverses opioid analgesia by acting at the level of the rostral ventromedial medulla (Mitchell, Lowe, & Fields, 1998; Heinricher, McGaraughty, & Tortorici, 2001) and activates pain-facilitating neurons within the rostral ventromedial medulla (Heinricher & Neubert, 2004). The similarity of the pain-facilitating action of CCK both on brain-stem neurons in animals and on nocebo mechanisms in humans may represent an interesting starting point for further research into the neurochemical mechanisms of nocebo-induced hyperalgesia.

It is worth pointing out that the discrepancy between anxiety-induced hyperalgesia and stress-induced analgesia may be only apparent. In fact, stress is known to induce analgesia in different situations, both in animals and in humans. Indeed, when one is under stress, the threshold of pain is increased. However, the nature of the stressor is likely to play a central role. In fact, whereas hyperalgesia may occur when the anticipatory anxiety is about the pain itself (Sawamoto et al. 2000; Koyama, McHaffie, Laurienti, & Coghill, 2005; Benedetti et al., 2006; Keltner et al., 2006), analgesia may occur when anxiety is about a stressor that shifts the attention from the pain (Willer & Albe-Fessard, 1980; Terman, Morgan, & Liebeskind, 1986; Flor & Grusser, 1999). We should therefore use these two definitions in two different ways (Colloca & Benedetti, 2007). In the case of anxiety-induced hyperalgesia, we are talking about anticipation of pain, in which attention is focused on the impending pain. We have seen that the biochemical link between this anticipatory anxiety and the pain increase is represented by the CCK-ergic systems. Conversely, we should refer to stress-induced analgesia whenever a general state of arousal stems from a stressful situation in the environment, so that attention is now focused on the environmental stressor. In this case, there is experimental evidence that analgesia results from the activation of the endogenous opioid systems (Willer & Albe-Fessard, 1980; Terman et al., 1986).

IMAGING THE BRAIN DURING NEGATIVE EXPECTATIONS

Modern brain imaging techniques have been fundamental to our understanding of the neurobiology of negative expectations. It should be noted that no inert substance is given in these studies, and the experimenter typically uses verbal suggestions. Therefore, in this case it is better to talk about nocebo-related effects. Typically, the experimenter tells the subject about the forthcoming pain so as to make the subject expect a painful stimulation, and both the anticipatory phase and the poststimulus phase are analyzed.

By using this experimental approach, Sawamoto et al. (2000) found that expectation of painful stimulation amplifies perceived unpleasantness of innocuous thermal stimulation. These psychophysical findings were correlated to enhanced transient brain responses to the nonpainful thermal stimulus in the anterior cingulate cortex (ACC), the parietal operculum, and the posterior insula. This enhancement consisted in both a higher intensity signal change (in the ACC) and a larger volume of activated voxels (in parietal operculum and posterior insula). Therefore, expecting a painful stimulus enhances both the subjective unpleasant experience of an innocuous stimulus and the objective responses in some brain regions.

Overall, negative expectations may result in the amplification of pain (Koyama, Tanaka, & Mikami, 1998; Price, 2000; Dannecker, Price, & Robinson, 2003), and several brain regions, like the ACC, the prefrontal cortex (PFC), and the insula, have been found to be activated during the anticipation of pain (Chua, Krams, Toni, Passingham, & Dolan, 1999; Hsieh, Stone-Elander, & Ingvar, 1999; Ploghaus et al., 1999; Porro et al., 2002, Porro, Cettolo, Francescato, Baraldi 2003; Koyama et al., 2005; Lorenz et al., 2005; Keltner et al., 2006). These effects are opposite to those elicited by positive expectations, whereby expectations of reduced pain are investigated. In fact, in some studies in which both positive and negative outcomes have been studied with the same experimental approach, modulation of both subjective experience and brain activation has been found. For example, in a study by Koyama et al. (2005), as the magnitude of expected pain increased, activation increased in the thalamus, insula, PFC, and ACC. By contrast, expectations of decreased pain reduced activation of pain-related brain regions, like the primary somatosensory cortex, the insular cortex, and the ACC. In a different magnetoelectroencephalographic study in which a source localization analysis was performed, Lorenz et al. (2005) found modulation of the dipole in the secondary somatosensory cortex by nocebo-like and placebo-like suggestions. The dipole was modulated in the same direction as expectations, shrinking when a decrease in pain was expected and expanding when an increase in pain was anticipated.

In another study, Keltner et al. (2006) found that the level of expected pain intensity alters perceived pain intensity, along with the activation of different brain regions. By using two visual cues, each conditioned to one of two noxious thermal stimuli (high and low), these investigators showed that subjects reported higher pain when the noxious stimulus was preceded by the high-intensity visual cue. By comparing the brain activation produced by the two visual cues, they found significant differences in the ipsilateral caudal ACC, the head of the caudate, the cerebellum, and the contralateral nucleus cuneiformis. Interestingly, the imaging results of this study indicate that expectation and noxious stimulus intensity act in an additive manner on afferent pathways activated by cutaneous noxious thermal stimulation.

Somewhat different from the previous studies, Kong et al. (2008) investigated nocebo responses by administering an inert treatment, which the subjects believed to be hyperalgesic. These investigators showed that, after administration of the inert treatment along with negative suggestions, subjective pain intensity ratings increased significantly more on nocebo regions compared with the control regions in which no expectation manipulation was performed. Functional magnetic resonance imaging analysis of hyperalgesic nocebo responses to identical calibrated noxious stimuli showed signal increases in brain regions including bilateral dorsal ACC, insula, superior temporal gyrus, left frontal and parietal operculum, medial frontal gyrus, orbital PFC, superior parietal lobule, and hippocampus; right claustrum/putamen, lateral prefrontal gyrus, and middle temporal gyrus. Functional connectivity analysis of spontaneous resting state showed a correlation between two seed regions (left frontal operculum and hippocampus) and a pain network including bilateral insula, operculum, ACC, and left primary somatosensory and motor cortices. Therefore, nocebo hyperalgesia may be predominantly produced through an affective–cognitive pain pathway (medial pain system), and the left hippocampus may play an important role in this process.

We have used activation likelihood estimation meta-analysis, a state-of-the-art approach, to search for the cortical areas involved in pain anticipation in human experimental pain models (Palermo, Benedetti, Costa, & Amanzio, 2015). What can we say about activated foci considering pain anticipation? During expectation of hyperalgesia, activated foci have been found in the dorsolateral PFC, inferior frontal gyrus, anterior insula (AI) cortex, midcingulate cortex (MCC), and medial dorsal nucleus of the thalamus. We further provided a meta-analytic connectivity model (MACM) within the MCC and AIC as selected seed region of interest. The identified networks of coactivation are largely overlapping and seem to have a common origin in the dorsolateral (BA 9,46) and medial PFC (BA 32). Importantly, the MACM allows meta-analyses to look for global coactivation patterns across a diverse range of tasks, thus responding to the question "for a given region what tasks elicit activation?" In particular, the specific preidentified seed regions (AI and ACC) were analyzed in terms of the functional activation behavioral domains. Interestingly, once again AI and ACC produced very consistent results. Behavioral domains embraced the main categories of action (imagination, inhibition, and execution), emotion, and perception (pain and interoception). Importantly, since the paradigms used in the selected studies analyzed the period of "expected hyperalgesia," as the time between the beginning of the scan and the beginning of the stimulus, and as the nocebo response also occurs through negative verbal suggestions when inert substances are not administered, the pain anticipation phenomenon may be considered as a way to elicit and study the nocebo response (Palermo et al., 2015) (see Figure 1(B)).

Early enhancement of pain signals in the dorsal horn of the spinal cord has also been found in a study in which nocebo hyperalgesia was investigated in combination with spinal functional magnetic resonance imaging in healthy volunteers (Geuter & Büchel, 2013). The local application of an inert nocebo cream on the forearm increased pain ratings compared with a control cream and also reduced pain thresholds on the nocebo-treated skin. Pain stimulation induced a strong activation in the spinal cord at the level of the stimulated dermatomes C5/C6, and comparison of the nocebo with the control condition revealed enhanced nocebo-related activity in the ipsilateral dorsal horn of the spinal cord. Therefore, the nocebo hyperalgesic effect envisages a pain-facilitating mechanism at a very early stage of pain processing, that is, in the spinal cord, well before cortical processing.

CONCLUSIONS

Nocebo is a frequent, clinically relevant phenomenon. A better understanding of the nocebo response and of nocebo-related effects is essential for physicians to mitigate its impact on clinical practice and to improve the therapeutic outcome. Translational research in this area is a future challenge and priority. The objective is to find a way to manage, and possibly treat, nocebo effects to reduce them to a minimum for the benefit of patients. All these findings highlight the important role of cognition and emotion in the therapeutic outcome. In particular, nocebo and nocebo-related effects may represent a vulnerable point that should be minimized when patients receive a treatment. Therefore, a better understanding of the psychological and biological underpinnings of nocebo is in order.

REFERENCES

Amanzio, M. (2011). Do we need a new procedure for the assessment of adverse events in anti-migraine clinical trials? *Recent Patents on CNS Drug Discovery, 6,* 41–47.

Amanzio, M., Corazzini, L. L., Vase, L., & Benedetti, F. (2009). A systematic review of adverse events in placebo groups of anti-migraine clinical trials. *Pain, 146,* 261–269.

Andre, J., Zeau, B., Pohl, M., Cesselin, F., Benoliel, J. J., & Becker, C. (2005). Involvement of cholecystokininergic systems in anxiety-induced hyperalgesia in male rats: behavioral and biochemical studies. *Journal of Neuroscience, 25,* 7896–7904.

Barsky, A. J., Saintfort, R., Rogers, M. P., & Borus, J. F. (2002). Nonspecific medication side effects and the nocebo phenomenon, *JAMA, 287,* 622–627.

Benedetti, F. (1997). Cholecystokinin type-A and type-B receptors and their modulation of opioid analgesia. *News in Physiological Sciences, 12,* 263–268.

Benedetti, F., & Amanzio, M. (1997). The neurobiology of placebo analgesia: from endogenous opioids to cholecystokinin. *Progress in Neurobiology, 52,* 109–125.

Benedetti, F., Amanzio, M., Casadio, C., Oliaro, A., & Maggi, G. (1997). Blockade of nocebo hyperalgesia by the cholecystokinin antagonist proglumide. *Pain, 71,* 135–140.

Benedetti, F., Amanzio, M., Vighetti, S., & Asteggiano, G. (2006). The biochemical and neuroendocrine bases of the hyperalgesic nocebo effect. *Journal of Neuroscience, 26,* 12014–12022.

Benedetti, F., & Colloca, L. (2004). Placebo-induced analgesia: methodology, neurobiology, clinical use, and ethics. *Reviews in Analgesia, 7,* 129–143.

Benedetti, F., Durando, J., & Vighetti, S. (2014). Nocebo and placebo modulation of hypobaric hypoxia headache involves the cyclooxygenase-prostaglandins pathway. *Pain, 155,* 921–928.

Benedetti, F., Lanotte, M., Lopiano, L., & Colloca, L. (2007). When words are painful—unraveling the mechanisms of the nocebo effect. *Neuroscience, 147,* 260–271.

Benedetti, F., Maggi, G., Lopiano, L., Lanotte, M., Rainero, I., Vighetti, S., et al. (2003). Open versus hidden medical treatments: the patient's knowledge about a therapy affects the therapy outcome. *Prevention and Treatment.* http://dx.doi.org/10.1037/1522-3736.6.1.61a. No Pagination Specified Article http://content2.apa.org/journals/pre/6/1/1.

van den Broeke, E. N., Geene, N., van Rijn, C. M., Wilder-Smith, O. H., & Oosterman, J. (2013). Negative expectations facilitate mechanical hyperalgesia after high-frequency electrical stimulation of human skin. *European Journal of Pain, 18*(1), 86–91.

Chua, P., Krams, M., Toni, I., Passingham, R., & Dolan, R. (1999). A functional anatomy of anticipatory anxiety. *Neuroimage, 9,* 563–571.

Colloca, L., & Benedetti, F. (2007). Nocebo hyperalgesia: how anxiety is turned into pain. *Current Opinion in Anaesthesiology, 20,* 435–439.

Colloca, L., Lopiano, L., Lanotte, M., & Benedetti, F. (2004). Overt versus covert treatment for pain, anxiety and Parkinson's disease. *Lancet Neurology, 3,* 679–684.

Colloca, L., Sigaudo, M., & Benedetti, F. (2008). The role of learning in nocebo and placebo effects. *Pain, 136,* 211–218.

Dannecker, E. A., Price, D. D., & Robinson, M. E. (2003). An examination of the relationships among recalled, expected, and actual intensity and unpleasantness of delayed onset muscle pain. *Journal of Pain, 4,* 74–81.

Dworkin, S. F., Chen, A. C., LeResche, L., & Clark, D. W. (1983). Cognitive reversal of expected nitrous oxide analgesia for acute pain. *Anesthesia and Analgesia, 62,* 1073–1077.

Elsenbruch, S., Schmid, J., Bäsler, M., Cesko, E., Schedlowski, M., & Benson, S. (2012). How positive and negative expectations shape the experience of visceral pain: an experimental pilot study in healthy women. *Neurogastroenterology and Motility, 24,* 914–e460.

Fields, H. L., & Levine, J. D. (1984). Pain–mechanics and management. *Western Journal of Medicine, 141,* 347–357.

Flaten, M. A., Simonsen, T., & Olsen, H. (1999). Drug-related information generates placebo and nocebo responses that modify the drug response. *Psychosomatic Medicine, 61,* 250–255.

Flor, H., & Grusser, S. M. (1999). Conditioned stress-induced analgesia in humans. *European Journal of Pain, 3,* 317–324.

Geuter, S., & Büchel, C. (2013). Facilitation of pain in the human spinal cord by nocebo treatment. *Journal of Neuroscience, 33,* 13784–13790.

Hahn, R. A. (1985). Culture-bound syndromes unbound. *Social Science and Medicine, 21*(2), 165–171.

Hahn, R. A. (1997). The nocebo phenomenon: concept, evidence, and implications for public health. *Preventive Medicine, 26,* 607–611.

Häuser, W., Bartram, C., Bartram-Wunn, E., & Tölle, T. (2012). Adverse events attributable to nocebo in randomized controlled drug trials in fibromyalgia syndrome and painful diabetic peripheral neuropathy: systematic review. *Clinical Journal of Pain, 28,* 437–451.

Hebb, A. L. O., Poulin, J. F., Roach, S. P., Zacharko, R. M., & Drolet, G. (2005). Cholecystokinin and endogenous opioid peptides: interactive influence on pain, cognition, and emotion. *Progress in Neuro-Psychopharmacology and Biological Psychiatry, 29,* 1225–1238.

Heinricher, M. M., McGaraughty, S., & Tortorici, V. (2001). Circuitry underlying antipioid actions of cholecystokinin within the rostral ventromedial medulla. *Journal of Neurophysiology, 85,* 280–286.

Heinricher, M. M., & Neubert, M. J. (2004). Neural basis for the hyperalgesic action of cholecystokinin in the rostral ventromedial medulla. *Journal of Neurophysiology, 92,* 1982–1989.

Holloway, R. G., Gramling, R., & Kelly, A. G. (2013). Estimating and communicating prognosis in advanced neurologic disease. *Neurology, 80,* 764–772.

Hsieh, J. C., Stone-Elander, S., & Ingvar, M. (1999). Anticipatory coping of pain expressed in the human anterior cingulated cortex: a positron emission tomography study. *Neuroscience Letters, 262*(1), 61–64.

Keltner, J. R., Furst, A., Fan, C., Redfern, R., Inglis, B., & Fields, H. L. (2006). Isolating the modulatory effect of expectation on pain transmission: a functional magnetic imaging study. *Journal of Neuroscience, 26,* 4437–4443.

Kennedy, W. P. (1961). The nocebo reaction. *The World Medical Journal, 95,* 203–205.

Kissel, P., & Barrucand, D. (1964). *Placebos et effet placebo en medecine.* Paris: Elsevier Masson.

Kong, J., Gollub, R. L., Polich, G., Kirsch, I., Laviolette, P., Vangel, M., et al. (2008). A functional magnetic resonance imaging study on the neural mechanisms of hyperalgesic nocebo effect. *Journal of Neuroscience, 28,* 13354–13362.

Koyama, T., McHaffie, J. G., Laurienti, P. J., & Coghill, R. C. (2005). The subjective experience of pain: where expectations become reality. *Proceedings of the National Academy of Sciences of the United States of America, 102*, 12950–12955.

Koyama, T., Tanaka, Y. Z., & Mikami, A. (1998). Nociceptive neurons in the macaque anterior cingulate activate during anticipation of pain. *Neuroreport, 9*, 2663–2667.

Leeuw, M., Goossens, M. E., Linton, S. J., Crombez, G., Boersma, K., & Vlaeyen, J. W. (2007). The fear-avoidance model of musculoskeletal pain: current state of scientific evidence. *Journal of Behavioral Medicine, 30*, 77–94.

Lorenz, J., Hauck, M., Paur, R. C., Nakamura, Y., Zimmermann, R., Bromm, B., et al. (2005). Cortical correlates of false expectations during pain intensity judgments—a possible manifestation of placebo/nocebo cognitions. *Brain, Behavior and Immunity, 19*, 283–295.

Manchikanti, L., Pampati, V., & Damron, K. (2005). The role of placebo and nocebo effects of perioperative administration of sedatives and opioids in interventional pain management. *Pain Physician, 8*, 349–355.

Mitchell, J. M., Lowe, D., & Fields, H. L. (1998). The contribution of the rostral ventromedial medulla to the antinociceptive effects of systemic morphine in restrained and unrestrained rats. *Neuroscience, 87*, 123–133.

Mitsikostas, D. D., Chalarakis, N. G., Mantonakis, L. I., Delicha, E. M., & Sfikakis, P. P. (2012). Nocebo in fibromyalgia: meta-analysis of placebo-controlled clinical trials and implications for practice. *European Journal of Neurology, 19*, 672–680.

Mitsikostas, D. D., Mantonakis, L. I., & Chalarakis, N. G. (2011). Nocebo is the enemy, not placebo. A meta-analysis of reported side effects after placebo treatment in headaches. *Cephalalgia, 31*, 550–561.

Oftedal, G., Straume, A., Johnsson, A., & Stovner, L. J. (2007). Mobile phone headache: a double blind, sham-controlled provocation study. *Cephalalgia, 27*, 447–455.

Palermo, S., Benedetti, F., Costa, T., & Amanzio, M. (2015). Pain anticipation: an activation likelihood estimation meta-analysis of brain imaging studies. *Human Brain Mapping, 36*, 1648–1661.

Papadopoulos, D., & Mitsikostas, D. D. (2012). A meta-analytic approach to estimating nocebo effects in neuropathic pain trials. *Journal of Neurology, 259*, 436–447.

Petersen, G. L., Finnerup, N. B., Colloca, L., Amanzio, M., Price, D. D., Staehelin Jensen, T., & Vase, L. (2014). The magnitude of nocebo effects in pain: a meta-analysis. *Pain, 155*(8), 1426–1434.

Ploghaus, A., Tracey, I., Gati, J. S., Clare, S., Menon, R. S., Matthews, P. M., et al. (1999). Dissociating pain from its anticipation in the human brain. *Science, 284*, 1979–1981.

Pogge, R. C. (1963). The toxic placebo, 1: side and toxic effects reported during the administration of placebo medicine. *Medical Times, 91*, 1–6.

Porro, C. A., Baraldi, P., Pagnoni, G., Serafini, M., Facchin, P., Maieron, M., et al. (2002). Does anticipation of pain affect cortical nociceptive systems? *Journal of Neuroscience, 22*, 3206–3214.

Porro, C. A., Cettolo, V., Francescato, M. P., & Baraldi, P. (2003). Functional activity mapping of the mesial hemispheric wall during anticipation of pain. *Neuroimage, 19*, 1738–1747.

Price, D. D. (2000). Psychological and neural mechanisms of the affective dimension of pain. *Science, 288*, 1769–1772.

Sanderson, C., Hardy, J., Spruyt, O., & Currow, D. C. (2013). Placebo and nocebo effects in randomized controlled trials: the implications for research and practice. *Journal of Pain and Symptom Management, 46*(5), 722–730.

Sawamoto, N., Honda, M., Okada, T., Hanakawa, T., Kanda, M., Fukuyama, H., et al. (2000). Expectation of pain enhances responses to nonpainful somatosensory stimulation in the anterior cingulated cortex and parietal operculum/posterior insula: an event-related functional magnetic resonance imaging study. *Journal of Neuroscience, 20*, 7438–7445.

Svedman, P., Ingvar, M., & Gordh, T. (2005). "Anxiebo", placebo, and postoperative pain. *BMC Anesthesiology, 5,* 9.

Swider, K., & Bąbel, P. (2013). The effect of the sex of a model in nocebo hyperalgesia induced by social observational learning. *Pain, 154,* 1312–1317.

Terman, G. W., Morgan, M. J., & Liebeskind, J. C. (1986). Opioid and non-opioid stress analgesia from cold water swim: importance of stress severity. *Brain Research, 372,* 167–171.

Varelmann, D., Pancaro, C., Cappiello, E. C., & Camann, W. R. (2010). Nocebo-induced hyperalgesia during local anesthetic injection. *Anesthesia and Analgesia, 110,* 868–870.

Vlaeyen, J. W., & Linton, S. J. (2000). Fear-avoidance and its consequences in chronic musculoskeletal pain: a state of the art. *Pain, 85,* 317–332.

Vögtle, E., Barke, A., & Kröner-Herwig, B. (2013). Nocebo hyperalgesia induced by social observational learning. *Pain, 154,* 1427–1433.

Wells, R. E., & Kaptchuk, T. J. (2012). To tell the truth, the whole truth, may do patients harm: the problem of the nocebo effect for informed consent. *American Journal of Bioethics, 12,* 22–29.

Willer, J. C., & Albe-Fessard, D. (1980). Electrophysiological evidence for a release of endogenous opiates in stress-induced "analgesia" in man. *Brain Research, 198,* 419–426.

CHAPTER 7

The Neuroscience of Pain and Fear

Emma E. Biggs[1,2] Ann Meulders[1,3], Johan W.S. Vlaeyen[1,3,4]
[1]Research Group Health Psychology, University of Leuven, Leuven, Belgium; [2]Department of Cognitive Neuroscience, Maastricht University, Maastricht, The Netherlands; [3]Center for Excellence on Generalization Research in Health and Psychopathology, University of Leuven, Leuven, Belgium; [4]Department of Clinical Psychological Science, Maastricht University, Maastricht, The Netherlands

INTRODUCTION TO PAIN AND FEAR

Pain is "[an] unpleasant sensory and emotional experience associated with actual or potential tissue damage, or described in terms of such damage" (Merskey & Bogduk, 1994). For this reason, both defensive and recuperative behaviors are evolutionarily advantageous, and optimizing learning about possible cues of imminent harm can be valuable. However, there are circumstances in which these behaviors and learning processes can become dysfunctional, a situation commonly seen among individuals who suffer from chronic pain. Clinical definitions of chronic pain conditions typically revolve around a critical time point, which marks a transition from a "healthy" pain response to a persisting pain that is not proportionate to the current state of injury (Merskey & Bogduk, 1994). A 2006 study of prevalence found that approximately 19% of Europeans suffer from chronic pain and that this condition has a severe impact on their social and work lives (Breivik, Collett, Ventafridda, Cohen, & Gallacher, 2006). The disability that patients experience has been shown to be largely mediated by fear of pain (for a review and meta-analysis of this relationship see Zale, Lange, Fields, & Ditre, 2013), and this specific fear can be even more disabling than the pain itself (Crombez, Vlaeyen, Heuts, & Lysens, 1999). In this chapter, we will discuss the relationship between pain and fear, including a number of pathways of influence through which they can interact.

Pain Processing

Contemporary models of pain processing emphasize the multifaceted nature of the pain experience (Garcia-Larrea & Peyron, 2013; Peyron,

Laurent, & García-Larrea, 2000). For instance, a three-tiered hierarchical model has been proposed, which divides neural pain processing into three networks: nociception, attentional–perceptive, and affective–reappraisive (Garcia-Larrea & Peyron, 2013). In this model, the first network (nociception) relates to the processing of incoming signals from the spinal cord that are projected to the posterior thalamus, and therefore refers to the activity that occurs before conscious perception (including transduction and transmission). The second network, attentional–perceptive, includes the mid- and anterior insula, anterior cingulate cortex (ACC), prefrontal cortex (PFC), and posterior parietal cortex. The role of this network is to perceive pain and to allocate attentional resources accordingly. The third network is the affective–reappraisive network. Including the orbitofrontal cortex, perigenual cingulate, and anterolateral PFC, this network is involved in assigning emotional value to the pain experience. It can also modulate pain perception via the descending pain modulatory system owing to direct links with the periaqueductal gray (PAG). For the purpose of this review, we note the predominance of affective and cognitive influences in the final pain percept. In addition, the flow of information is bidirectional, with many connections between networks, consistent with the idea of a generative model: constantly in flux and updating with new input (Figure 1).

Fear Processing

There are a number of neuroimaging studies that have tried to elucidate the neural correlates of fear in humans; a 2009 systematic review identified 46 studies that used either functional magnetic resonance imaging (fMRI) or positron emission tomography to compare the brain's response to a threatening versus safe stimulus (Sehlmeyer et al., 2009). The authors identified three core regions that were consistently activated: amygdala, ACC, and insula (Figure 2). The amygdala is a region that has received much attention in studies of fear conditioning and is the focus of much debate. While research with animals and early research with humans identified the amygdala as a "hub" for fear, the specificity and necessity of the amygdala for the experience of fear have been questioned (Adolphs, 2013; Barrett & Satpute, 2013; Guillory & Bujarski, 2014). For example, a review of intracranial electrophysiology research reported that while stimulation of the amygdala often does result in self-reported fear, it is not the only region to elicit this response (insula and parahippocampal gyrus also evoked a similar response). In addition, it is possible that self-reported

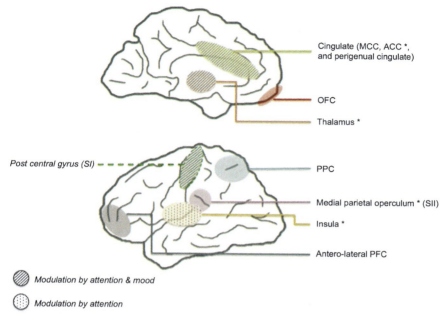

Post central gyrus (SI)

Cingulate (MCC, ACC *, and perigenual cingulate)

OFC

Thalamus *

PPC

Medial parietal operculum * (SII)

Insula *

Antero-lateral PFC

Modulation by attention & mood

Modulation by attention

Figure 1 Summary of brain regions commonly implicated in pain processing. Regions labeled are those described by contemporary models of pain processing (Garcia-Larrea & Peyron, 2013). Regions marked with (*) are also part of the neurologic pain signature (NPS; Wager et al., 2013). The postcentral gyrus (SI) is not part of the NPS (Wager et al., 2013), nor the pain matrices described by Garcia-Larrea and Peyron (2013); however, it has traditionally been included in neurological models of pain processing (Peyron et al., 2000) and shows modulated activity in response to pain during changes in both attention and mood (Villemure & Bushnell, 2009; Wiech et al., 2008).

fear is associated with another region being activated because of its connections with the amygdala (Guillory & Bujarski, 2014). Furthermore, meta-analytic approaches using neuroimaging data show that the amygdala is also part of a salience network, which is in line with its activation by most arousing stimuli (both positive and negative; Barrett & Satpute, 2013). While in animal research amygdala activation is the hallmark of fear processing, it has been suggested that drawing the same conclusion from human data should be done cautiously. The alternative view to a localized and specific region for fear processing is a distributed network of regions, which will vary depending on the content of the threatening stimulus (Adolphs, 2013; Gross & Canteras, 2012). In addition to activation of the amygdala, insula activation is commonly reported in human studies of fear, and it has been proposed that this region is differentially activated depending on the

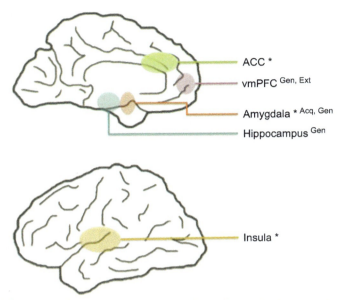

Figure 2 Summary of brain regions commonly implicated in fear learning. Regions marked with (*) were identified by a systematic review of human fear conditioning studies (Sehlmeyer et al., 2009). Regions marked with "Acq" are commonly implicated in fear acquisition memory, regions marked with "Gen" are involved in the generalization of fear, and regions marked with "Ext" are implicated in fear extinction memory.

uncertainty of the feared event, whilst the ACC has been associated with approach and avoidance learning (Sehlmeyer et al., 2009). However, further research is still needed before a consensus on the nodes within this network may be reached, as well as their respective roles in the fear experience.

Pain and Fear

In the perceptual–defensive–recuperative (PDR) model of Bolles and Fanselow (1980), pain and fear are conceptualized as antagonistic motivational states. The role of fear is to organize defensive behavior when pain is expected, while pain motivates recuperative behaviors with the aim of promoting recovery. Critically, in this model, pain does not elicit fear. Rather it is the expectancy of pain that elicits fear. This expectancy is formed by a perceptual system that identifies the salient features of an aversive event and associates them, via associative learning mechanisms, with a cue. The model consists of three sequential phases: perceptual, defensive, and recuperative. In the perceptual phase, the salient features of the painful stimulus are detected and associated with contingent cues or contexts. This association is formed with the aim of constructing a predictor for the painful event. Future presentations of the painful event will be compared to the expectation and any discrepancy is incorporated and used to refine future predictions. When pain is expected, fear is elicited. Fear is a motivational system that organizes behavior and perception, for example, by selectively facilitating the perception of escape pathways and the selection of a behavior given the current environment. In addition, fear can inhibit other motivational systems by competition. This competition can take the form of response competition (e.g., we perform an action for defense, which prevents us from simultaneously carrying out a different action), motivation competition (e.g., fear might outweigh our motivation for socializing), or perceptual competition (e.g., we no longer notice other stimuli that are not relevant for defense). The final stage of the model occurs once pain has occurred: recuperation. This stage is characterized by behaviors that promote recovery and take precedence over other motivational systems.

Thus, in the PDR model fear precedes pain and can have an inhibitory effect on pain (i.e., stress–induced analgesia (SIA)). However, if fear is prolonged (which Bolles and Fanselow (1980) refer to as anxiety), then it can have the opposite effect and increase perceived pain intensity (i.e., hyperalgesia) (see the Section Psychophysiological Response: Stress). The other side of the bidirectional relationship, that is, the effect of pain on fear, is less clear, although Bolles and Fanselow (1980) do emphasize that pain does not elicit fear, stating that they "… reject the idea … that a noxious US [unconditioned stimulus] can arouse the fear motivational system" (Bolles & Fanselow, 1980, p. 295). Instead, fear can be elicited by worries about pain, such as the cause of pain or a misinterpretation about the level of bodily injury signaled by the pain. This specific fear—fear of pain due to the beliefs about pain or possible reinjury—has been termed "pain-related fear" and features heavily in the fear–avoidance model of chronic musculoskeletal pain (Lethem, Slade, Troup, & Bentley, 1983; Vlaeyen & Linton, 2000, 2012).

Pain-Related Fear

Chronic pain refers to pain that persists beyond the expected point of healing (Merskey & Bogduk, 1994) and current fear–avoidance models posit possible pathways through which this can occur. It is proposed that individuals who have catastrophic pain beliefs and misinterpret their pain as being highly threatening are more prone to become afraid of movements that they believe will worsen their pain (or result in reinjury). These negative pain beliefs can stem from threatening pain-related information (Houben et al., 2005) or a predisposing negative affectivity. The fear they experience (i.e., pain-related fear), as posited by Bolles and Fanselow (1980), is a motivator for defensive behavior that can lead to disuse and disability (Crombez et al., 1999; Leeuw, Goossens, et al., 2007; Swinkels-Meewisse, Roelofs, Oostendorp, Verbeek, & Vlaeyen, 2006).

A growing number of studies are providing evidence that pain-related fear is a key factor in maintaining chronicity and, therefore, an essential consideration for therapy (den Hollander et al., 2010; de Jong, Vlaeyen, Onghena, Goossens, et al., 2005; Vlaeyen, de Jong, Sieben, & Crombez, 2002). However, less commonly discussed is the conceptualization and definition of pain-related fear, which has stimulated debate over its assessment and its proposed role in chronic pain (Wideman et al., 2013). The term is typically used to refer to beliefs about damage and/or pain caused by movement, fear of certain movements and activities, and avoidance of such movements and activities (Pincus, Smeets, Simmonds, & Sullivan, 2010). If fear is defined as an emotional state that evokes three response systems, cognitive, psychophysiological, and behavioral (Lang, Davis, & Ohman, 2000), then the same template can be applied to pain-related fear: an emotional state experienced when the threat of pain is present. This results in a cognitive, psychophysiological, and behavioral response. The strength of the fearful state is dependent on pain-related beliefs and expectations about the likelihood of pain.

An important distinction to consider is between pain-related fear and pain-related anxiety. Fear is a response to a specific threat, which is characterized by escape behaviors, while anxiety refers to a prolonged affective state in response to an uncertain environment and is characterized by avoidance (Gray & McNaughton, 2000; McNaughton & Corr, 2004; Sylvers, Lilienfeld, & LaPrairie, 2011). Another distinction is between pain-related fear and phobia, the latter being characterized by the recognition that the fear is irrational—this is not the case in pain-related fear, during which patients are convinced that avoidance is necessary to protect them against further injury (Vlaeyen, de Jong, Sieben, et al., 2002) (Box 1).

Box 1 Fear and Anxiety

Fear and anxiety commonly share several characteristics. They are future-oriented negative affective states, and they both refer to anticipation of danger or discomfort with tense apprehensiveness. There are also differences, and fear and anxiety can be placed at opposing ends of several conceptual spectra: duration, cue specificity, and function. The view proposed by Bolles and Fanselow (1980) is that anxiety is a "prolonged-duration, ill-defined variety" (p. 300) of fear, whereas Lang et al. (2000) distinguish fear and anxiety by the instigating event: an explicit and identifiable stimulus evokes fear, whereas a less explicit or more generalized cue results in anxiety. Furthermore, McNaughton and Corr (2004) emphasize a "sharp (functional, behavioral and pharmacological) distinction between fear and anxiety" (p. 286), in that the function of fear is to move an individual away from danger and the function of anxiety is to facilitate approaching danger.

In addition to these conceptual differences it has been shown that the expression of fear, compared to the expression of anxiety, relies on different neural structures. Specifically, the fear-potentiated startle response to cue-induced fear relies on the central nucleus, while sustained anxiety (from contextual conditioning) relies on the bed nucleus of the stria terminalis (Lang et al., 2000). Cued and contextual conditioning are well-established paradigms to investigate fear and anxiety in humans (e.g., the NPU-threat test (Schmitz & Grillon, 2012)), and therefore in some cases a shift in terminology to cued and contextual fear (see Meulders et al., 2011, 2013) may be more informative. These terms are more closely related to the phenomena under investigation in experimental settings and allow us to disentangle and focus upon specific elements of complex states such as fear and anxiety.

The Acquisition of Pain-Related Fear

Pain-related fear can be acquired and extinguished via associative learning mechanisms, such as classical (Pavlovian) conditioning (Pavlov, 1927). In a typical classical conditioning procedure a neutral stimulus (conditioned stimulus: CS) is paired with an aversive stimulus (unconditioned stimulus: US) so that, after repeated pairings, this initially neutral stimulus starts to elicit a conditioned response (CR) that can share similarities with the unconditioned response (UR) to the US, but which may also be quite different. The idea is that the CS–US association is stored in memory, so that the presence of the CS activates the memory representation of the US, thereby eliciting a CR. In a differential conditioning paradigm the response to this CS+ is compared to the response evoked by a control stimulus that is never paired with the US (CS−). This CS–US association can be formed through direct experience, by observing someone else experiencing the association, or by being verbally instructed about the association (Olsson & Phelps, 2007; Rachman & Crespigny, 1977). The formation of these associations occurs in the lateral nuclei of the amygdala, from which projections via the central nuclei evoke a fear response (Gross & Canteras, 2012; Maren, 2001). This pathway underlies learning through direct experience and observation, but learning through language (i.e., instructional conditioning) is also reliant upon higher-order regions (Olsson & Phelps, 2007). Learning by instruction seems to require a cortical representation of the aversive stimulus that is conveyed to the amygdala via the insula (Phelps et al., 2001), and also relies more heavily on the left amygdala nuclei, consistent with the laterality of language processing (Olsson & Phelps, 2007).

While there are a number of studies investigating the mechanisms and neural correlates of fear learning, the studies described below have focused specifically on the acquisition of pain-related fear by associative learning. *First*, acquisition of pain-related fear through direct experience has been demonstrated using a range of paradigms. For example, in the voluntary joystick movement paradigm (Meulders, Vansteenwegen, & Vlaeyen, 2011), movements in one plane (e.g., horizontal) were part of a predictable condition, while movements in the other plane (e.g., vertical) were part of an unpredictable condition. In the predictable condition, one movement was paired with a painful electrocutaneous stimulus (CSp+), while the other was never paired with a pain-US (CSp−). Results showed that participants were more afraid of making the CSp+ movement than the CSp− movement. During the unpredictable condition, neither movement was paired with painful stimuli; instead they occurred during the intertrial interval at random time points. Despite these two movements (CSu1, CSu2) never being paired with a painful stimulus, participants were still more fearful of these movements than the CSp− movement. This experiment demonstrates the difference between a cued pain-related fear elicited by the CSp+ movement and a more generalized pain-related anxiety elicited by the CSu1 and CSu2 movements. *Second*, the observation of painful expressions can also serve as a US to condition pain-related fear toward a previously neutral stimulus (Goubert, Vlaeyen, Crombez, & Craig, 2011). Using both a cold pressor task and warm water immersion task, Helsen et al. (Helsen, Goubert, Peters, & Vlaeyen, 2011; Helsen, Goubert, & Vlaeyen, 2013) found that when a participant views a model displaying a painful facial expression during either task, he or she will rate more pain-related fear than when he or she views a model with a neutral facial expression. *Third*, learning by instruction is perhaps the least researched of these three pathways (Olsson & Phelps, 2007). However, it may be of particular relevance in chronic pain conditions, when we consider the possible effect of health care information communication. Research has demonstrated that simply being informed about the contingency between two events can result in a fear response being elicited by the CS+ (Phelps et al., 2001; Van Dessel, de Houwer, Gast, & Smith, 2014), and thus informing patients that a certain movement will be painful may be sufficient to lead to avoidance of that movement. This might be the reason there is often an association between patients' and their health care providers' fears (Houben et al., 2005).

The Generalization of Pain-Related Fear

Novel stimuli that are similar to the CS+ can evoke the same response as the CS+, despite never being paired with the US. The strength of the response diminishes as similarity to the CS+ decreases: a phenomenon termed stimulus generalization (Ghirlanda & Enquist, 2003; Honig & Urcuioli, 1981; Kalish, 1969; Lissek, 2012). In an extension of the voluntary joystick movement paradigm (Meulders, Vandebroek, Vervliet, & Vlaeyen, 2013) participants carried out movements with varying degrees of similarity to the CS+ and CS− and results showed a generalization gradient in which pain-related fear was generalized to the movements that were proprioceptively similar to the original CS+ movement, but not to those that were similar to the CS−. In the unpredictable condition (in which CSs did not predict the pain) participants showed generalized fear of all of the novel movements, which demonstrates the effect of the context on the generalization of the response. Similar findings were obtained in a study with fibromyalgia patients (Meulders, Jans, & Vlaeyen, 2015). Generalization of fear of painful movement is not only based on perceptual equivalence between stimuli, but can also occur by virtue of the *symbolic* relationship between movements and pain-relevant stimuli (Bennett, Meulders, Baeyens, & Vlaeyen, 2015).

Evidence for the neurobiological mechanisms underlying generalization is largely from animal studies, although an fMRI study acquired data that are in line with the current view from animal literature: pattern separation or completion (i.e., determining whether the CS+ and a novel stimulus are different or similar, respectively) is the result of a mediating effect of the hippocampus on either the ventromedial PFC (for separation) or the amygdala (for completion) (Lissek, 2012).

The Extinction of Pain-Related Fear

Extinction of fear learning takes place when a CS+ is repeatedly presented in the absence of the US, resulting in a decrease in the CR. Extinction is not the unlearning of the previously acquired association—instead a new association is formed that inhibits the behavioral expression of the previous association (Hermans, Craske, Mineka, & Lovibond, 2006; Milad & Quirk, 2012). This process occurs by regulation of amygdala activity by prefrontal regions (ventromedial PFC), specifically, the connection between the lateral and the central nuclei, so that the CS is no longer able to evoke a CR via the central nucleus (Milad, Rosenbaum, & Simon, 2014; Sotres-Bayon, Cain, & LeDoux, 2006).

The clinical analog of extinction, used as a treatment to reduce pain-related disability in chronic pain patients, is graded exposure in vivo (GEXP). By exposing patients to their feared movements (CS+) the expected US (a catastrophic outcome such as reinjury) is challenged and disconfirmed. Thus, when the feared consequence does not occur, patients may reevaluate the threat value of the movement. The main principles of GEXP are (1) informing patients of the paradoxical effects of avoiding pain, (2) gradual exposure to feared movements, and (3) challenging catastrophic thoughts (mental representations of US) by activating the fear network and presenting new information that disconfirms the initial expectation (de Jong, Vlaeyen, Onghena, Goossens, et al., 2005; Vlaeyen, de Jong, Sieben, et al., 2002).

The main aim of GEXP is to reduce functional disability. However, pain-related fear and even pain severity have also been shown to improve after treatment, despite not being a main therapeutic target. Studies have so far demonstrated that GEXP is effective for chronic low back pain (CLBP) (Vlaeyen, de Jong, Geilen, Heuts, & van Breukelen, 2001; Vlaeyen, de Jong, Geilen, Heuts, & van Breukelen, 2002; Woods & Asmundson, 2008), complex regional pain syndrome (CRPS) type I (de Jong, Vlaeyen, Onghena, Cuypers, et al., 2005), upper extremity pain (de Jong, Vlaeyen, van Eijsden, Loo, & Onghena, 2012), and post-traumatic neck pain (de Jong et al., 2008). The single-case experimental design studies of CLBP (Vlaeyen et al., 2001; Vlaeyen, de Jong, Geilen, et al., 2002) and CRPS (de Jong, Vlaeyen, Onghena, Cuypers, et al., 2005) both showed a significant reduction in pain-related fear. This change was still present at follow-up (6 months for CRPS, 1 year for CLBP). In a randomized controlled trial similar results were found: 93% of

CLBP patients were no longer categorized as having "high" fear post-treatment, a criterion of clinical significance (Woods & Asmundson, 2008). In addition, a therapy with similar principles has also been shown to be effective at normalizing neural circuits in pediatric CRPS patients (Becerra et al., 2014).

Further research is needed to bridge the gap between experimental research into extinction and graded exposure in clinical populations. The experimental evidence is usually highly controlled, yet in clinical settings there are numerous confounds and complexities. Therefore, given that the behavioral evidence shows that GEXP can be effective at reducing pain-related fear, a better understanding of the mechanisms that drives this change may contribute to more effective and customized treatments for patients with chronic pain.

THE MODULATION OF SELF-REPORTED PAIN BY PAIN-RELATED FEAR

A number of experimental studies have demonstrated that there is a strong predictive relationship between pain-related fear and pain intensity (Etherton, Lawson, & Graham, 2014; George, Dannecker, & Robinson, 2006; Hirsh, George, Bialosky, & Robinson, 2008; Sullivan, Thorn, Rodgers, & Ward, 2004). However, this relationship is not consistently replicated (Gheldof et al., 2010; Sullivan et al., 2009; Wideman et al., 2013; Wideman & Sullivan, 2011), and a 2013 meta-analysis found that the relationship between pain-related fear and disability is not mediated by pain intensity, despite pain intensity being related to a number of negative outcomes, such as depression and disability (Zale et al., 2013).

While this evidence shows that pain-related fear can affect pain experience (in some circumstances), it does not explain *how* this modulation occurs. Perhaps the difficulty in defining the link between pain-related fear and pain experience is due to the fact that pain-related fear is a complex construct, with many possible pathways of influence. To further explore this issue it might be helpful to examine the various components of pain-related fear. As defined earlier pain-related fear is an emotional state that evokes a response, which can be cognitive, behavioral, and psychophysiological. Each of these components may influence pain perception in a unique way and will therefore be discussed individually.

Emotion: The Fearful State

Pain-related fear is first and foremost an emotional state. In general, negative emotion leads to higher pain intensity ratings and reduced pain tolerance, while positive mood decreases perceived pain intensity (Wiech & Tracey, 2013). Research has largely focused on the effect of stress or anxiety on pain processing (Wiech & Tracey, 2009) and has struggled to dissociate the contribution of emotion and attention on the observed effects (Villemure & Bushnell, 2009; Villemure, Slotnick, & Bushnell, 2003). Nonetheless, by combining odors with painful stimulation, Villemure et al. (2003) could induce either a pleasant or an unpleasant mood, and by changing task demands they could direct attention toward either the painful stimulation or the odor. They found that attention affected the perceived intensity of pain, while mood affected the perceived unpleasantness of pain. In a replication of this study using fMRI, it was found that mood modulated pain-related activity in a number of regions of interest: ACC, medial thalamus, and primary and secondary somatosensory cortex (SI and SII). Further functional connectivity analyses indicated that attention and mood modulation involve dissociable neural networks, with the mood-related network including the ACC, lateral inferior frontal cortex, and PAG (Villemure & Bushnell, 2009). Furthermore, it has been demonstrated that viewing unpleasant pictures is associated with lower pain tolerance, and this effect is more pronounced when the unpleasant picture is injury related (de Wied & Verbaten, 2001). This research implies that mood and attention influence pain perception via dissociable networks. However, if a stimulus is feared, then its capture of attention is (almost) automatic (Pessoa, Kastner, & Ungerleider, 2003) and, consequently, whilst it may be theoretically interesting to consider the effect of fear as an emotional state separate from the contribution of attention, it may not be practically relevant.

Cognitive Response: Attributions, Expectations, and Attention

Inherent to pain-related fear is the concept of pain beliefs; to fear pain, one must also believe that it is harmful. Within certain limits this is adaptive; however, if an individual has a tendency to believe that the pain he or she feels is indicative of something terrible, then he or she is likely to show higher levels of pain-related fear than an individual who does not feel that pain is a sign of bodily damage (Arntz & Claassens, 2004). This magnification of the threat value of pain is a defining characteristic of pain catastrophizing, along with a feeling of helplessness and a lack of inhibition of pain-related thoughts (Quartana, Campbell, & Edwards, 2009). The fear–avoidance model (Vlaeyen & Linton, 2000) proposes that pain catastrophizing is a risk factor for the development of pain-related fear. Indeed, research has shown that an individual who scores high in pain catastrophizing—who thinks that pain is highly threatening—will also develop high pain-related fear (Leeuw, Houben, et al., 2007; Vlaeyen et al., 2004).

As posited by Bolles and Fanselow (1980), another prerequisite for pain-related fear is the expectancy of imminent pain. This expectancy is a prediction made on the basis of previous experience and with an associated degree of certainty (Bubic, von Cramon, & Schubotz, 2010; Büchel, Geuter, Sprenger, & Eippert, 2014). Considering that it has been advanced to consider the brain as containing a generative model of the world, which is constantly updating its predictions based on the discrepancy (or prediction error) between its expectations and the sensory input (Friston, 2010). These prediction errors have been shown to drive fear conditioning and are an integral part of most learning models (McNally, Johansen, & Blair, 2011). Therefore, our previous experiences lead us to construct predictions about the future, when these predictions are tested any discrepancy leads us to update our model. In addition, when our prediction about the future is that pain is imminent, we will mobilize a defensive response that includes components that influence our experience, feeding back into our generative model.

The second phase of the PDR model (Bolles & Fanselow, 1980) is the defensive response that is organized by the motivational state of fear. This defensive response includes a perceptual component that will aid us in escaping threat. For example, attention can be used to filter relevant and irrelevant information. It is well established that painful stimuli capture attention, especially if they are perceived as highly threatening (Crombez, Eccleston, Baeyens, & Eelen, 1998). This effect has been demonstrated using a modified dot–probe task: a task that uses reaction times to a visual target to quantify the time taken to either engage attention (when a target is spatially congruent) or disengage attention (when a target is spatially incongruent) from a visual cue. In the modified version of this task used by Van Damme et al. (Van Damme, Crombez, Eccleston, & Goubert, 2004; Van Damme, Lorenz, et al., 2004; Van Damme, Crombez, Eccleston, & Koster, 2006; Van Damme, Crombez, Hermans, Koster, & Eccleston, 2006) the cue took two forms: one was associated with pain (CS+) and one was not (CS−). When the cueing procedure was exogenous (that is, the cue was not a reliable predictor of target location), then participants showed greater attentional engagement but no differences in attentional disengagement. However, when the cue was a good predictor of the target location (an endogenous cueing procedure), then both increased attentional engagement and increased disengagement were present on CS+ compared to CS− trials. Van Damme, Crombez, Hermans, et al. (2006) suggest that the difference in findings between the two cueing procedures is due to attentional disengagement requiring top-down processes that can be engaged only by a predictive cue.

This research establishes the phasic effects of fear on attention; however, the relationship between pain-related fear (as a trait) and attention is still debated. Studies have shown that pain-related fear is related to an attention bias to threatening stimuli (Goubert, Crombez, & Van Damme, 2004; Keogh, Ellery, Hunt, & Hannent, 2001; Peters, Vlaeyen, & van Drunen, 2000; Yang, Jackson, & Chen, 2013; Yang, Jackson, Gao, & Chen, 2012), although this relationship has not consistently been replicated (Asmundson, Wright, & Hadjistavropoulos, 2005; Roelofs, Peters, Fassaert, & Vlaeyen, 2005; Roelofs, Peters, & Vlaeyen, 2002). These inconsistencies highlight the need for further research in this area. In addition, current empirical methods allow us only to infer attentional shifts based on behavioral changes and therefore, it is possible that the variability in results is due, at least in part, to differences in the underlying mechanism being measured or the sensitivity of the measures. Another possibility is that the allocation of attention to painful stimuli may be inhibited in the presence of competing nonpain goals (Schrooten et al., 2012).

Whether or not it is pain-related fear that increases attention, the consequence of increased attention to pain (as a response of the defensive system activated when pain is expected) is altered pain perception. When a noxious stimulus is attended to it is often perceived as more intense than when it is ignored, and neuroimaging studies have shown that when a participant is distracted from noxious stimulation, pain-processing areas (e.g., SI and SII, thalamus, insula, and ACC) show decreased activity (Wiech, Ploner, & Tracey, 2008), and a top-down modulation from the cingulofrontal cortex on the PAG and posterior thalamus has been proposed (Valet et al., 2004). Attention can modulate sensory perception via top-down mechanisms that include changes in functional connectivity between sensory regions, modulation of the spatial integration of sensory inputs, and baseline shifts in neuronal firing rates (Pessoa et al., 2003; Wiech et al., 2008). Research in this area is mostly on other sensory modalities (such as visual processing), as the experimental manipulation of attention to pain is inherently problematic—pain is highly salient and will almost always be prioritized over other incoming stimuli. However, research does suggest that many attentional mechanisms are not modality-specific and so may influence pain perception in the same way that they influence, for example, visual perception (Pessoa et al., 2003).

One such mechanism is the so-called "baseline shift," in which frontal and parietal regions generate top-down biasing signals. These signals result in an increase in baseline firing rates in the target neuronal population—single-cell recording studies have reported rates of 30–40% higher—resulting in an increased likelihood that the stimulus will "win" the competition for resources (Pessoa et al., 2003). Second, and in addition to this baseline shift, changes in functional connectivity between sensory pain-processing areas can occur (Ohara, Crone, Weiss, & Lenz, 2006). This suggests that during the anticipation and experience of pain, directed attention results in increased synchrony between regions involved in the encoding of the sensory properties of the painful stimulus. A third mechanism by which attention can modulate pain perception is via spatial summation of painful stimulation. This is characterized by an increase in pain intensity when the area being stimulated increases, possibly owing to task-dependent changes in receptive field sizes. To test this hypothesis, Quevedo and Coghill (2007) presented participants with pairs of painful stimuli and asked them to rate the intensity of the stimuli using different rating strategies (to manipulate the focus of attention). Results indicated that during directed attention there was a spatial summation of the two pain stimuli that led to higher pain intensity ratings compared to divided attention.

In sum, we tend to engage our attention more strongly to, and are more resistant to disengaging our attention from, a pain cue compared to a "safe" stimulus. A result of this increased attention to cues of pain is an increase in perceived pain intensity, due to mechanisms that alter the activity of pain-processing regions. One caveat to this conclusion is that in our natural environment threatening stimuli do not occur in isolation—we are usually engaged in an ongoing task. Research has demonstrated that slowed attentional disengagement from threatening stimuli can be overridden by the current task (Schrooten et al., 2012; Vromen, Lipp, & Remington, 2014).

Behavioral Response: Selecting the Best Course of Action

The behavioral component of the defensive response evoked by fear involves selecting the best course of action given the current environment (Bolles & Fanselow, 1980). A key cortical structure in the selection of aversively motivated action is the anterior midcingulate cortex (aMCC), a region implicated in pain, negative affect, and cognitive control processes (Shackman et al., 2011). This region is active during both anticipation and escape from pain, its activity is amplified by action–outcome uncertainty, and it encodes punishment prediction errors during the reversal of learned fear. Therefore, Shackman et al. (2011) propose the "adaptive control hypothesis," which considers the aMCC a "hub" that uses information about punishment to control aversive-motivated action. This function is crucial when automatic responses conflict with current goals. For example, a 2014 study used a voluntary joystick movement paradigm, in which one movement is consistently paired with a painful electric shock (CS+) and one movement is not (CS−), to demonstrate that a concurrent reward can attenuate avoidance behavior during the CS+ movement. During the CS+ movement participants were significantly slower compared to the CS− movement; however, if a monetary reward was also paired with the CS+ movement, then this slowing was no longer present—although participants still reported being fearful of the CS+ movement (Claes, Karos, Meulders, Crombez, & Vlaeyen, 2014). Studies with chronic pain patients have found that in situations of high goal–conflict patients report higher levels of pain intensity (Hardy, Crofford, & Segerstrom, 2011) and pain-related fear (Karoly, Okun, Ruehlman, & Pugliese, 2007). However, experimental research of different conflicting situations indicates that the relationship between goal–conflict and pain-related fear and pain perception may be mediated by perceived control (Schrooten, Wiech, & Vlaeyen, 2014).

Psychophysiological Response: Stress

The amygdala, a primary region of interest in fear processing, receives many inputs from the central nucleus and targets a number of regions that eventually result in a wide variety of physiological responses, including a stress response (Lang et al., 2000). While an acute stress response can result in increased pain thresholds, a phenomenon termed SIA (Bolles & Fanselow, 1980; Butler et al., 2005), chronic stress can have the opposite effect, stress-induced hyperalgesia (SIH) (Jennings, Okine, Roche, & Finn, 2014), depending on whether stress is acute (SIA) or chronic (SIH). The pathways underlying both SIA and SIH are thought to be highly similar, although owing to their complexity further research is needed to elucidate the exact mechanisms. Both human and animal studies have implicated descending pain-facilitation pathways, from ACC through amygdala, PAG, and rostral ventromedial medulla. In addition, many neurotransmitter imbalances have been shown to facilitate the processing of noxious stimuli in states of stress. The main pathway underlying the stress response is the hypothalamic–pituitary–adrenal axis. The primary stress hormone of this axis is cortisol (a glucocorticoid), which self-regulates via a negative feedback loop including the amygdala (Blackburn-Munro & Blackburn-Munro, 2003; Dedovic, Duchesne, Andrews, Engert, & Pruessner, 2009). Research has demonstrated that in a chronic stress state cortisol dysfunction can lead to increased pain sensitivity, that is, SIH (Hannibal & Bishop, 2014). For example, a 2013 study compared cortisol measures with neuroimaging in both a chronic pain and a healthy population (Vachon-Presseau et al., 2013). Patients had significantly higher basal cortisol levels than healthy controls and cortisol levels were positively related to pain-related activity in the anterior parahippocampal gyrus, which was in turn related to patients' pain intensity ratings. A path analysis suggested that hippocampal volume was a risk factor for increased levels of cortisol, this increased cortisol enhanced the parahippocampal activity, and the increased activity then led to higher pain intensity ratings (Vachon-Presseau et al., 2013).

CONCLUSIONS AND EMERGING ISSUES

There is a body of research supporting the idea that pain-related fear is a factor in developing and maintaining disability in chronic pain. However, the impact of pain-related fear on pain perception, specifically perceived intensity of pain, has not been as heavily researched. Considering the significant role of affective processes in the pathway from nociception to pain, it is worth exploring the influence pain-related fear can have in this pathway. The difficulty in exploring these interactions is that both fear and pain processing rely on a widely distributed network of regions. Characterizing the bidirectional direct and indirect connections between these networks and subnetworks is inherently problematic.

The approach to this complex interaction taken here is to view each component of fear separately and focus on self-reported perceived pain intensity. A number of possible pathways of influence have been identified, such as decreased pain tolerance and increased perceived pain unpleasantness as a result of mood manipulation, an effect that is even stronger when primed with pain-related negative images (de Wied & Verbaten, 2001). With regard to the effect of attention, a number of possible mechanisms have been proposed that could explain why increased attention to painful stimulation may result in increased perceived pain intensity. These mechanisms include an increase in baseline firing rates, increased functional connectivity, and spatial summation of incoming sensory signals (Pessoa et al., 2003). The psychological side of the pain-related fear and attention relationship is still unclear, mainly limited by available methods for inferring attentional changes. However, one tentative conclusion is that the threat of pain results in increased attentional engagement and decreased disengagement, unless this would conflict with the current task demands (Legrain et al., 2009; Van Damme, Crombez, et al., 2004; Vromen et al., 2014). This effect of higher-order functions, such as prioritizing goal achievement, is also apparent in the selection of appropriate action in the face of a perceived threat (Claes et al., 2014). The effect of behavioral responses to fear on perceived pain intensity seems to be largely indirect—possibly mediated by perceived control (Crombez, Eccleston, De Vlieger, Van Damme, & De Clercq, 2008; Wiech et al., 2008). The final pathway discussed was stress, a clear illustrator of the distinction between an acute (adaptive: SIA) response versus a chronic (maladaptive: SIH) response (Butler & Finn, 2009; Jennings et al., 2014).

There are still many unanswered questions, however, the first of which being the role of unpredictability. It has been proposed that we are constantly making predictions about future events, and this "predictive brain" theory has grown increasingly popular in the neuroscientific and psychological fields of research (Bubic et al., 2010). If the expectancy of pain results in fear, then the remaining question is, what is the effect of varying certainty in our pain expectancy? If our predictions are often erroneous, then there is high uncertainty in the environment; the construct of psychological entropy has been introduced to explain the occurrence of anxiety as a result of this uncertainty (Hirsh, Mar, & Peterson, 2012). Hirsh et al. (2012) propose that uncertainty is subjectively experienced as anxiety and that an individual, as in any self-organizing system, will strive to reduce uncertainty by acquiring beliefs and rules that constrain the system. The idea that we try to constrain uncertainty is also relevant to chronic pain patients who may engage in the acquisition of rules to help them reduce anxiety in the face of uncontrollable, spontaneous pain (Grupe & Nitschke, 2011; Whitson & Galinsky, 2008).

A second emerging issue is related to our currently available methodologies. An increasing body of evidence is utilizing methods such as functional or effective connectivity to investigate the relationship between brain regions and create a more "network-focused" approach to investigate the neural basis of pain and fear. However, these methods typically do not allow for the dynamic nature of these networks, and the emergence of time varying connectivity methods has demonstrated that the correlation between networks (such as the default mode and default attention networks) is related to fluctuations in mental state (as assessed using concurrent electroencephalography–fMRI) (Chang, Liu, Chen, Liu, & Duyn, 2013). These methods are still new, and there is debate about the best approach to assess these internetwork relationships (Cribben, Wager, & Lindquist, 2013). However, they do raise new research questions that we can tackle concerning the role of intra- and internetwork coherence in the interaction between widely distributed and variable networks, such as those in fear and pain.

In conclusion, there has been much progress since the seminal work by Bolles and Fanselow (1980) on the relationship between fear and pain. In addition, understanding the mechanisms mediating the bidirectional influence has aided in the development of therapies for chronic pain. However, there are still outstanding issues that require investigation, such as the role of unpredictability and controllability, which could add to our current understanding of the interaction between fear and pain. In addition, methodological and statistical advancements allow increasingly complex models of the neural activity that may underlie the interactions between fear and pain that we observe on a behavioral and physiological level.

REFERENCES

Adolphs, R. (2013). The biology of fear. *Current Biology, 23*(2), R79–R93.
Arntz, A., & Claassens, L. (2004). The meaning of pain influences its experienced intensity. *Pain, 109*(1–2), 20–25.
Asmundson, G., Wright, K., & Hadjistavropoulos, H. (2005). Hypervigilance and attentional fixedness in chronic musculoskeletal pain: consistency of findings across modified stroop and dot-probe tasks. *The Journal of Pain, 6*(8), 497–506.
Barrett, L., & Satpute, A. (2013). Large-scale brain networks in affective and social neuroscience: towards an integrative functional architecture of the brain. *Current Opinion in Neurobiology, 23*(3), 361–372.
Becerra, L., Sava, S., Simons, L., Drosos, A., Sethna, N., Berde, C., et al. (2014). Intrinsic brain networks normalize with treatment in pediatric complex regional pain syndrome. *NeuroImage, 6*, 347–369.
Bennett, M., Meulders, A., Baeyens, F., & Vlaeyen, J. W. (2015). Words putting pain in motion: the generalization of pain-related fear within an artificial stimulus category. *Frontiers in Psychology, 6*, 520.
Blackburn-Munro, G., & Blackburn-Munro, R. (2003). Pain in the brain: are hormones to blame? *Trends in Endocrinology & Metabolism, 14*(1), 20–27.

Bolles, R., & Fanselow, M. (1980). A perceptual-defensive-recuperative model of fear and pain. *The Behavioral and Brain Sciences, 3*, 291–323.

Breivik, H., Collett, B., Ventafridda, V., Cohen, R., & Gallacher, D. (2006). Survey of chronic pain in Europe: prevalence, impact on daily life, and treatment. *European Journal of Pain, 10*(4), 287–333.

Bubic, A., von Cramon, D., & Schubotz, R. (2010). Prediction, cognition and the brain. *Frontiers in Human Neuroscience, 4*, 25.

Büchel, C., Geuter, S., Sprenger, C., & Eippert, F. (2014). Placebo analgesia: a predictive coding perspective. *Neuron, 81*(6), 1223–1239.

Butler, R., & Finn, D. (2009). Stress-induced analgesia. *Progress in Neurobiology, 88*(3), 184–202.

Butler, T., Pan, H., Epstein, J., Protopopescu, X., Tuescher, O., Goldstein, M., et al. (2005). Fear-related activity in subgenual anterior cingulate differs between men and women. *Neuroreport, 16*(11), 1233–1236.

Chang, C., Liu, Z., Chen, M. C., Liu, X., & Duyn, J. H. (2013). EEG correlates of time-varying BOLD functional connectivity. *NeuroImage, 72*, 227–236.

Claes, N., Karos, K., Meulders, A., Crombez, G., & Vlaeyen, J. (2014). Competing goals attenuate avoidance behavior in the context of pain. *The Journal of Pain, 15*(11), 1120–1129.

Cribben, I., Wager, T. D., & Lindquist, M. A. (2013). Detecting functional connectivity change points for single-subject fMRI data. *Frontiers in Computational Neuroscience, 7*.

Crombez, G., Eccleston, C., Baeyens, F., & Eelen, P. (1998). When somatic information threatens, catastrophic thinking enhances attentional interference. *Pain, 75*(2–3), 187–198.

Crombez, G., Eccleston, C., De Vlieger, P., Van Damme, S., & De Clercq, A. (2008). Is it better to have controlled and lost than never to have controlled at all? An experimental investigation of control over pain. *Pain, 137*(3), 631–639.

Crombez, G., Vlaeyen, J., Heuts, P., & Lysens, R. (1999). Pain-related fear is more disabling than pain itself: evidence on the role of pain-related fear in chronic back pain disability. *Pain, 80*(1–2), 329–339.

Dedovic, K., Duchesne, A., Andrews, J., Engert, V., & Pruessner, J. (2009). The brain and the stress axis: the neural correlates of cortisol regulation in response to stress. *NeuroImage, 47*(3), 864–871.

Etherton, J., Lawson, M., & Graham, R. (2014). Individual and gender differences in subjective and objective indices of pain: gender, fear of pain, pain catastrophizing and cardiovascular reactivity. *Applied Psychophysiology and Biofeedback, 39*(2), 89–97.

Friston, K. (2010). The free-energy principle: a unified brain theory? *Nature Reviews. Neuroscience, 11*(2), 127–138.

Garcia-Larrea, L., & Peyron, R. (2013). Pain matrices and neuropathic pain matrices: a review. *Pain, 154*(Suppl), S29–S43.

George, S. Z., Dannecker, E. A., & Robinson, M. E. (2006). Fear of pain, not pain catastrophizing, predicts acute pain intensity, but neither factor predicts tolerance or blood pressure reactivity: an experimental investigation in pain-free individuals. *European Journal of Pain, 10*(5), 457–465.

Gheldof, E., Crombez, G., Van den Bussche, E., Vinck, J., Van Nieuwenhuyse, A., Moens, G., et al. (2010). Pain-related fear predicts disability, but not pain severity: a path analytic approach of the fear-avoidance model. *European Journal of Pain, 14*(8), 870.e1–870.e9.

Ghirlanda, S., & Enquist, M. (2003). A century of generalization. *Animal Behaviour, 66*(1), 15–36.

Goubert, L., Crombez, G., & Van Damme, S. (2004). The role of neuroticism, pain catastrophizing and pain-related fear in vigilance to pain: a structural equations approach. *Pain, 107*(3), 234–241.

Goubert, L., Vlaeyen, J., Crombez, G., & Craig, K. (2011). Learning about pain from others: an observational learning account. *The Journal of Pain, 12*(2), 167–174.

Gray, J., & McNaughton, N. (2000). *The neuropsychology of anxiety: An enquiry into the functions of the septo-hippocampal system* (2nd ed.). New York, NY: Oxford University Press.

Gross, C., & Canteras, N. (2012). The many paths to fear. *Nature Reviews. Neuroscience, 13*(9), 651–658.

Grupe, D., & Nitschke, J. (2011). Uncertainty is associated with biased expectancies and heightened responses to aversion. *Emotion, 11*(2), 413–424.

Guillory, S., & Bujarski, K. (2014). Exploring emotions using invasive methods: review of 60 years of human intracranial electrophysiology. *Social Cognitive and Affective Neuroscience,* 1880–1889.

Hannibal, K., & Bishop, M. (2014). Chronic stress, cortisol dysfunction, and pain: a psychoneuroendocrine rationale for stress management in pain rehabilitation. *Physical Therapy.*

Hardy, J., Crofford, L., & Segerstrom, S. (2011). Goal conflict, distress, and pain in women with fibromyalgia: a daily diary study. *Journal of Psychosomatic Research, 70*(6), 534–540.

Helsen, K., Goubert, L., Peters, M., & Vlaeyen, J. (2011). Observational learning and pain-related fear: an experimental study with colored cold pressor tasks. *The Journal of Pain, 12*(12), 1230–1239.

Helsen, K., Goubert, L., & Vlaeyen, J. (2013). Observational learning and pain-related fear: exploring contingency learning in an experimental study using colored warm water immersions. *The Journal of Pain, 14*(7), 676–688.

Hermans, D., Craske, M., Mineka, S., & Lovibond, P. (2006). Extinction in human fear conditioning. *Biological Psychiatry, 60*(4), 361–368.

Hirsh, A., George, S., Bialosky, J., & Robinson, M. (2008). Fear of pain, pain catastrophizing, and acute pain perception: relative prediction and timing of assessment. *The Journal of Pain, 9*(9), 806–812.

Hirsh, J., Mar, R., & Peterson, J. (2012). Psychological entropy: a framework for understanding uncertainty-related anxiety. *Psychological Review, 119*(2), 304–320.

den Hollander, M., de Jong, J. R., Volders, S., Goossens, M., Smeets, R., & Vlaeyen, J. (2010). Fear reduction in patients with chronic pain: a learning theory perspective. *Expert Review of Neurotherapeutics, 10*(11), 1733–1745.

Honig, W., & Urcuioli, P. (1981). The legacy of Guttman and Kalish (1956): twenty-five years of research on stimulus generalization. *Journal of the Experimental Analysis of Behavior, 36*(3), 405–445.

Houben, R., Ostelo, R., Vlaeyen, J., Wolters, P., Peters, M., & Stomp-van den Berg, S. (2005). Health care providers' orientations towards common low back pain predict perceived harmfulness of physical activities and recommendations regarding return to normal activity. *European Journal of Pain, 9*(2), 173–183.

Jennings, E., Okine, B., Roche, M., & Finn, D. (2014). Stress-induced hyperalgesia. *Progress in Neurobiology, 121*, 1–18.

de Jong, J., Vangronsveld, K., Peters, M., Goossens, M., Onghena, P., Bulté, I., et al. (2008). Reduction of pain-related fear and disability in post-traumatic neck pain: a replicated single-case experimental study of exposure in vivo. *The Journal of Pain, 9*(12), 1123–1134.

de Jong, J., Vlaeyen, J., van Eijsden, M., Loo, C., & Onghena, P. (2012). Reduction of pain-related fear and increased function and participation in work-related upper extremity pain (WRUEP): effects of exposure in vivo. *Pain, 153*(10), 2109–2118.

de Jong, J., Vlaeyen, J., Onghena, P., Cuypers, C., den Hollander, M., & Ruijgrok, J. (2005). Reduction of pain-related fear in complex regional pain syndrome type I: the application of graded exposure in vivo. *Pain, 116*(3), 264–275.

de Jong, J., Vlaeyen, J., Onghena, P., Goossens, M., Geilen, M., & Mulder, H. (2005). Fear of movement/(re)injury in chronic low back pain: education or exposure in vivo as mediator to fear reduction? *The Clinical Journal of Pain, 21*(1), 9–17.

Kalish, H. (1969). Stimulus generalization. *Learning: Processes,* 207–297.

Karoly, P., Okun, M., Ruehlman, L., & Pugliese, J. (2007). The impact of goal cognition and pain severity on disability and depression in adults with chronic pain: an examination of direct effects and mediated effects via pain-induced fear. *Cognitive Therapy and Research, 32*(3), 418–433.

Keogh, E., Ellery, D., Hunt, C., & Hannent, I. (2001). Selective attentional bias for pain-related stimuli amongst pain fearful individuals. *Pain, 91*(1–2), 91–100.

Lang, P., Davis, M., & Ohman, A. (2000). Fear and anxiety: animal models and human cognitive psychophysiology. *Journal of Affective Disorders, 61*(3), 137–159.

Leeuw, M., Goossens, M., Linton, S., Crombez, G., Boersma, K., & Vlaeyen, J. (2007). The fear-avoidance model of musculoskeletal pain: current state of scientific evidence. *Journal of Behavioral Medicine, 30*(1), 77–94.

Leeuw, M., Houben, R., Severeijns, R., Picavet, H., Schouten, E., & Vlaeyen, J. (2007). Pain-related fear in low back pain: a prospective study in the general population. *European Journal of Pain, 11*(3), 256–266.

Legrain, V., Damme, S. V., Eccleston, C., Davis, K. D., Seminowicz, D. A., & Crombez, G. (2009). A neurocognitive model of attention to pain: behavioral and neuroimaging evidence. *Pain, 144*(3), 230–232.

Lethem, J., Slade, P. D., Troup, J. D., & Bentley, G. (1983). Outline of a fear-avoidance model of exaggerated pain perception–I. *Behaviour Research and Therapy, 21*(4), 401–408.

Lissek, S. (2012). Toward an account of clinical anxiety predicated on basic, neurally mapped mechanisms of Pavlovian fear-learning: the case for conditioned over-generalization. *Depression and Anxiety, 29*(4), 257–263.

Maren, S. (2001). Neurobiology of Pavlovian fear conditioning. *Annual Review of Neuroscience, 24*, 897–931.

McNally, G., Johansen, J., & Blair, H. (2011). Placing prediction into the fear circuit. *Trends in Neurosciences, 34*(6), 283–292.

McNaughton, N., & Corr, P. (2004). A two-dimensional neuropsychology of defense: fear/anxiety and defensive distance. *Neuroscience and Biobehavioral Reviews, 28*(3), 285–305.

Merskey, H., & Bogduk, N. (1994). *Classification of chronic pain* (2nd ed.) Seattle.

Meulders, A., Jans, A., & Vlaeyen, J. (2015). Differences in pain-related fear acquisition and generalization: an experimental study comparing fibromyalgia patients and healthy controls. *Pain, 156*(1), 108–122.

Meulders, A., Vandebroek, N., Vervliet, B., & Vlaeyen, J. (2013). Generalization gradients in cued and contextual pain-related fear: an experimental study in healthy participants. *Frontiers in Human Neuroscience, 7*, 345.

Meulders, A., Vansteenwegen, D., & Vlaeyen, J. (2011). The acquisition of fear of movement-related pain and associative learning: a novel pain-relevant human fear conditioning paradigm. *Pain, 152*(11), 2460–2469.

Milad, M., & Quirk, G. (2012). Fear extinction as a model for translational neuroscience: ten years of progress. *Annual Review of Psychology, 63*, 129–151.

Milad, M., Rosenbaum, B., & Simon, N. (2014). Neuroscience of fear extinction: implications for assessment and treatment of fear-based and anxiety related disorders. *Behaviour Research and Therapy, 62*, 17–23.

Ohara, S., Crone, N., Weiss, N., & Lenz, F. (2006). Analysis of synchrony demonstrates "pain networks" defined by rapidly switching, task-specific, functional connectivity between pain-related cortical structures. *Pain, 123*(3), 244–253.

Olsson, A., & Phelps, E. (2007). Social learning of fear. *Nature Neuroscience, 10*(9), 1095–1102.

Pavlov, I. (1927). Conditioned reflexes: an investigation of the physiological activity of the cerebral cortex (G. V Anrep, Trans.) *Annals of Neurosciences, 17*, 136–141, 2010 ed..

Pessoa, L., Kastner, S., & Ungerleider, L. (2003). Neuroimaging studies of attention: from modulation of sensory processing to top-down control. *The Journal of Neuroscience, 23*(10), 3990–3998.

Peters, M., Vlaeyen, J., & van Drunen, C. (2000). Do fibromyalgia patients display hypervigilance for innocuous somatosensory stimuli? Application of a body scanning reaction time paradigm. *Pain, 86*, 283–292.

Peyron, R., Laurent, B., & García-Larrea, L. (2000). Functional imaging of brain responses to pain. A review and meta-analysis. *Clinical Neurophysiology, 30*(5), 263–288.

Phelps, E., Connor, K., Gatenby, J., Gore, J., Davis, M., & O'Connor, K. (2001). Activation of the left amygdala to a cognitive representation of fear. *Nature, 4*(4), 437–441.

Pincus, T., Smeets, R., Simmonds, M., & Sullivan, M. (2010). The fear avoidance model disentangled: improving the clinical utility of the fear avoidance model. *The Clinical Journal of Pain, 26*(9), 739–746.

Quartana, P., Campbell, C., & Edwards, R. (2009). Pain catastrophizing: a critical review. *Expert Review of Neurotherapeutics, 9*(5), 745–758.

Quevedo, A., & Coghill, R. (2007). Attentional modulation of spatial integration of pain: evidence for dynamic spatial tuning. *The Journal of Neuroscience, 27*(43), 11635–11640.

Rachman, S., & Crespigny, D. (1977). The conditioning theory of fear-acquisition: a critical examination. *Behavior Research and Therapy, 15*, 375–387.

Roelofs, J., Peters, M., Fassaert, T., & Vlaeyen, J. (2005). The role of fear of movement and injury in selective attentional processing in patients with chronic low back pain: a dot-probe evaluation. *The Journal of Pain, 6*(5), 294–300.

Roelofs, J., Peters, M., & Vlaeyen, J. (2002). Selective attention for pain-related information in healthy individuals: the role of pain and fear. *European Journal of Pain, 6*(5), 331–339.

Schmitz, A., & Grillon, C. (2012). Assessing fear and anxiety in humans using the threat of predictable and unpredictable aversive events (the NPU-threat test). *Nature Protocols, 7*(3), 527–532.

Schrooten, M., Van Damme, S., Crombez, G., Peters, M., Vogt, J., & Vlaeyen, J. (2012). Nonpain goal pursuit inhibits attentional bias to pain. *Pain, 153*(6), 1180–1186.

Schrooten, M., Wiech, K., & Vlaeyen, J. (2014). When pain meets ... pain-related choice behavior and pain perception in different goal conflict situations. *The Journal of Pain, 15*(11), 1166–1178.

Sehlmeyer, C., Schöning, S., Zwitserlood, P., Pfleiderer, B., Kircher, T., Arolt, V., et al. (2009). Human fear conditioning and extinction in neuroimaging: a systematic review. *PloS One, 4*(6), e5865.

Shackman, A., Salomons, T., Slagter, H., Andrew, S., Winter, J., & Davidson, R. (2011). The integration of negative affect, pain, and cognitive control in the cingulate cortex. *Nature Reviews. Neuroscience, 12*(3), 154–167.

Sotres-Bayon, F., Cain, C., & LeDoux, J. (2006). Brain mechanisms of fear extinction: historical perspectives on the contribution of prefrontal cortex. *Biological Psychiatry, 60*(4), 329–336.

Sullivan, M., Tanzer, M., Stanish, W., Fallaha, M., Keefe, F., Simmonds, M., et al. (2009). Psychological determinants of problematic outcomes following Total Knee Arthroplasty. *Pain, 143*(1–2), 123–129.

Sullivan, M., Thorn, B., Rodgers, W., & Ward, L. (2004). Path model of psychological antecedents to pain experience: experimental and clinical findings. *The Clinical Journal of Pain, 20*(3), 164–173.

Swinkels-Meewisse, I., Roelofs, J., Oostendorp, R., Verbeek, A., & Vlaeyen, J. (2006). Acute low back pain: pain-related fear and pain catastrophizing influence physical performance and perceived disability. *Pain, 120*(1–2), 36–43.

Sylvers, P., Lilienfeld, S., & LaPrairie, J. (2011). Differences between trait fear and trait anxiety: implications for psychopathology. *Clinical Psychology Review, 31*(1), 122–137.

Vachon-Presseau, E., Roy, M., Martel, M., Caron, E., Marin, M., Chen, J., et al. (2013). The stress model of chronic pain: evidence from basal cortisol and hippocampal structure and function in humans. *Brain, 136*(Pt 3), 815–827.

Valet, M., Sprenger, T., Boecker, H., Willoch, F., Rummeny, E., Conrad, B., et al. (2004). Distraction modulates connectivity of the cingulo-frontal cortex and the midbrain during pain–an fMRI analysis. *Pain, 109*(3), 399–408.

Van Damme, S., Crombez, G., Eccleston, C., & Goubert, L. (2004). Impaired disengagement from threatening cues of impending pain in a crossmodal cueing paradigm. *European Journal of Pain, 8*(3), 227–236.

Van Damme, S., Crombez, G., Eccleston, C., & Koster, E. (2006). Hypervigilance to learned pain signals: a componential analysis. *The Journal of Pain, 7*(5), 346–357.

Van Damme, S., Crombez, G., Hermans, D., Koster, E., & Eccleston, C. (2006). The role of extinction and reinstatement in attentional bias to threat: a conditioning approach. *Behaviour Research and Therapy, 44*(11), 1555–1563.

Van Damme, S., Lorenz, J., Eccleston, C., Koster, E., de Clercq, A., & Crombez, G. (2004). Fear-conditioned cues of impending pain facilitate attentional engagement. *Clinical Neurophysiology, 34*, 33–39.

Van Dessel, P., de Houwer, J., Gast, A., & Smith, C. (2014). Instruction-based approach-avoidance effects: changing stimulus evaluation via the mere instruction to approach or avoid stimuli. *Experimental Psychology*, 1–33.

Villemure, C., & Bushnell, M. (2009). Mood influences supraspinal pain processing separately from attention. *The Journal of Neuroscience, 29*(3), 705–715.

Villemure, C., Slotnick, B., & Bushnell, M. (2003). Effects of odors on pain perception: deciphering the roles of emotion and attention. *Pain, 106*(1–2), 101–108.

Vlaeyen, J., de Jong, J., Geilen, M., Heuts, P., & van Breukelen, G. (2001). Graded exposure in vivo in the treatment of pain-related fear: a replicated single-case experimental design in four patients with chronic low back pain. *Behaviour Research and Therapy, 39*(2), 151–166.

Vlaeyen, J., de Jong, J., Geilen, M., Heuts, P., & van Breukelen, G. (2002). The treatment of fear of movement/(re)injury in chronic low back pain: further evidence on the effectiveness of exposure in vivo. *The Clinical Journal of Pain, 18*(4), 251–261.

Vlaeyen, J., de Jong, J., Sieben, J., & Crombez, G. (2002). Graded exposure in vivo for pain-related fear. In D. Turk, & R. Gatchel (Eds.), *Psychological approaches to pain management* (2nd ed., pp. 210–233). New York, NY: The Guilford Press.

Vlaeyen, J., & Linton, S. (2000). Fear-avoidance and its consequences in chronic musculoskeletal pain: a state of the art. *Pain, 85*(3), 317–332.

Vlaeyen, J., & Linton, S. (2012). Fear-avoidance model of chronic musculoskeletal pain: 12 years on. *Pain*, 10–13.

Vlaeyen, J., Timmermans, C., Rodriguez, L., Crombez, G., van Horne, W., Ayers, G., et al. (2004). Catastrophic thinking about pain increases discomfort during internal atrial cardioversion. *Journal of Psychosomatic Research, 56*(1), 139–144.

Vromen, J., Lipp, O., & Remington, R. (November 2014). The spider does not always win the fight for attention: disengagement from threat is modulated by goal set. *Cognition & Emotion*, 1–12.

Wager, T. D., Atlas, L. Y., Lindquist, M. A., Roy, M., Woo, C. W., & Kross, E. (2013). An fMRI-based neurologic signature of physical pain. *New England Journal of Medicine, 368*(15), 1388–1397.

Whitson, J., & Galinsky, A. (2008). Lacking control increases illusory pattern perception. *Science, 322*, 115–117.

Wideman, T., Asmundson, G., Smeets, R., Zautra, A., Simmonds, M., Sullivan, M., et al. (2013). Rethinking the fear avoidance model: toward a multidimensional framework of pain-related disability. *Pain, 154*(11), 2262–2265.

Wideman, T., & Sullivan, M. (2011). Differential predictors of the long-term levels of pain intensity, work disability, healthcare use, and medication use in a sample of workers' compensation claimants. *Pain, 152*(2), 376–383.

Wiech, K., Ploner, M., & Tracey, I. (2008). Neurocognitive aspects of pain perception. *Trends in Cognitive Sciences, 12*(8), 306–313.

Wiech, K., & Tracey, I. (2009). The influence of negative emotions on pain: behavioral effects and neural mechanisms. *NeuroImage, 47*(3), 987–994.

Wiech, K., & Tracey, I. (2013). Pain, decisions, and actions: a motivational perspective. *Frontiers in Neuroscience, 7*, 46.

de Wied, M., & Verbaten, M. (2001). Affective pictures processing, attention, and pain tolerance. *Pain, 90*(1–2), 163–172.

Woods, M., & Asmundson, G. (2008). Evaluating the efficacy of graded in vivo exposure for the treatment of fear in patients with chronic back pain: a randomized controlled clinical trial. *Pain, 136*(3), 271–280.

Yang, Z., Jackson, T., & Chen, H. (2013). Effects of chronic pain and pain-related fear on orienting and maintenance of attention: an eye movement study. *The Journal of Pain, 14*(10), 1148–1157.

Yang, Z., Jackson, T., Gao, X., & Chen, H. (2012). Identifying selective visual attention biases related to fear of pain by tracking eye movements within a dot-probe paradigm. *Pain, 153*(8), 1742–1748.

Zale, E., Lange, K., Fields, S., & Ditre, J. (2013). The relation between pain-related fear and disability: a meta-analysis. *The Journal of Pain, 14*(10), 1019–1030.

CHAPTER 8

Integrating Memory, Meaning, and Emotions during Placebo Analgesia and Nocebo Hyperalgesia

Donald D. Price[1], Lene Vase[2]
[1]Division of Neuroscience, Department of Oral and Maxillofacial Surgery, University of Florida, Gainesville, FL, USA; [2]Department of Psychology and Behavioural Sciences, School of Business and Social Sciences, Aarhus University, Aarhus, Denmark

The history of placebo analgesia is marked by controversy about the magnitude of its effects and whether placebo (and nocebo) phenomena are best understood as statistical problems or as biological/psychological processes. Claims about the efficacy of placebos have ranged from "extremely powerful" (Beecher, 1955) to almost negligible (Hrobjartsson & Gøtzsche, 2001) since the 1950s. It is generally agreed that the magnitudes of placebo and nocebo effects are highly variable across studies (Petersen et al., 2014; Vase, Riley III, & Price, 2002; Vase, Petersen, Riley III, & Price, 2009). Yet the sources of this variability remain somewhat mysterious—do they arise from the physical and psychosocial setting or within the subjective experiences of those who have placebo and nocebo responses. The resolution of this question would make placebo much less of a nuisance for industry and more importantly a potential advance for health care professionals who want to enhance the efficacy of their treatments. After all, placebo and nocebo components are potentially embedded in all types of treatments. This chapter explores this mystery, beginning with questions about possible environmental and physical causes of placebo responses. Learning mechanisms, such as classical conditioning, are explored in relation to these environmental factors. However, the main focus of this chapter is on causes that exist *within* the experience of someone receiving a placebo, starting with dimensions such as "expectation," "desire for relief," and possible distortions in memory. Particular emphasis is given to placebo and nocebo effects that are instantiated by verbal suggestion without conditioning, because they provide ideal instances of how phenomenal

The Neuroscience of Pain, Stress, and Emotion
http://dx.doi.org/10.1016/B978-0-12-800538-5.00008-X

experience is a major cause of changes in pain and its associated neural mechanisms. We also consider the possibility that nocebo responses can be partly mediated by verbal suggestion and have dynamics similar to that of placebo responses. We think these considerations are extremely important because of their value in understanding mind–brain–body relationships and their practical influence in health care practice.

ENVIRONMENTAL AND PHYSICAL CAUSES OF PLACEBO AND NOCEBO RESPONSES

Although it is clear that the simulation of an active medical treatment, such as sham treatment, is sometimes followed by large reductions in symptoms in both individuals and groups of patients, it is usually not obvious whether the improvement is due to the effect of placebo. The reduction in symptoms may simply reflect the natural course of a disease or condition. Failure to appreciate this point has bedeviled and confused placebo research from its beginning. The *physical placebo agent* itself is a dummy treatment such as sham surgery, a sugar pill, and magnets. The *placebo effect* is the difference in mean treatment effect between sham and no treatment control conditions across two groups of patients or at different times within the same group of patients (crossover studies) (Fields & Price, 1997). The *placebo response* refers to the improvement in symptoms in an individual that results from the experience of receiving a therapeutic intervention, regardless of whether the intervention is a "real" treatment or just a simulation (Vase, Price, Verne, & Robinson, 2004; Vase, Nørskov, Petersen, & Price, 2011).

EXTERNAL CAUSES

Conditioning

After patients or pain-free volunteers are given repeated effective treatments, subsequent administration of a placebo treatment is often sufficient to produce an analgesic effect. Some have proposed a stimulus substitution model of classical conditioning (e.g., Pavlovian model) (Jensen et al., 2012; Wickramasekera, 1985). This model of learning emphasizes environmental "stimuli" and responses and does not require a conscious association between the "inert" aspects of the treatment or medication (e.g., shape and color of pill) and the results of a biologically active agent. Others are neutral as to whether a conscious association is necessary (Amanzio & Benedetti, 1999; Laska & Sunshine, 1973). However,

Montgomery and Kirsch (1997) provide evidence that although placebo analgesia can be partly explained by conditioning, it requires a conscious expectation of pain reduction because, in contrast to participants who remain deceived, participants who are informed about the real causes of their pain reduction during conditioning trials do not have subsequent placebo responses. Moreover, conditioning may be sufficient for placebo effects, yet it can also be produced by verbal statements alone (Amanzio & Benedetti, 1999; Price, Craggs, Verne, Perlstein, & Robinson, 2007; Vase, Robinson, Verne, & Price, 2003; Vase, Robinson, Verne, & Price, 2005) and by all of the psychosocial factors that are present in the context of the treatment. Finally, verbal suggestion and conditioning have been shown to make additive contributions to placebo analgesia (Amanzio & Benedetti, 1999).

Simulation of Active Therapies and Social Observational Learning

One has to wonder what constitutes "conditioning stimuli" (CS), for which there are endless candidates. After all, when patients receive a treatment, there are many cues to which they can attend and these cues are embedded in the behavior and appearance of the persons carrying out the treatment, the physical aspects of the treatment itself, and the overall environment. It might appear convenient to pick out the most salient cues and call them CS, but this approach would always involve presuppositions and would ignore the enormous variability in the manner and degree to which people attend to specific cues. *Most critically, it would ignore the meanings that patients give to the therapeutic context.* Benedetti and his colleagues suggest that placebo phenomena reflect *simulation* of an active treatment (Amanzio, Pollo, Maggi, & Benedetti, 2001; Price, Finniss, & Benedetti, 2008). Studies that compare analgesic effects across "open" and "hidden" conditions illustrate the notion of simulation. The overall effectiveness of analgesic drugs was tested in clinical postoperative settings using open and hidden injections of traditional painkillers such as buprenorphine (Amanzio et al., 2001; Benedetti et al., 2003; Levine, Gordon, & Fields, 1978). When patient groups were given an injection in a standard open manner, pain ratings and/or amount of analgesics needed for effective relief were considerably less in comparison to administration by a hidden drug infusion pump. In the hidden condition, the clinician is not present and the patient is unaware that the treatment is being administered (Levine et al., 1978). Open–hidden differences directly reflect placebo analgesic effects

(Amanzio et al., 2001; Benedetti et al., 2003; Colloca, Lopiano, Lanotte, & Benedetti, 2004; Levine et al., 1978). Verbal suggestion was not included in some of these studies and so it is not a necessary condition for a placebo response. Verbal suggestion is also unnecessary when placebo effects are induced in study participants as a result of observing others receiving an effective analgesic treatment, a form of social observational learning (Colloca & Benedetti, 2009). Finally, placebo analgesic responses can be induced when *only* verbal suggestions are given during a treatment that the patient has never experienced before (Amanzio & Benedetti, 1999; Price et al., 2007; Vase et al., 2003, 2005).

Thus, it is noteworthy that placebo analgesic responses can be instantiated in multiple ways, through conditioning, simulation of a treatment, observing someone else receiving an analgesic treatment (Colloca & Benedetti, 2009), and verbal suggestion alone (Amanzio & Benedetti, 1999; Vase et al., 2003, 2005). Some of these external means of inducing placebo analgesia can be combined and have been shown to be additive (Amanzio & Benedetti, 1999). Given multiple external causes of placebo analgesia, perhaps the proximal causes are within the experience of the persons receiving a treatment or medication.

EXPERIENTIAL CAUSES OF PLACEBO ANALGESIC RESPONSES: EXPECTATION, DESIRE FOR RELIEF, AND EMOTIONS

Several studies provide converging lines of evidence that expected pain intensity and desire for relief and emotional feelings of relief ("reward") serve as proximate mediators of placebo responses, as has been reviewed elsewhere (Price et al., 2008; Zubieta et al., 2005; Zubieta, Yau, Scott, & Stohler, 2006). Expectation and desire for a specific outcome are two factors that determine the magnitudes of some types of positive and negative emotional feelings (Price & Barrell, 1984; Price, Barrell, & Barrell, 1985; Price et al., 2008; Price & Barrell, 2012). Since desire and expectation also constitute dimensions of emotions related to receiving and expecting results from medical treatments, then desire and expectation and hence emotions and emotional regulation may well be pivotal in mediating placebo analgesia (Price et al., 2008; Price & Barrell, 2012). A series of studies of evoked rectal pain in patients with irritable bowel syndrome (IBS) provided support for this general hypothesis (Craggs, Price, & Robinson, 2014; Price et al., 2007; Vase et al., 2003, 2004, 2005;

Verne, Robinson, Vase, & Price, 2003). Except for one study that used a standard clinical trial design (Verne et al., 2003), each study used a single verbal suggestion to enhance placebo analgesia: "The agent you have just received is known to powerfully reduce pain in some patients." These studies used repeated rectal distension stimuli (seven stimuli, 20 s each) and an experimental design involving baseline, placebo (rectal saline gel), and, in some studies, active analgesic treatment (rectal lidocaine gel) as shown in Figure 1. As discussed elsewhere (Price et al., 2008; Vase et al., 2003, 2004), ratings of expected pain and desire for relief accounted for large

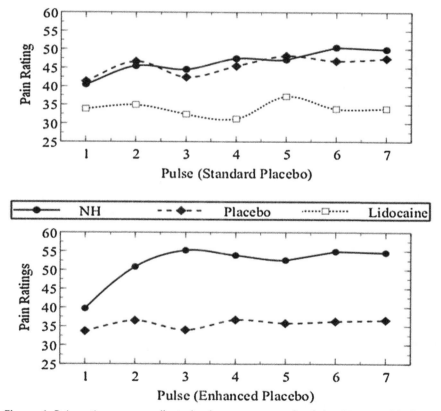

Figure 1 Pain ratings were collected subsequent to each of the 20-s rectal balloon distensions. The mean pain ratings in response to each of the seven rectal distensions are shown for the group given the standard placebo instructions (top) and the enhanced placebo instructions (bottom). Pain ratings after intrarectal lidocaine gel application are shown in the top panel. *(Based on data presented by Craggs et al. (2014) and Price et al. (2007).)*

amounts of variability in pain ratings (e.g., 77%) during the placebo condition (Vase et al., 2003, 2005). In another analysis of IBS patients, changes in desire/expectancy ratings predicted changes in pain ratings across natural history and placebo conditions (i.e., placebo responses) (Vase et al., 2004). Changes in expectation and desire along with the multiplicative interaction between them (i.e., desire × expectation) accounted for 38% of the variability in placebo responses (corresponding to a correlation coefficient of $r = 0.62$). This analysis suggests that both desire for pain relief and expected pain intensity contribute to placebo analgesia, and a main factor is a multiplicative interaction between desire for pain reduction and expected pain intensity. This interaction is consistent with a desire–expectation model of emotions in which ratings of negative and positive emotional feelings are predicted by multiplicative interactions between ratings of desire and expectation (Price & Barrell, 1984; Price et al., 1985, 2008). When patients with IBS rated desire, expectation, and anxiety during placebo analgesia, all three variables *decreased* during the same time that the placebo effect *increased* (Vase et al., 2005). These three mediating variables of placebo analgesia are not static, but change dynamically over time, possibly as a result of feedback from early results and perception of the dynamic aspects of the treatment procedure itself. The experiences of the process of being treated may be integrated with experiencing the results of treatment.

Qualitative results that corroborate the rating scale data were obtained by interviews of patients of this earlier (Vase et al., 2005) study (Vase et al., 2011). Patients' reports of their direct experiences showed that they considered their prospects of treatment as well as their attitudes toward the treatment provider soon after the beginning of treatment but to a lesser extent later on.

A MODEL OF SOMATIC SELF-REINFORCING FEEDBACK IN PLACEBO (NOCEBO) EFFECTS ON PATIENTS WITH IBS

Emotions, Somatic Focus, and Feedback

Based on several interrelated experiments, Geers and his colleagues argue that the placebo effect is most likely to occur when individuals have a goal that can be fulfilled by confirmation of the placebo expectation, consistent with the desire–emotion model and the explanation just given (Geers, Weiland, Kosbab, Landry, & Helfer, 2005; Geers, Helfer, Weiland, & Kosbab, 2006). The results of Geers and colleagues demonstrated a role for desire for an effect across a variety of symptom domains, including those related to approach and avoidance goals. They also found that the degree of somatic focus has a moderating influence on desire and expectation in the context of placebo effects. Somatic focus reflects the disposition to focus on body functions and to be vigilant to changes in them. In an experiment that induced expectations of unpleasant symptoms, individuals who expected they were taking a drug but given placebo tablets reported more placebo symptoms when they closely focused on their symptoms (Geers et al., 2005, 2006). This type of interaction also has been proposed for approach or appetitive goals. Thus, Lundh (1987) proposed a cognitive–emotional model of the placebo effect in which *positive* suggestions for improvement in physical health led individuals to attend selectively to signs of improvement. This idea is supported by Jensen and Karoly's (1991) observation that placebo effects related to pleasant symptoms (e.g., feeling arousal or energized) are supported by *increases* in desire for an effect. Focusing more closely on symptoms can enhance their significance as well as their implications. In the case of approach goals such as focusing on "improvement in physical health" (Lundh, 1987) or "feeling energized" (Jensen & Karoly, 1991) an increased desire for an effect would facilitate placebo responses. In contrast, *decreases* in desire for an effect would be more likely to contribute to placebo responses associated with avoidance goals such as terminating or reducing pain. In the case of avoidance goals, decreased desire is generally accompanied by decreased negative emotions (Price & Barrell, 1984; Price et al., 1985). Nocebo responses may have similar dynamics. Thus, if catastrophic meanings are enhanced as a result of somatic focusing, nocebo effects could be developed in association with increased desire to avoid negative consequences. These types of influences can occur during both explicit placebo or nocebo treatments, but more importantly, even when active treatments are given. For example, when patients closely notice signs of pain relief, this perception provides "evidence" that the treatment has been effective regardless of whether the treatment is a placebo or an active medication. Placebo effects, and for that matter nocebo effects, are potentially embedded in active treatments depending on what patients are told, the behavior and appearance of the caregivers, and numerous other psychosocial contextual factors that occur during treatment.

If focusing on bodily symptoms or cues operates as a kind of feedback that supports factors underlying placebo responding, increasing the degree or frequency of somatic focusing could increase the magnitudes of placebo responses over time. One way to increase somatic focusing is to increase the frequency of test stimuli during experiments that utilize evoked pain. As discussed above, ratings of desire, expectation, and anxiety decrease over time along with the increase in placebo effect (Vase et al., 2005). As shown in Figure 1, it took 3–4 min for the placebo effect to increase to its maximum level under conditions wherein stimuli were applied seven times during 10 min (Price et al., 2007). This same pattern of increase was found in two previous experiments that applied stimuli at much longer intervals of once every 10 min (Vase et al., 2003, 2005), taking 15–20 min to reach a maximum placebo effect. In all three experiments the placebo effect increased to its maximum level during the first three stimuli, suggesting that feedback from stimuli, not just the passage of time, is critical. Thus, feedback from the test stimuli serve as cues that signal increasing pain relief, and more frequent test stimuli lead to more rapid pain reduction. Taken together, the studies of Geers, Vase, Price, and their colleagues support a placebo mechanism wherein goals, desire, expectation, and consequent emotional feelings codetermine the placebo response. Somatic focus provides a self-confirming feedback that facilitates these factors over time, leading to less negative emotional feelings and higher expectations of avoiding aversive experiences. In other contexts, somatic focus could lead to positive feelings about obtaining pleasant consequences, such as feeling healthy, invigorated, or energized (Lundh, 1987; Price et al., 2008). In any case, the stimuli of the experiment can help confirm that the treatment is working if someone is expecting it to work. Since the stimuli self-reinforce expectations of pain reduction, reduce desire for relief, and consequently reduce negative emotions, the placebo effect increases more rapidly over time with higher frequencies of test stimulation. A similar dynamic may work for nocebo responses, such as the increase in symptoms over time as a result of catastrophic thinking and expectations related to threatening cues.

NEUROIMAGING EVIDENCE FOR A SELF-REINFORCING PLACEBO ANALGESIC MECHANISM

The account just made for a self-reinforcing mechanism suggests that the placebo response can develop quickly as a result of active psychological factors (somatic feedback, desire, expectation, and emotions) and then is maintained by self-confirmation of treatment effectiveness. If so, then brain mechanisms that generate the placebo response should be active in close temporal proximity to the treatment administration and less active later on. Since the above account also demonstrates that the stimuli themselves, and not just time, generate the critical feedback, then brain mechanisms that generate the placebo response should be triggered by the test stimuli. We provide support for both predictions.

This discussion should be prefaced by acknowledging that many brain areas decrease or increase their activity in relationship to placebo analgesia. Thus, several studies have shown that several pain-processing areas of the brain and spinal cord dorsal horn *decrease* their neural activity during placebo analgesia (Amanzio, Benedetti, Porro, Palermo, & Cauda, 2013; Eippert, Finsterbuch, & Bingel, 2009; Eippert & Büchel, 2013). Similarly, many brain areas that are likely to be involved in generating placebo analgesia *increase* their neural activity during placebo analgesia (Amanzio et al., 2013; Büchel, Geuter, & Eippert, 2014; Craggs, Price, Perlstein, Verne, & Robinson, 2008; Craggs et al., 2014). These areas include those known to be involved in reward/aversion, emotions, and the classical descending pain-inhibitory pathway (Basbaum & Fields, 1978). The last includes a core rostral anterior cingulate cortex (rACC)–amygdala–periaqueductal gray (PAG)–-rostroventral medulla–spinal cord connection, wherein pain-related signals are inhibited in the dorsal horn of the spinal cord (Basbaum & Fields, 1978; Mayer & Price, 1976).

Decreases in Neural Activity during Placebo Responses of Patients with IBS

Using the experimental paradigm discussed above for analysis of placebo effects in patients with IBS, a large placebo was produced in patients with IBS by a verbal suggestion ("The treatment you are being given …") and this effect was accompanied by large reductions in visceral-evoked neural activity (as measured by BOLD) in the thalamus; first and second somatosensory cortices (i.e., S-1 and S-2); anterior, mid-, and posterior insular cortices; and ACC, all areas that are part of the pain matrix (Price et al., 2007). The widespread reduction in these areas, including those at early levels of processing (e.g., thalamus, S-1), is consistent with a descending brain-to-spinal cord mechanism. Clearly, more direct measures of spinal cord processing, such as that provided by Eippert et al. (2009), are needed. In any case, widespread reduction of neural activity in pain-related areas tends to rule out a mechanism of modulation that would involve only *selective* effects on forebrain areas involved in cognitive processing of pain without effects at earlier stages.

Increases in Placebo-Generating Brain Activity in IBS ("Early" vs "Late" Periods of the Placebo Response)

In our studies of patients with IBS and patients with neuropathic pain large placebo effects were induced when a verbal suggestion was given combined with visual information associated with this suggestion (i.e., coating the rectal catheter with saline gel while verbally suggesting that "The agent you have just received is known to powerfully reduce pain in some patients") (Petersen et al., 2012; Price et al., 2007; Vase et al., 2003, 2005; Verne et al., 2003). Neuroimaging of the patients with IBS provided analysis of brain regions that were activated more during placebo analgesia than during the untreated baseline natural history condition (Craggs et al., 2008). Activated areas known to be involved in the classic brain–spinal cord modulatory system included the rACC and bilateral amygdalae, consistent with the classic descending control mechanism (Figure 2). These same placebo-activated regions are also known to be involved in emotions and emotional regulation, functions that are currently considered to be a part of endogenous pain modulation (Flaten, Aslaksen, & Lyby, 2013; Petrovic et al., 2005). However, a later study showed that increased activation also occurred in relation to other phenomena likely to be involved in maintaining memory for the placebo suggestion, developing meanings associated with the suggestion and treatment, and linking these meanings to expectations of pain reduction (Craggs et al., 2014). Thus, some placebo-activated regions were those involved in neurolinguistic processes and memory, such as the parahippocampal gyrus, medial aspects of the left temporal lobe, and left lentiform nucleus. Other regions activated by placebo are known to comprise a network involved in associative thinking and included the left precuneus, posterior cingulate, and aspects of the temporal lobe (Craggs et al., 2008, 2014). These regions were most active during the first 4 min of the placebo condition, presumably at a time wherein subjects were attending to the memory of the placebo suggestions and to somatic feedback, as described earlier. This is also the same time during which the placebo effect increased to its maximum level (Figure 1, lower panel). This temporal profile of placebo-induced brain activations is consistent with the idea that the placebo effect increases early in its development as a result of a self-reinforcing confirmation of the efficacy of the treatment (Craggs et al., 2008, 2014; Geers et al., 2005, 2006; Vase et al., 2003, 2005, 2011).

Verbal suggestions and/or simulation of treatment

Semantic processing and memory network

1. Angular gyrus
2. Superior temporal gyrus
3. Parahippocampal gyrus
4. Middle frontal gyrus
5. Postcentral gyrus

Expectation, desire, and emotion network

1. Dorsolateral prefrontal cortex
2. Orbitofrontal cortex
3. Rostral anterior cingulate cortex
4. Mid and dorsal anterior cingulate cortex
5. Amygdala
6. Hypothalamus
7. Nucleus Accumbens
8. Periacqueductal gray

Pain modulation network (Placebo and nocebo)

1. *Rostral anterior cingulate cortex*
2. *Amygdala*
3. *Hypothalamus*
4. *Periacqueductal grey*
5. Rostroventral medulla ("On" and "Off" cells)
6. Spinal cord dorsal horn

Figure 2 Schematic of general relationships between three central nervous system networks that interact during placebo analgesia that result from verbal suggestion and/or simulation of an effective treatment (top box): (1) Semantic processing and memory (Craggs et al., 2014 (1–5)); (2) expectation, desire, and emotion (Wager et al., 2004 (1–2); Büchel et al., 2014 (3–8)); (3) pain modulation (placebo and nocebo) (Amanzio et al., 2011; Kong et al., 2008; Price et al., 2007). Many of the regions of the brain related to each network are listed inside each box. These regions overlap, for example, many of the regions of 2 overlap with 3 and are designated by italics.

This profile is partially consistent with another imaging study of placebo analgesia that used electrical and heat stimulation (Wager et al., 2004). Neural activity increased in several brain areas involved in generating placebo responses in this study, including the orbitofrontal cortex (OFC), dorsolateral prefrontal cortex (DLPFC), rACC, and midbrain PAG, during periods of anticipation and/or stimulation. These areas have been suggested to have roles in expectation and working memory (DLPFC) (Miller & Cohen, 2001; Wager et al., 2004); motivation, desire, and reward (nucleus accumbens) (Wager et al., 2004; Zubieta et al., 2006); and descending modulation (PAG). Thus, all of these activated areas of the central nervous system are likely to be involved in expectation, motivation, and emotion and many of these areas overlap with those involved in pain modulation (Figure 2).

Our analysis of increased neural activity in patients with IBS showed changes over time (Craggs et al., 2008). During the first 5 min of the placebo condition there was increased activity in areas of the temporal lobe (involved in memory) and the precuneus. These areas are involved in associative thinking, during which one makes unconstrained associations unrelated to the immediate external environment (Bar, Aminoff, Mason, & Fenske, 2007). There was also increased activity in the left and right amygdalae, areas involved in emotions and in inhibition of pain. Activity in all of these areas subsided somewhat during the latter 5 min of the placebo condition. Apparently, the greatest neurophysiological "work" in generating the placebo effect occurred during the early part of the placebo condition. This is a time when patients were likely to make associations between remembered suggestions about the placebo agent, somatic cues that suggest whether or not the agent is working, and their expectations about pain reduction. This is likely to involve associative thinking (Bar et al., 2007; Craggs et al., 2008). It is during the time period immediately after the placebo administration that the placebo effect is self-enhancing. Once the placebo effect is established, it may be more passively maintained later.

Neural Activities that Link Verbal Suggestion, Memory, and Meaning to Pain Modulation

The critical role of somatic feedback over time is further demonstrated by comparing placebo-generating brain activity across two groups of patients with IBS, one that received standard instructions about possibly receiving placebo, similar to a clinical trial, and the other that received a verbally enhanced placebo suggestion (i.e., "The agent that you are being given is known to powerfully reduce pain in some people.") (Craggs et al., 2014). The pain ratings of the former and latter are shown in the top and bottom panels of Figure 1, respectively. In comparison to the group receiving standard instruction, the group that received a verbal suggestion showed large increases in neural activity in areas involved in memory and semantic processing, areas that are likely to process the placebo suggestions. These areas, in turn, are also linked to brain areas involved in emotions and expectations, and consequently placebo/nocebo effects (Figure 2).

The functional magnetic resonance imaging contrast of brain areas showing greater activity during verbally enhanced placebo compared to standard placebo treatment revealed a network of brain areas that has established roles in recent and long-term memory as well as semantic/linguistic processing (hippocampus, parahippocampal gyrus, angular gyrus, BA 39, superior temporal gyrus) (Figure 2). Thus, the angular gyrus is an integrative region involved in heteromodal semantic processing, including verbal processing (Bonner, Peele, Cook, & Grossman, 2013), and the parahippocampal gyrus has been shown to participate in paralinguistic elements of verbal communication and in semantic memory encoding (Rankin et al., 2009). In the case of enhancement of placebo analgesia by a verbal suggestion, this memory–semantic processing network is likely to sustain the memory of the recent placebo suggestions and their meaning. *Patients have to hear the suggestion(s), understand what it means, retain a memory of it, and then link the meaning to expectations and feelings about reduced pain.* The sequence of these steps is accompanied by corresponding activation within areas of the brain that generate and maintain placebo analgesia (Figure 2).

Neural Responses Linking Test Stimuli to Somatic Feedback

Comparison of results between these two groups also supports the somatic feedback hypothesis in showing that the differences in placebo-generating areas occurred in close association with the onset of each of the test stimuli (Figure 3). Thus, areas of the memory–semantic network have greater activity in the enhanced placebo condition in comparison to the standard placebo condition. Yet this difference begins immediately or within the first 4–5 s after the onset of the test stimulus (e.g., parahippocampal gyrus, left and right superior temporal gyri) (Figure 3). Average BOLD activity from 15 brain regions also shows this group difference in temporal development (Figure 3, lower right panel). This pattern of results further confirms that the onset of the test stimulus itself serves as a cue for activating brain activity

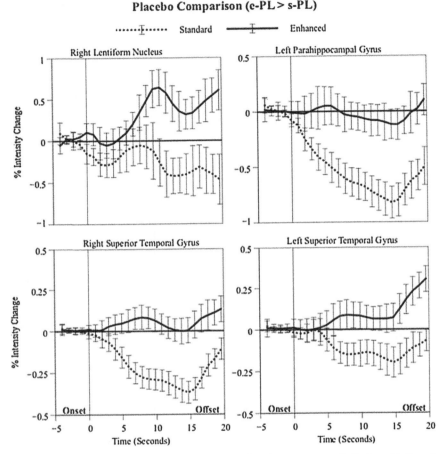

Figure 3 Representative BOLD activity curves showing greater activity in e-PL than in s-PL (right lentiform nucleus at top left, right and left superior temporal gyrus at lower left and right, respectively). The lower right graph shows average activity from the 15 areas. Many of these regions are typically associated with language-related functions, semantic processing, and memory. Note that in all cases the separation of the curves for the e-PL condition (solid line) and s-PL condition (dashed line) begins very near the stimulus onset and becomes increasing larger as the stimulus continues. *(Based on data presented by Craggs et al. (2014).)*

associated with memory and meaning of the placebo suggestion. The cuing of the meaning of the placebo suggestion by the stimulus also helps explain why the placebo analgesic effect develops more rapidly when test stimuli are given more rapidly as described earlier. These results extend the explanation that somatic focus and feedback from the stimuli themselves act to reinforce and enhance placebo analgesia over time. The role of test stimuli as signaling impending pain reduction also was evident in pain-processing brain areas of the brain, including posterior thalamus, insular cortex, and ACC (Craggs et al., 2014). Large reductions in neural activity of these areas emerged within seconds after the onset of the test stimulus, again supporting the somatic feedback hypothesis.

NOCEBO RESPONSE

The nocebo response is also influenced by verbal suggestions, for example, "this treatment will increase pain" (Benedetti et al., 2003; Johansen, Brox, & Flaten, 2003; Vase et al., 2003). In line with placebo effects, nocebo effects can be induced by conditioning (Benedetti, Amanzio, Vighetti, & Asteggiano, 2006; Colloca, Sigaudo, & Benedetti, 2008; Colloca, Petrovic, Wager, Ingvar, & Benedetti, 2010; Elsenbruch et al., 2012; Kong et al., 2008) and social observations (Vögtle, Barke, & Kröner-Herwig, 2013), but verbal suggestions alone may be highly efficient in inducing nocebo effects (Benedetti, Amanzio, Casadio, Oliaro, & Maggi, 1997; Benedetti et al., 2003).

The dynamics of nocebo and placebo effects appear to be largely similar. In the first of the series of IBS studies described above, patients were exposed not only to baseline and placebo but also to a nocebo condition, in which the rectal saline gel was combined with a verbal suggestion to enhance pain levels: "the agent you have just been given is known to significantly increase pain in some patients" (Vase et al., 2003). In this study, there was a trend for the pain levels to be higher in the nocebo condition compared to the baseline condition, but the nocebo effect was not quite statistically significant, probably because of the relatively low number of patients. Interestingly, however, the pain levels in the nocebo condition remained high over the entire 50 min of testing and were higher toward the end of testing, which is similar to the growth of the placebo effect over time. The contribution of expected pain levels and emotional feelings has been investigated less in relation to nocebo compared to placebo effects. Still, in a study of healthy volunteers exposed to rectal balloon distention Schmid et al. (2013) found that expected pain levels measured on a visual analogue scale prior to treatment administration significantly predicted pain levels in the nocebo group and accounted for 37% of the variance in the pain level. In this study, state-anxiety levels were not increased in the nocebo group, but anxiety levels have previously been found to be significantly enhanced in the nocebo condition compared to a control condition (Elsenbruch et al., 2012). This finding is consistent with studies showing that cortisol levels increase during a nocebo effect, indirectly suggesting that anxiety and stress responses related to hyperactivity of the hypothalamic–pituitary–adrenal axis are implicated in the nocebo effect (Benedetti et al., 2006; Johansen et al., 2003).

Brain imaging studies have shown that the nocebo effect is associated with enhanced activity in the superior temporal gyrus (Kong et al., 2008), which is involved in semantic processing, and the hippocampus, which is involved in working memory (Bingel et al., 2011; Kong et al., 2008). The nocebo effect is also associated with enhanced activity in the left OFC, bilateral ACC, and insula, all of which are involved in affective–cognitive pain modulation (Bingel et al., 2011; Kong et al., 2008; Schmid et al., 2013). These findings suggest that participants may be integrating verbal suggestions for increased pain with previous experiences as well as with present perceptions of threat and expectation of pain increase, thereby leading to enhanced pain levels. Thus, overall dynamics of the psychological mediators and the brain areas involved in nocebo and placebo responses appear to share similar features. Studies that differentiate placebo and nocebo responses need to be further investigated.

CONCLUSIONS: FUTURE DIRECTIONS IN RELATING BRAIN ACTIVITY TO PSYCHOLOGICAL VARIABLES ASSOCIATED WITH PLACEBO AND NOCEBO

Large placebo effects that accompany corresponding decreases in activity within symptom-related areas of the brain highlight both the psychological and the biological reality of the placebo response. However, elucidating the relationships between cognitive and emotional factors to placebo responses is an enormous challenge, as is determining their neurobiological underpinnings. Psychological studies of placebo analgesic responses have included progressively more variables, such as expectancy, desire, somatic focus, and type of goal. Measures of these variables can be potentially incorporated into brain imaging and other types of neurobiological studies, so that explicit mechanistic hypotheses about these factors can be tested at more refined psychological and neurobiological levels. Such improvements should provide increasing potential for utilizing knowledge of these mechanisms in clinical research and practice. However, beyond this relatively straightforward approach, there remains a need to characterize placebo responses and effects in a much more refined manner. Thus, the following questions could serve as guidelines for studies of placebo/nocebo responses that are mediated by suggestion: (1) How is the placebo suggestion experienced? (2) How do the suggestions, context, and somatic feedback lead to increased expectations of relief? (3) How do expectations coupled with desires lead to emotions that evoke the placebo response and, for that matter, the nocebo response? (4) How do emotional feelings change the experience of symptoms such as pain and anxiety? (5) What are the neural causes and correlates of (1–4)?

Adding a verbal suggestion to a medication or treatment can sometimes add significant increases in linguistic and semantic processing associated with the suggestion, and these increases are very likely linked to placebo/nocebo effects. Brain regions associated with this processing include those that process the memory and meaning of a verbal placebo suggestion. Suggestion also adds a significant decrease in the activity of brain areas that process pain. The test stimulus itself seems to cue these effects and is consistent with previous explanations that somatic focus and sensory feedback reinforce expectations and other factors that mediate placebo analgesic effects. Nocebo modulation may work along similar lines. Placebo and nocebo responses are not static or passive but reflect enactive cognitive processes that change dynamically over time and with somatic feedback. These processes can be learned and enhanced, suggesting a potential wealth of opportunity to use placebo factors to enhance the efficacy of treatments and medications and to diminish nocebo factors. Manipulations of both placebo and nocebo responses of course need to be constrained by ethical considerations.

REFERENCES

Amanzio, M., & Benedetti, F. (1999). Neuropharmacological dissection of placebo analgesia: expectation-activated opioid systems versus conditioning-activated specific subsystems. *The Journal of Neuroscience, 19*(1), 484–494.

Amanzio, M., Benedetti, F., Porro, C. A., Palermo, S., & Cauda, F. (2013). Activation likelihood estimation meta-analysis of brain correlates of placebo analgesia in human experimental pain. *Human Brain Mapping, 34*, 738–752.

Amanzio, M., Pollo, A., Maggi, G., & Benedetti, F. (2001). Response variability to analgesics: a role for non-specific activation of endogenous opioids. *Pain, 90*(3), 205–215.

Bar, M., Aminoff, E., Mason, M., & Fenske, M. (2007). The units of thought. *Hippocampus, 17*, 420–428.

Basbaum, A. I., & Fields, H. L. (1978). Endogenous pain control mechanisms: review and hypothesis. *Annals of Neurology, 4*(5), 451–462. http://dx.doi.org/10.1002/ana.410040511.

Beecher, H. K. (1955). The powerful placebo. *Journal of the American Medical Association, 159*(17), 1602–1606.

Benedetti, F., Amanzio, M., Casadio, O., Oliaro, A., & Maggi, G. (1997). Blockade of nocebo hyperalgesia by the cholecystokinin antagonist roglumide. *Pain, 71*, 135–140.

Benedetti, F., Amanzio, M., Vighetti, S., & Asteggiano, G. (2006). The biochemical and neuroendocrine basis of the hyperalgesic nocebo effect. *The Journal of Neuroscience, 26*, 12014–12022.

Benedetti, F., Pollo, A., Lopiano, L., Lanotte, M., Vighetti, S., & Rainero, I. (2003). Conscious expectation and unconscious conditioning in analgesic, motor, and hormonal placebo/nocebo responses. *The Journal of Neuroscience, 23*, 4315–4323.

Bingel, U., Wanigasekera, V., Wiech, K., Mhuircheartaigh, R. N., Lee, M. C., Ploner, M., et al. (2011). The effect of treatment expectation on drug efficacy: imaging the analgesic benefit of the opioid remifentanil. *Science Translational Medicine, 3*, 70ra14.

Bonner, M. F., Peele, J. E., Cook, P. A., & Grossman, M. (2013). Heteromodal conceptual processing in the angular gyrus. *Neuroimage, 71*, 175–186.

Büchel, C., Geuter, S., & Eippert, F. (2014). Placebo analgesia: a predictive coding perspective. *Neuron, 81*, 1223–1239.

Colloca, L., & Benedetti, F. (2009). Placebo analgesia induced by social observational learning. *Pain, 3*, 679–684.

Colloca, L., Lopiano, L., Lanotte, M., & Benedetti, F. (2004). Overt versus covert treatment for pain, anxiety, and Parkinson's disease. *Lancet Neurol, 3*(11), 679–684. http://dx.doi.org/10.1016/S1474-4422(04)00908-1.

Colloca, L., Petrovic, P., Wager, T. D., Ingvar, M., & Benedetti, F. (2010). How the number of learning trials affects placebo and nocebo responses. *Pain, 151*, 430–439.

Colloca, L., Sigaudo, M., & Benedetti, F. (2008). The role of learning in nocebo and placebo effects. *Pain, 136*, 211–218.

Craggs, J. G., Price, D. D., Perlstein, W. M., Verne, G. N., & Robinson, M. E. (2008). The dynamic mechanisms of placebo induced analgesia: evidence of sustained and transient regional involvement. *Pain, 139*(3), 660–669. http://dx.doi.org/10.1016/j.pain.2008.07.025.

Craggs, J. G., Price, D. D., & Robinson, M. E. (2014). Enhancing the placebo response: functional resonance imaging evidence of memory and semantic processing in placebo analgesia. *The Journal of Pain, 15*(4), 435–446.

Eippert, F., & Büchel, C. (2013). Spinal and supraspinal mechanisms of placebo analgesia. In L. Colloca, M. A. Flaten, & K. Meissner (Eds.), *Placebo and pain. From bench to bedside* (pp. 53–71). Elsevier.

Eippert, F., Finsterbuch, J., & Bingel, U. (2009). Direct evidence for spinal cord involvement in placebo analgesia. *Science, 326*(5951), 404.

Elsenbruch, S., Schmid, J., Bäsler, M., Cesko, E., Schedlowski, M., & Benson, S. (2012). How positive and negative expectations shape the experience of visceral pain: an experimental pilot study in healthy women. *Neurogastroenterology and Motility, 24*, 914–e460. doi:10.1111/j.1365-2982.2012.01950.x.

Fields, H. L., & Price, D. D. (1997). Toward a neurobiology of placebo analgesia. In A. Harrington (Ed.), *The placebo effect* (pp. 93–116). Boston, MA: Harvard University Press.

Flaten, M. A., Aslaksen, P. M., & Lyby, P. S. (2013). Positive and negative emotions and placebo analgesia. In L. Colloca, M. A. Flaten, & K. Meissner (Eds.), *Placebo and pain. From bench to bedside* (pp. 73–81). Elsevier.

Geers, A. L., Helfer, S. G., Weiland, P. E., & Kosbab, K. (2006). Expectations and placebo response: a laboratory investigation into the role of somatic focus. *Journal of Behavioral Medicine, 29*(2), 171–178. http://dx.doi.org/10.1007/s10865-005-9040-5.

Geers, A. L., Weiland, P. E., Kosbab, K., Landry, S. J., & Helfer, S. G. (2005). Goal activation, expectations, and the placebo effect. *Journal of Personality and Social Psychology, 89*(2), 143–159. http://dx.doi.org/10.1037/0022-3514.89.2.143.

Hrobjartsson, A., & Gøtzsche, P. C. (2001). Is the placebo effect powerless? An analysis of clinical trials comparing placebo with no treatment. *The New England Journal of Medicine, 344,* 1594–1602.

Jensen, K. B., Kaptchuk, T. J., Kirsch, I., Raicek, J., Lindstrom, K. M., Berna, C., et al. (2012). Nonconscious activation of placebo and nocebo pain responses. *Proceedings of National Academy of Sciences of USA, 109*(39), 15959–15964.

Jensen, M. P., & Karoly, P. (1991). Motivation and expectancy factors in symptom perception: a laboratory study of the placebo effect. *Psychosomatic Medicine, 53*(2), 144–152.

Johansen, O., Brox, J., & Flaten, M. A. (2003). Placebo and nocebo responses, cortisol and circulating beta-endorphin. *Psychosomatic Medicine, 65,* 786–790.

Kong, J., Gollub, R. L., Polic, G., Kirsch, I., LaViolette, P., Vangen, M., et al. (2008). A functional magnetic resonance imaging study on the neural mechanisms of hyperalgesic nocebo effect. *The Journal of Neuroscience, 28,* 13354–13362.

Laska, E., & Sunshine, A. (1973). Anticipation of analgesia. A placebo effect. *Headache, 13*(1), 1–11.

Levine, J. D., Gordon, N. C., & Fields, H. L. (1978). The mechanism of placebo analgesia. *Lancet, 2*(8091), 654–657.

Lundh, L. G. (1987). Placebo, belief, and health. A cognitive-emotional model. *Scandinavian Journal of Psychology, 28*(2), 128–143.

Mayer, D. J., & Price, D. D. (1976). Central nervous system mechanisms of analgesia. *Pain, 2*(4), 379–404.

Miller, E. K., & Cohen, J. D. (2001). An integrative theory of prefrontal cortex function. *Annual Review of Neuroscience, 24,* 167–202. http://dx.doi.org/10.1146/annurev.neuro.24.1.167.

Montgomery, G. H., & Kirsch, I. (1997). Classical conditioning and the placebo effect. *Pain, 72*(1–2), 107–113.

Petersen, G. L., Finnerup, N. B., Colloca, L., Amanzio, M., Price, D. D., Jensen, T. S., et al. (2014). The magnitude of nocebo effects in relation to pain: a meta-analysis. *Pain, 155,* 1426–1434.

Petersen, G. L., Finnerup, N. B., Nørskov, K. N., Grosen, K., Pilegaard, H., Benedetti, F., et al. (2012). Placebo manipulations reduce hyperalgesia in neuropathic pain. *Pain, 153,* 1292–1300.

Petrovic, P., Dietrich, T., Fransson, P., Andersson, J., Carlsson, K., & Ingvar, M. (2005). Placebo in emotional processing–induced expectations of anxiety relief activate a generalized modulatory network. *Neuron, 46*(6), 957–969. http://dx.doi.org/10.1016/j.neuron.2005.05.023.

Price, D. D., & Barrell, J. J. (1984). Some general laws of human emotion: interrelationships between intensities of desire, expectation, and emotional feeling. *Journal of Personality, 52*(4), 389–409. http://dx.doi.org/10.1111/j.1467-6494.1984.tb00359.x.

Price, D. D., & Barrell, J. J. (2012). *Inner experience and neuroscience: Merging both perspectives.* Cambridge, Mass: MIT Press.

Price, D. D., Barrell, J. E., & Barrell, J. J. (1985). A quantitative-experiential analysis of human emotions. *Motivation and Emotion, 9*(1), 19–38. http://dx.doi.org/10.1007/BF00991548.

Price, D. D., Craggs, J., Verne, G. N., Perlstein, W. M., & Robinson, M. E. (2007). Placebo analgesia is accompanied by large reductions in pain-related brain activity in irritable bowel syndrome patients. *Pain, 127*(1–2), 63–72. http://dx.doi.org/10.1016/j.pain.2006.08.001.

Price, D. D., Finniss, D. G., & Benedetti, F. (2008). A comprehensive review of the placebo effect: recent advances and current thought. *Annual Review of Psychology, 59,* 565–590. http://dx.doi.org/10.1146/annurev.psych.59.113006.095941.

Rankin, K. P., Salazar, A., Gorno-Tempini, M. L., Sollberger, M., Wilson, S. M., Pavlic, D., et al. (2009). Detecting sarcasm from paralinguistic cues: anatomic and cognitive correlates in neurodegenerative disease. *Neuroimage, 47*, 2005–2015.

Schmid, J., Theysohn, N., Gass, F., Benson, S., Gramsch, C., Forsting, M., et al. (2013). Neural mechanisms mediating positive and negative treatment expectations in visceral pain: a functional magnetic resonance imaging study on placebo and nocebo effects in healthy volunteers. *Pain, 154*, 2372–2380.

Vase, L., Nørskov, K., Petersen, G. L., & Price, D. D. (2011). Patients' direct experiences as central elements of placebo analgesia. *Philosophical Transactions of the Royal Society B: Biological Sciences, 366*(1572), 1913–1921. http://dx.doi.org/10.1098/rstb.2010.0402.

Vase, L., Petersen, G. L., Riley, J. L., III, & Price, D. D. (2009). Factors contributing to large analgesic effects in placebo mechanism studies conducted between 2002 and 2007. *Pain, 145*(1–2), 36–44. http://dx.doi.org/10.1016/j.pain.2009.04.008.

Vase, L., Price, D. D., Verne, G. N., & Robinson, M. E. (2004). The contribution of changes in expected pain levels and desire for pain relief to placebo analgesia. In D. D. Price, & M. C. Bushnell (Eds.), *Psychological methods of pain control: Basic science and clinical perspectives* (pp. 207–234). Seattle: IAPS Press.

Vase, L., Riley, J. L., III, & Price, D. D. (2002). A comparison of placebo effects in clinical analgesic trials versus studies of placebo analgesia. *Pain, 99*(3), 443–452.

Vase, L., Robinson, M. E., Verne, G. N., & Price, D. D. (2003). The contributions of suggestion, desire, and expectation to placebo effects in irritable bowel syndrome patients. An empirical investigation. *Pain, 105*(1–2), 17–25.

Vase, L., Robinson, M. E., Verne, G. N., & Price, D. D. (2005). Increased placebo analgesia over time in irritable bowel syndrome (IBS) patients is associated with desire and expectation but not endogenous opioid mechanisms. *Pain, 115*(3), 338–347. http:// dx.doi.org/10.1016/j.pain.2005.03.014.

Verne, G. N., Robinson, M. E., Vase, L., & Price, D. D. (2003). Reversal of visceral and cutaneous hyperalgesia by local rectal anesthesia in irritable bowel syndrome (IBS) patients. *Pain, 105*(1–2), 223–230.

Vögtle, E., Barke, A., & Kröner-Herwig, B. (2013). Nocebo hyperalgesia induced by social observational learning. *Pain, 154*, 1427–1432. http://dx.doi.org/10.1016/j.pain.2013. 04.041.

Wager, T. D., Rilling, J. K., Smith, E. E., Sokolik, A., Casey, K. L., Davidson, R. J., et al. (2004). Placebo-induced changes in FMRI in the anticipation and experience of pain. *Science (New York, NY), 303*(5661), 1162–1167. http://dx.doi.org/10.1126/science.1093065.

Wickramasekera, I. (1985). A conditioned response model of the placebo effect: predictions from the model. In L. White, B. Tursky, & G. E. Schwartz (Eds.), *Placebo: Theory, research and mechanisms*. New York: Guilford Press.

Zubieta, J. K., Bueller, J. A., Jackson, L. R., Scott, D. J., Xu, Y., Koeppe, R. A., et al. (2005). Placebo effects mediated by endogenous opioid activity on mu-opioid receptors. *The Journal of Neuroscience, 25*(34), 7754–7762. http://dx.doi.org/10.1523/JNEUROSCI.0439-05.2005.

Zubieta, J. K., Yau, W. Y., Scott, D. J., & Stohler, C. S. (2006). Belief or need? Accounting for individual variations in the neurochemistry of the placebo effect. *Brain, Behavior, and Immunity, 20*(1), 15–26. http://dx.doi.org/10.1016/j.bbi.2005.08.006.

PART 3

Clinical Implications

CHAPTER 9

Chronic Pain and Depression: Vulnerability and Resilience

Akiko Okifuji[1], Dennis C. Turk[2]

[1]Department of Anesthesiology, University of Utah, Salt Lake City, UT, USA; [2]Department of Anesthesiology, University of Washington, Seattle, WA, USA

Chronic pain is one of the most significant public health issues from the perspectives of prevalence, quality of life (QOL), and costs. The Institute of Medicine (2011) estimates that over 100 million adults in the United States experience chronic pain, costing the nation up to $635 million annually. The problem of chronic pain is not unique to the United States. A Canadian National Population Health Survey of over 17,000 adults estimates the cumulative incidence of chronic pain over 12 months to be about 36% (Reitsma, Tranmer, Buchanan, & VanDenKerkhof, 2012), and an international survey covering 18 countries (42,249 people) estimates the 12-month prevalence of chronic pain as 37% in developed countries and 41% in developing countries (Tsang et al., 2008). Chronic pain is also prevalent in children. A systematic review evaluating the prevalence of pediatric chronic and recurrent pain (King et al., 2011) estimates a prevalence ranging from 4% to 40% depending on the type of pain reported.

The adverse impact of chronic pain is ubiquitous in the lives of those afflicted. It can compromise not only physical ability but also maintenance of enjoyable life activities (Gatchel & Schultz, 2014), interfere with sleep (Onen, Onen, Courpron, & Dubray, 2005), have an impact on social relationships (Schwartz, Slater, Birchler, & Atkinson, 1991; Turk, 2000), and disturb mood (Banks & Kerns, 1996; Gureje, 2007), and it is a significant determinant of pain-related disability (Tripp, VanDenKerkhof, & McAlister, 2006). In this chapter, we will specifically focus on depression, a common psychological comorbidity of chronic pain estimated to affect 40–60% of people seeking treatment for chronic pain (Banks & Kerns, 1996). This is not to suggest that other affective factors are not important. For discussion of other negative mood states that have been extensively examined in chronic pain, namely anxiety and anger, the interested reader should see Fernandez (2002) and Keefe et al. (2001). We will review the

The Neuroscience of Pain, Stress, and Emotion
http://dx.doi.org/10.1016/B978-0-12-800538-5.00009-1

epidemiology of depression in chronic pain and the sequential relationship between the two.

EPIDEMIOLOGY

Although it is generally agreed upon that depression is a common co-occurring condition for chronic pain patients, the exact prevalence of depression as a comorbid psychological condition in chronic pain varies greatly depending on how and where patients are assessed and the criteria for depression used, such as how it is defined, method of assessment, and particularly where samples are selected.

A large international survey of 85,088 people (Demyttenaere et al., 2007) yields the odds ratio of having a mood disorder to be 2.2 [95% CI = 2.1–2.5] for community samples of people with chronic pain (Gureje et al., 2008). The large-scale population studies typically report that people with migraine headaches are 2.2–4 times more likely to have depression (Hamelsky & Lipton, 2006) than those without migraine. The population-based survey and interview studies typically report a range of 5–25% of people with chronic pain also experiencing depression (Breivik, Collett, Ventafridda, Cohen, & Gallacher, 2006; Carroll, Cassidy, & Cote, 2000; Currie & Wang, 2004; Demyttenaere, et al., 2007; Magni, Caldieron, Rigatti-Luchini, & Merskey, 1990). In the large Canadian population survey of 118,533 people, depression was reported by 6% of pain-free individuals, whereas 20% of those with persistent back pain reported depression (Currie & Wang, 2004). The likelihood of having depression increases as the number of painful sites increases (Gerrits, van Oppen, van Marwijk, Penninx, & van der Horst, 2014).

Among those who present to specialized pain treatment centers, the prevalence of depression appears to be greater. The prevalence of depression, for example, is estimated to range from 40% to 60% in the specialized pain center setting (Bair, Robinson, Katon, & Kroenke, 2003; Banks & Kerns, 1996; Haley, Turner, & Romano, 1985), whereas it ranges from 6% to 10% in the pain patients seeking treatment in the primary care setting (Arnow et al., 2009; Von Korff, Dworkin, LeResche, & Kruger, 1988). A 2011 study (Wong et al., 2011) showed the prevalence of significant depressive symptoms based on the standardized self-report measures in orthopedic clinics and pain clinics in Hong Kong to be 20.2% and 57.8%, respectively. Specialized pain clinics tend to receive patients whose pain is refractory to conventional therapies and the persistence and severity of pain may be particularly important amplifiers of depression. The epidemiology studies (Crook, Weir, & Tunks, 1989; Weir, Browne, Tunks, Gafni, & Roberts, 1992) indicate that chronic pain patients who are referred to specialized pain centers are likely to have greater pain, functional impairment, emotional distress, and health care utilization, as well as greater use of opioid analgesics.

Depression adds a significant burden to chronic pain patients, their significant others, and society. Depression in chronic pain also drives the costs associated with disability and health care utilization upwards (Katon, 2009).

DEPRESSION AND SUICIDE

One of the significant concerns related to depression is suicide. Depression in chronic pain presents a particularly difficult concern for clinicians given the recent increase in misuse of potent opioid analgesics and unintentional as well as intentional poisoning from them. Fatalistic thoughts and wishes are common in chronic pain patients.

The available evidence indicates that persons living with chronic pain may be at greater risk of engaging in suicidal behaviors. An early study evaluating clinic cases over 6 years (Fishbain, Goldberg, Rosomoff, & Rosomoff, 1991) showed a greater rate of completed suicide in chronic pain patients relative to the general population. The risk of suicidality in chronic pain seems to be compounded by disability and legal issues (Fishbain, Bruns, Disorbio, & Lewis, 2009). Up to 23% of treatment-seeking chronic pain patients report suicidal ideation (Edwards, Smith, Kudel, & Haythornthwaite, 2006; Okifuji & Benham, 2011; Smith, Perlis, & Haythornthwaite, 2004).

PAIN–DEPRESSION RELATIONSHIPS

There has been much debate about the causal attribution between depression and pain. An earlier theory suggested that chronic pain is a form of "masked depression" (Blumer & Heilbronn, 1982). That is, patients' reports of pain reflect underlying depression because it may be more acceptable to complain of pain than to acknowledge depression, although this judgment process does not necessarily occur at a conscious level.

Although there is no scientific evidence to substantiate it, the claim remains a popular notion in public and very unfortunately even among some clinicians. Many patients experience undue distress upon facing the assumption that their chronic pain is "all in their head" or that their pain is not taken seriously because "it is just your depression."

Alternatively, there is some support that depression follows the development of chronic pain (Brown, 1990). A recent study following people with a history of remitted depression (Gerrits et al., 2014) revealed that the recurrence of depression was predicted by pain severity but not by chronic disease status per se. Some studies also suggest that the pain–depression relationship is not linear but rather is mediated by how individuals with chronic pain view their plight. For example, we (Rudy, Kerns, & Turk, 1988; Turk, Okifuji, & Scharff, 1995) demonstrated that the relationship was mediated by a cognitive appraisal that patients exercise in evaluating their condition. The interaction between cognition and mood in chronic pain makes sense given the presence of individual differences in depression among patients with the same diagnoses and comparable pain and physical findings and led us to ask, given the impact of pain on all aspects of functioning, "Why aren't they all depressed?" (Okifuji, Turk, & Sherman, 2000).

There is also some support that the presence of depression places people at risk of developing chronic pain. It is well established that depressed people report significant degrees of pain (Stahl, 2002). Longitudinal studies (Dworkin et al., 1992; Gureje, Simon, & Von Korff, 2001; Jarvik et al., 2005) suggest that depression may be a risk factor for reporting chronic pain. One study (Leino & Magni, 1993) followed 607 individuals and found that their depressed mood at the baseline and 5-year follow-up was related to the development of pain symptoms at the 10-year follow-up. However, these results do not necessarily represent a causal relationship; they simply show the sequential association. It is also likely that pain and depression influence one another reciprocally. Hamelsky and Lipton (2006) reported a bidirectional increase in the likelihood of predicting one from the other between migraine pain and depression. There are a number of factors that present vulnerability and protective factors that mediate the relationship (see Figure 1 for a pictorial representation and Table 1 for a list of the factors). We will now review specific factors.

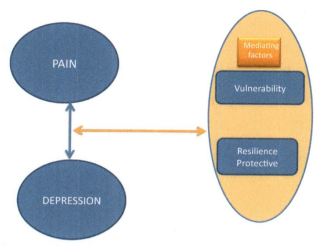

Figure 1 Heuristic model of the pain–depression relationship.

Table 1 Vulnerability and Resilience Factors for Depression in Chronic Pain

Vulnerability/Exacerbating Factors	Resilience/Protective Factors
• Helplessness	• Resourcefulness
• Feelings of no self-control	• Sense of control
• Low self-efficacy	• High self-efficacy
• Catastrophizing	• Optimism
• Rigid thinking	• Psychological flexibility
• Defeated/overwhelmed	• Resilient
• Lack or perceived lack of social support	• Availability of positive social support

VULNERABILITY

As the prevalence rates we presented demonstrate, not all chronic pain patients become depressed. A range of research has attempted to better understand this individual difference and to delineate specific factors that may mediate the pain–depression relationship.

A longitudinal study of over 1000 chronic pain patients with depression and/or anxiety (Gerrits et al., 2012) showed that the worsening of their psychological symptoms was predicted by baseline pain severity, number of pain sites, use of pain medications, and joint pain, although the odds ratios were quite modest (all <2.0). The literature generally presents that pain itself is not a very strong predictor of depression but it is often mediated by psychological variables (Gillanders, Ferreira, Bose, & Esrich, 2013). There are several cognitive factors that are implicated in depression in chronic pain, as well as physical and medication factors.

Cognitive Factor: Catastrophizing

Catastrophizing is a cognitive process whereby a person exhibits an exaggerated notion of negativity, assuming the worst outcomes and interpreting even minor problems as major calamities. Catastrophizing has been found to be instrumental in exacerbating the chronic pain experience. It is related to worsening pain experience in various situations including experimentally induced pain in pain-free children (Lu, Tsao, Myers, Kim, & Zeltzer, 2007) and adults (Edwards, Smith, Stonerock, & Haythornthwaite, 2006), as well as people with acute and chronic pain (Geisser et al., 2003; George et al., 2008; Somers, Keefe, Carson, Pells, & Lacaille, 2008; Sterling, Hodkinson, Pettiford, Souvlis, & Curatolo, 2008).

Catastrophizing has been shown to have significant association with emotional distress in pain patients with a range of diagnoses (Osborne, Jensen, Ehde, Hanley, & Kraft, 2007; Shelby et al., 2009; Somers et al., 2009; Turner, Jensen, & Romano, 2000). This has prompted a question as to whether catastrophizing is a symptom of emotional distress itself, rather than a separate construct. Research generally supports the idea that catastrophizing and depression are fundamentally different and relatively independent concepts. For example, a study (Arnow et al., 2011) indicates that both depression and catastrophizing contribute independently to pain-related disability in chronic pain patients.

A number of studies have reported results supporting the mediating role of catastrophizing between pain and depression (Jensen et al., 2002; Richardson et al., 2009; Wood, Nicholas, Blyth, Asghari, & Gibson, 2013). A 2014 study (Sturgeon, Zautra, & Arewasikporn, 2014) followed 260 women with fibromyalgia or osteoarthritis who recorded negative and positive affect for 30 days nightly. The multilevel analyses suggest that the day-to-day changes in pain catastrophizing mediate the relationship between pain and affect. Furthermore, catastrophizing and depression seem to have an additive impact on pain; Linton et al. (2011) reported that having one or the other was associated with current pain problems and outcome, while having both increased the associations substantially.

Cognitive Factor: Self-Efficacy

A self-efficacy belief is defined as a personal conviction that one can successfully execute a course of action to produce a desired outcome in a given situation. Experimental studies have shown that pain-related self-efficacy is associated with reports of pain sensitivity in response to noxious stimulation (Bandura, 1977). Self-efficacy belief also plays a role in clinical presentation of chronic pain. Lower self-efficacy is consistently related to greater clinical pain ratings in various chronic pain conditions (Buckelew, Murray, Hewett, Johnson, & Huyser, 1995; Chong, Cogan, Randolph, & Racz, 2001).

Research has consistently reported the mediating role of self-efficacy belief in the relationship between pain and depression (Arnstein, 2000; Miro, Martinez, Sanchez, Prados, & Medina, 2011) in chronic pain. Furthermore, it is possible that a low level of self-efficacy belief initiates a chain of adverse sequences by facilitating deactivation and functional disability that would reduce the level of satisfaction with life and social reinforcement. There is ample evidence showing that a low level of perceived self-efficacy is related to disability (Benyon, Hill, Zadurian, & Mallen, 2010; Sarda, Nicholas, Asghari, & Pimenta, 2009). Low levels of self-efficacy belief also appear to have a direct impact on sleep quality, which in turn may have an impact on the physical ability of the patient (Miro et al., 2011). We will return to the role of physical functioning in depression later in this chapter.

Whereas low self-efficacy beliefs are associated with greater pain and physical as well as emotional dysfunction, improvement in self-efficacy is one of the best predictors for successful rehabilitation for pain patients. An elevated level of self-efficacy belief at pretreatment tends to predict better treatment outcome (Buckelew et al., 1996; Kores, Murphy, Rosenthal, Elias, & North, 1990). Furthermore, successful outcomes of pain therapy typically show associated improvement in self-efficacy, along with an improvement in depression and anxiety (Garnefski et al., 2013; Wells-Federman, Arnstein, & Caudill, 2002).

Cognitive Factor: Sense of Control/Helplessness

A sense of control represents the perceived ability to manage pain or pain-related problems. How individuals conceptualize their ability to control pain and associated stress seems to be an important determinant for how they actually cope with pain. Indeed, increased sense of control has been shown to be linearly related to greater functionality in chronic pain patients

(Turner et al., 2000). Furthermore, improvement in control beliefs following treatment typically has been shown to result in reduction in pain and disability (Jensen, Turner, & Romano, 2007). The opposite end of the control spectrum is a sense of lack of control—helplessness. Helplessness is a central variable in the cognitive–behavioral framework of depression (Overmier & Seligman, 1967).

Because chronic pain often presents persistent pain despite attempts to control it, it is not surprising that a sense of helplessness is widely experienced by people with chronic pain. A number of studies have demonstrated the importance of helplessness and sense of control in influencing the mental health of pain patients (Keefe, Rumble, Scipio, Giordano, & Perri, 2004). Several studies (Maxwell, Gatchel, & Mayer, 1998; Palomino, Nicassio, Greenberg, & Medina, 2007; Turk et al., 1995) have demonstrated that although depression is common in chronic pain, the relationship between them is not linear but may be mediated by a poor sense of control and helplessness. The effects of perceived control are not limited to chronic pain but they significantly influence how people experience pain and emotional response following an acute pain episode. For example, perceived controllability of pain during childbirth has been shown to be associated with lower pain report and distressed emotion up to 6 months following the delivery (Tinti, Schmidt, & Businaro, 2011).

Since learned helplessness can be experimentally and acutely presented by creating an inescapable and uncontrollable aversive situation, this particular cognitive concept has been extensively studied in animals, pain-free humans, and people with depression. There is a substantial amount of evidence supporting the relationship between helplessness and depression in humans as well as animals (Henkel, Bussfeld, Moller, & Hegerl, 2002; Pryce et al., 2011). There is also an increasing volume of empirical data suggesting a neurobiological link between the two. Some studies show the neural correlates in various specific areas of the brain (e.g., prefrontal cortex, dorsal raphe nucleus, lateral habenula) (Christianson & Greenwood, 2014; Li et al., 2011; Wang, Perova, Arenkiel, & Li, 2014). Peng et al. (2014) demonstrated the relationship between helplessness in depression and decreased efficiency in functional connectivity among various regions of the brain.

Functioning Factors

Physical functioning is reduced in many people with chronic pain. Inability to do things that are essential, that one values and used to enjoy, is understandably frustrating. Decreased functioning is a significant predictor of depression for many disease statuses (e.g., cancer, stroke) (Landreville, Desrosiers, Vincent, Verreault, & Boudreault, 2009; Williamson, 2000). Indeed, reduced ability to engage in activities seems to play a significant role in depression in chronic pain patients. A longitudinal study (Williamson & Schulz, 1995) showed that declining level of physical activity as pain persisted over time predicted the level of depression later. Similarly, long-term functional compromise over time in people with osteoarthritis increases depressive symptoms (Parmelee, Harralson, Smith, & Schumacher, 2007). The results from a 2014 study evaluating this relationship in the elderly, both community residing and those in nursing homes (Lopez–Lopez, Gonzalez, Alonso-Fernandez, Cuidad, & Matias, 2014), suggest that although the role of pain itself in depression may be relatively modest, the perception of how much activity is restricted by pain may mediate the relationship.

A perhaps less studied area of disability is sexual functioning. A 2014 study of chronic low back pain implicated a significant mediating role of sexuality for depression in this population (Pakpour, Nikoobakht, & Campbell, 2014). It is also important to recognize that the physical activity that shapes one's lifestyle also contributes to how one views the world and oneself. A low level of functioning in back pain patients has been found to relate to catastrophizing (Elfving, Andersson, & Grooten, 2007). Improved ability to engage in physical activity is known to positively influence self-efficacy (Cataldo, John, Chandran, Pati, & Shroyer, 2013; McAuley et al., 2006). Thus, physical and cognitive vulnerability factors of depression in chronic pain patients are likely to have a rather complex, dynamically interacting relationship.

RESILIENCY

Resilience is broadly defined as an ability to encompass and exhibit adaptive coping within a context of significant adversity. There is a wide range of variability in the amount and nature of adverse effects in response to stress. This is clearly true in chronic pain patients; a substantial minority of treatment seekers for chronic pain do not appear to be depressed, and even lower rates of depression are observed in community samples of people with persistent pain. A large individual variability in emotional distress and QOL can be found in chronic pain patients at similar pain levels with similar pain durations (Okifuji, et al., 2000). In this section, we will focus on factors that, despite persistent pain, appear to protect or inoculate patients from depression and promote more adaptive coping and accommodation despite the presence of persistent pain.

The literature points to three protective factors that are particularly important in building resilience: positive emotion, perceptions of life control, and social support. Fredrickson, Mancuso, Branigan, and Tugade (2000) theorized that action tendencies associated with emotion may play a role in regulating well-being. According to their theory, negative emotion tends to restrict the focus of the behavioral response to escape or avoidance, whereas positive emotion enhances the behavioral and coping options. Moreover, the presence of positive emotion seems critical in modulating the coping experience whereby resilient people seek ways to enhance positive emotion that seems to disrupt the relationship between stress and distress (Affleck & Tennen, 1996; Ong, Bergeman, & Bisconti, 2004).

In the resilience research, positive and negative emotions are considered related but distinct entities, rather than a continuum. The absence of positive emotion appears to increase vulnerability to emotional distress during severe pain. Zautra et al., 2005 conducted 10- to 12-weekly interviews with women with chronic pain. The multilevel analyses of pain, mood, and stress yielded that patients with trait-like positivity tend to experience less negative affect during a high pain period. However, the situational positive affect, regardless of trait-like positive affect, seems to protect people from experiencing the negative consequences of high pain. The results suggest a protective property of the ability to experience positivity in the face of stressors.

Although it is generally considered that being able to employ positive affect at a time of difficulty (e.g., pain) offers the basis of resilience, the emotional experience of both positive and negative valence may modify how resilience affects pain patients. Mediational model analyses using the structural equation modeling of 858 chronic pain patients (fibromyalgia) (McAllister et al., 2015) showed that both positive and negative affects seem to mediate the effect of resilience on symptom burden.

Karoly and Ruehlman (2006) operationally defined pain resilience as having low pain interference and emotional distress despite high pain. Of 2407 chronic pain patients who completed the screening inventories, approximately 30% scored 1 standard deviation above the mean on pain severity, whereas their emotional and interference scores were 1 standard deviation below (resilient patients). Those who scored 1 standard deviation above the mean on all scales (high pain, emotional distress, and interference) were considered nonresilient patients. Resilient patients showed significantly lower levels of pain-related fear, catastrophizing, expectation of medical cure, and disability than nonresilient patients.

Social support has also been indicated to be an important factor in building resilience. Marital satisfaction and depression are significantly related in chronic pain patients (Kerns & Turk, 1984). Negative spousal response to patients' pain report is also related to depression in chronic pain patients (Cano, Weisberg, & Gallagher, 2000). On the other hand, spousal solicitous response to patients' pain, although it was related to greater functional interference, appears to be related to positive emotional consequence (Flor, Kerns, & Turk, 1987; Turk, Kerns, & Rosenberg, 1992). It is not just the presence of support but how patients value the support that may also be important. When chronic pain patients experience a high level of satisfaction with their social support, they are likely to experience less depression and use active coping strategies (Lopez-Martinez, Esteve-Zarazaga, & Ramirez-Maestre, 2008).

Resilience may also help people experience less pain particularly when stress is greater. Friborg et al. (2006) measured pain response to ischemic pain testing in pain-free people under two stress conditions, which were manipulated by the nature of the interaction with an experimenter. Those who scored high on the resilience scale reported significantly lower pain intensity under high stress than those with a low resilience score, although the difference was not observed when the stress level was low.

Despite the significant concern of suicide and depression among people with chronic pain, very little is known about resilience factors that may protect patients from self-harm. In a longitudinal study of returning veterans who were deployed to Iraq and Afghanistan (Youssef, Green, Beckham, & Elbogen, 2013), baseline level of resilience was significantly related to suicidal ideation at the 3-year follow-up. Given the prevalence of suicidal ideation and recent increase in opioid-related deaths, an evaluation of protective factors in the chronic pain population seems warranted.

Posttraumatic stress disorder (PTSD) has been shown to be elevated in people with chronic pain (Morasco et al., 2013; Sherman, Turk, & Okifuji, 2000). There is some evidence of the neurobiological correlates of resilience. The data on neuroimaging of resilience mostly come from studies examining PTSD. In those studies, "resilient individuals" are typically defined as those who were exposed to trauma but did not develop PTSD, whereas those who developed PTSD are labeled as people with a low level of resilience. A comprehensive review on the structural and functional neural circuitries of resilience (van der Werff, van den Berg, Pannekoek,

Elzinga, & van der Wee, 2013) suggests that resilient people indeed differ from those who are not resilient in the brain regions known to regulate emotional and stress experience. For depression, depression-free people, despite a significant family history ("resilient"), showed smaller volumes of right hippocampus and dorsomedial prefrontal cortex compared to depressed people with a family history (Amico et al., 2011). A functional magnetic resonance imaging study of police officers who were involved in gunfire attack (Peres et al., 2011) showed a significantly increased activity in the medial prefrontal cortex and decreased amygdala activity in response to trauma-related cues in resilient (officers with trauma without PTSD) and in those with PTSD who received benefit from therapy compared to officers with significant PTSD symptoms. Research on the neural basis of psychological resilience is still in its infancy; however, the available evidence thus far seems to demonstrate the ability of resilience to regulate emotion in response to stress.

PSYCHOLOGICAL FLEXIBILITY

Related to the concept of resilience is the notion of psychological flexibility. The definition of psychological flexibility reflects a multifactorial process of how a person deals with stress, situations, and people. According to a comprehensive review of this topic in the context of health (Kashdan & Rottenberg, 2010), the concept reflects multiple aspects of how persons contextualize their psychological responses, including (1) flexible accommodation of fluctuating situational demands, (2) reconfiguration of psychological resources, (3) modification of perspective, and (4) balancing competing desires, needs, and life domains. In the domain of chronic pain management, several factors are considered critical in psychological flexibility: acceptance, mindfulness, value-based processes, and cognitive defusion.

Acceptance may often be confused with resignation to having pain. Acceptance of pain is not the same thing as giving up on life because of pain. Instead, it requires a mental framework to feel pain with realistic expectation but without avoiding it and without judgmental disapproval (McCracken & Eccleston, 2003). What seems important is balance between acceptance and control. The serenity prayer attributed to Reinhold Niebuhr (2014) captures the need to strike a balance between accepting what we cannot change and striving to change what we can and asking for the wisdom to know the difference. Thus, acceptance not only encompasses "taking what it is" but also extends it to identifying what can be changed and committing oneself to the change. Acceptance of pain seems to be positively related to psychological well-being in chronic pain patients (Viane et al., 2003). Longitudinally, high acceptance early on predicts low depression at later times in chronic pain (McCracken & Eccleston, 2005).

A value-based process refers to the ability to identify valued life domains (activities, relationships, self-image) that can be used to build a set of goals for an individual to strive to achieve. It is fundamentally an individualized "wants" list that directs a person's commitment and priority. In chronic pain, positive emotional well-being is reported when a person perceives that he or she lives in accordance with his or her valued commitments (McCracken & Yang, 2006). Their subsequent prospective study (McCracken & Vowles, 2008) showed that acceptance and value-based processes, after controlling for pain severity, predicted 27% of the variance in depression at later times.

Cognitive fusion refers to the maladaptive thought process in which a person is constrained in his or her own thought process in experiencing emotion and directing behaviors. McCracken, DaSilva, Skillicorn, and Doherty (2014) describe it as "similar to the more familiar concept of believing a thought versus having a thought and not believing it" (pp. 894). For example, when a pain flare occurs, one may have the thought "I will never get better" (fusion) or place the thought in the context of "I am having a thought that I will never get better" (defusion). The ability to defuse such thoughts may be protective; indeed, the level of defusion in chronic pain patients is significantly related to depression after controlling for age, education, and pain level (McCracken, et al., 2014).

The concept of psychological flexibility is relatively new. However, the evidence seems to strongly point to it as an important, clinically relevant factor that may help us understand how people adapt or fail to adapt in a context of stress associated with chronic pain.

SUMMARY

In this chapter, we reviewed the relationship between chronic pain and depression. Depression is one of the most prevalent emotional comorbidities in chronic pain. Depression is not just common but also augments the suffering of people with chronic pain, compromises the quality of their lives, and raises the costs of health care and disability. There is a modest degree of relationship between depression and pain itself, but the relationship between them seems likely to be mediated by several cognitive factors as well as physical and medication variables. Those mediating variables, however, are not independent but interrelated and dynamically interact with one another to affect the emotional well-being of chronic pain patients. These are also the variables that are included as treatment targets in cognitive behavioral therapy of chronic pain; this implicates the clinical significance of understanding emotion relevant to chronic pain.

We also reviewed the psychological factors that may have a protective influence on depressive mood in chronic pain, with particular attention to the concepts of resilience and psychological flexibility. Evidence is quite encouraging that these positive sides of psychological factors protect patients from the negative emotional sequelae of pain as well as improving depression. The neurobiological data also suggest that these protective factors work on the neural circuitry and responses that are involved in emotional regulation.

Chronic pain is a complicated condition that is quite challenging as it is a multidimensional disorder involving biological, physical, and psychosocial domains. A better understanding of how these factors relate to one another should lead to further delineation of specific treatment targets, thereby helping develop effective interventions.

REFERENCES

Affleck, G., & Tennen, H. (1996). Construing benefits from adversity: adaptational significance and dispositional underpinnings. *Journal of Personality, 64*(4), 899–922.
Amico, F., Meisenzahl, E., Koutsouleris, N., Reiser, M., Moller, H. J., & Frodl, T. (2011). Structural MRI correlates for vulnerability and resilience to major depressive disorder. *Journal of Psychiatry and Neuroscience, 36*(1), 15–22.
Arnow, B. A., Blasey, C. M., Constantino, M. J., Robinson, R., Hunkeler, E., Lee, J., et al. (2011). Catastrophizing, depression and pain-related disability. *General Hospital Psychiatry, 33*(2), 150–156.
Arnow, B. A., Blasey, C. M., Lee, J., Fireman, B., Hunkeler, E. M., Dea, R., et al. (2009). Relationships among depression, chronic pain, chronic disabling pain, and medical costs. *Psychiatric Services, 60*(3), 344–350.
Arnstein, P. (2000). The mediation of disability by self efficacy in different samples of chronic pain patients. *Disability and Rehabilitation, 22*(17), 794–801.
Bair, M. J., Robinson, R. L., Katon, W., & Kroenke, K. (2003). Depression and pain comorbidity: a literature review. *Archives of Internal Medicine, 163*(20), 2433–2445.
Bandura, A. (1977). Self-efficacy: toward a unifying theory of behavioral change. *Psychological Review, 84*(2), 191–215.
Banks, S., & Kerns, R. (1996). Explaining high rates of depression in chronic pain: a diathesis-stress framework. *Psychological Bulletin, 119*, 95–110.

Benyon, K., Hill, S., Zadurian, N., & Mallen, C. (2010). Coping strategies and self-efficacy as predictors of outcome in osteoarthritis: a systematic review. *Musculoskeletal Care, 8*(4), 224–236.

Blumer, D., & Heilbronn, M. (1982). Chronic pain as a variant of depressive disease: the pain-prone disorder. *The Journal of Nervous and Mental Disease, 170*(7), 381–406.

Breivik, H., Collett, B., Ventafridda, V., Cohen, R., & Gallacher, D. (2006). Survey of chronic pain in Europe: prevalence, impact on daily life, and treatment. *European Journal of Pain, 10*(4), 287–333.

Brown, G. K. (1990). A causal analysis of chronic pain and depression. *Journal of Abnormal Psychology, 99*(2), 127–137.

Buckelew, S. P., Huyser, B., Hewett, J. E., Parker, J. C., Johnson, J. C., Conway, R., et al. (1996). Self-efficacy predicting outcome among fibromyalgia subjects. *Arthritis Care and Research, 9*(2), 97–104.

Buckelew, S. P., Murray, S. E., Hewett, J. E., Johnson, J., & Huyser, B. (1995). Self-efficacy, pain, and physical activity among fibromyalgia subjects. *Arthritis Care and Research, 8*(1), 43–50.

Cano, A., Weisberg, J. N., & Gallagher, R. M. (2000). Marital satisfaction and pain severity mediate the association between negative spouse responses to pain and depressive symptoms in a chronic pain patient sample. *Pain Medicine, 1*(1), 35–43.

Carroll, L. J., Cassidy, J. D., & Cote, P. (2000). The Saskatchewan health and back pain survey: the prevalence and factors associated with depressive symptomatology in Saskatchewan adults. *Canadian Journal of Public Health, 91*(6), 459–464.

Cataldo, R., John, J., Chandran, L., Pati, S., & Shroyer, A. L. (2013). Impact of physical activity intervention programs on self-efficacy in youths: a systematic review. *ISRN Obesity, 2013*, 586497.

Chong, G. S., Cogan, D., Randolph, P., & Racz, G. (2001). Chronic pain and self-efficacy: the effects of age, sex, and chronicity. *Pain Practice, 1*(4), 338–343.

Christianson, J. P., & Greenwood, B. N. (2014). Stress-protective neural circuits: not all roads lead through the prefrontal cortex. *Stress, 17*(1), 1–12.

Crook, J., Weir, R., & Tunks, E. (1989). An epidemiological follow-up survey of persistent pain sufferers in a group family practice and specialty pain clinic. *Pain, 36*(1), 49–61.

Currie, S. R., & Wang, J. (2004). Chronic back pain and major depression in the general Canadian population. *Pain, 107*(1–2), 54–60.

Demyttenaere, K., Bruffaerts, R., Lee, S., Posada-Villa, J., Kovess, V., Angermeyer, M. C., et al. (2007). Mental disorders among persons with chronic back or neck pain: results from the world mental health surveys. *Pain, 129*(3), 332–342.

Dworkin, R. H., Hartstein, G., Rosner, H. L., Walther, R. R., Sweeney, E. W., & Brand, L. (1992). A high-risk method for studying psychosocial antecedents of chronic pain: the prospective investigation of herpes zoster. *Journal of Abnormal Psychology, 101*(1), 200–205.

Edwards, R. R., Smith, M. T., Kudel, I., & Haythornthwaite, J. (2006). Pain-related catastrophizing as a risk factor for suicidal ideation in chronic pain. *Pain, 126*(1–3), 272–279.

Edwards, R. R., Smith, M. T., Stonerock, G., & Haythornthwaite, J. A. (2006). Pain-related catastrophizing in healthy women is associated with greater temporal summation of and reduced habituation to thermal pain. *The Clinical Journal of Pain, 22*(8), 730–737.

Elfving, B., Andersson, T., & Grooten, W. J. (2007). Low levels of physical activity in back pain patients are associated with high levels of fear-avoidance beliefs and pain catastrophizing. *Physiotherapy Research International, 12*(1), 14–24.

Fernandez, E. (2002). *Anxiety, depression, and anger in pain: Research implications.* Dallas, TX: Advanced Psychology Resources.

Fishbain, D. A., Bruns, D., Disorbio, J. M., & Lewis, J. E. (2009). Risk for five forms of suicidality in acute pain patients and chronic pain patients vs pain-free community controls. *Pain Medicine, 10*(6), 1095–1105.

Fishbain, D. A., Goldberg, M., Rosomoff, R. S., & Rosomoff, H. (1991). Completed suicide in chronic pain. *The Clinical Journal of Pain, 7*(1), 29–36.

Flor, H., Kerns, R. D., & Turk, D. C. (1987). The role of spouse reinforcement, perceived pain, and activity levels of chronic pain patients. *Journal of Psychosomatic Research, 31*(2), 251–259.

Fredrickson, B. L., Mancuso, R. A., Branigan, C., & Tugade, M. M. (2000). The undoing effect of positive emotions. *Motivation and Emotion, 24*(4), 237–258.

Friborg, O., Hjemdal, O., Rosenvinge, J. H., Martinussen, M., Aslaksen, P. M., & Flaten, M. A. (2006). Resilience as a moderator of pain and stress. *Journal of Psychosomatic Research, 61*(2), 213–219.

Garnefski, N., Kraaij, V., Benoist, M., Bout, Z., Karels, E., & Smit, A. (2013). Effect of a cognitive behavioral self-help intervention on depression, anxiety, and coping self-efficacy in people with rheumatic disease. *Arthritis Care Research (Hoboken), 65*(7), 1077–1084.

Gatchel, R., & Schultz, I. (Eds.). (2014). *Handbook of musculoskeletal pain and disability disorders in the workplace.* New York, NY: Springer.

Geisser, M. E., Casey, K. L., Brucksch, C. B., Ribbens, C. M., Appleton, B. B., & Crofford, L. J. (2003). Perception of noxious and innocuous heat stimulation among healthy women and women with fibromyalgia: association with mood, somatic focus, and catastrophizing. *Pain, 102*(3), 243–250.

George, S. Z., Wallace, M. R., Wright, T. W., Moser, M. W., Greenfield, W. H., 3rd, Sack, B. K., et al. (2008). Evidence for a biopsychosocial influence on shoulder pain: pain catastrophizing and catechol-O-methyltransferase (COMT) diplotype predict clinical pain ratings. *Pain, 136*(1–2), 53–61.

Gerrits, M. M., van Oppen, P., Leone, S. S., van Marwijk, H. W., van der Horst, H. E., & Penninx, B. W. (2014). Pain, not chronic disease, is associated with the recurrence of depressive and anxiety disorders. *BMC Psychiatry, 14*, 187.

Gerrits, M. M., van Oppen, P., van Marwijk, H. W., Penninx, B. W., & van der Horst, H. E. (2014). Pain and the onset of depressive and anxiety disorders. *Pain, 155*(1), 53–59.

Gerrits, M. M., Vogelzangs, N., van Oppen, P., van Marwijk, H. W., van der Horst, H., & Penninx, B. W. (2012). Impact of pain on the course of depressive and anxiety disorders. *Pain, 153*(2), 429–436.

Gillanders, D. T., Ferreira, N. B., Bose, S., & Esrich, T. (2013). The relationship between acceptance, catastrophizing and illness representations in chronic pain. *European Journal of Pain, 17*(6), 893–902.

Gureje, O. (2007). Psychiatric aspects of pain. *Current Opinion in Psychiatry, 20*(1), 42–46.

Gureje, O., Simon, G. E., & Von Korff, M. (2001). A cross-national study of the course of persistent pain in primary care. *Pain, 92*(1–2), 195–200.

Gureje, O., Von Korff, M., Kola, L., Demyttenaere, K., He, Y., Posada-Villa, J., et al. (2008). The relation between multiple pains and mental disorders: results from the World Mental Health Surveys. *Pain, 135*(1–2), 82–91.

Haley, W. E., Turner, J. A., & Romano, J. M. (1985). Depression in chronic pain patients: relation to pain, activity, and sex differences. *Pain, 23*(4), 337–343.

Hamelsky, S. W., & Lipton, R. B. (2006). Psychiatric comorbidity of migraine. *Headache, 46*(9), 1327–1333.

Henkel, V., Bussfeld, P., Moller, H. J., & Hegerl, U. (2002). Cognitive-behavioural theories of helplessness/hopelessness: valid models of depression? *European Archives of Psychiatry and Clinical Neuroscience, 252*(5), 240–249.

Institute of Medicine. (2011). *Relieving pain in America: A blueprint for transforming prevention, care, education, and research* (Washington, DC).

Jarvik, J. G., Hollingworth, W., Heagerty, P. J., Haynor, D. R., Boyko, E. J., & Deyo, R. A. (2005). Three-year incidence of low back pain in an initially asymptomatic cohort: clinical and imaging risk factors. *Spine (Phila Pa 1976), 30*(13), 1541–1548. discussion 1549.

Jensen, M. P., Ehde, D. M., Hoffman, A. J., Patterson, D. R., Czerniecki, J. M., & Robinson, L. R. (2002). Cognitions, coping and social environment predict adjustment to phantom limb pain. *Pain, 95*(1–2), 133–142.

Jensen, M. P., Turner, J. A., & Romano, J. M. (2007). Changes after multidisciplinary pain treatment in patient pain beliefs and coping are associated with concurrent changes in patient functioning. *Pain, 131*(1–2), 38–47.

Karoly, P., & Ruehlman, L. S. (2006). Psychological "resilience" and its correlates in chronic pain: findings from a national community sample. *Pain, 123*(1–2), 90–97.

Kashdan, T. B., & Rottenberg, J. (2010). Psychological flexibility as a fundamental aspect of health. *Clinical Psychology Review, 30*(7), 865–878.

Katon, W. (2009). The impact of depression on workplace functioning and disability costs. *American Journal of Managed Care, 15*(Suppl. 11), S322–S327.

Keefe, F. J., Lumley, M., Anderson, T., Lynch, T., Studts, J. L., & Carson, K. L. (2001). Pain and emotion: new research directions. *Journal of Clinical Psychology, 57*(4), 587–607.

Keefe, F. J., Rumble, M. E., Scipio, C. D., Giordano, L. A., & Perri, L. M. (2004). Psychological aspects of persistent pain: current state of the science. *Journal of Pain, 5*(4), 195–211.

Kerns, R., & Turk, D. C. (1984). Depression and chronic pain: the mediating role of the spouse. *Journal of Marriage and Family, 46*(4), 845–852.

King, S., Chambers, C. T., Huguet, A., MacNevin, R. C., McGrath, P. J., Parker, L., et al. (2011). The epidemiology of chronic pain in children and adolescents revisited: a systematic review. *Pain, 152*(12), 2729–2738.

Kores, R. C., Murphy, W. D., Rosenthal, T. L., Elias, D. B., & North, W. C. (1990). Predicting outcome of chronic pain treatment via a modified self-efficacy scale. *Behaviour Research and Therapy, 28*(2), 165–169.

Landreville, P., Desrosiers, J., Vincent, C., Verreault, R., & Boudreault, V. (2009). The role of activity restriction in poststroke depressive symptoms. *Rehabilitation Psychology, 54*(3), 315–322.

Leino, P., & Magni, G. (1993). Depressive and distress symptoms as predictors of low back pain, neck-shoulder pain, and other musculoskeletal morbidity: a 10-year follow-up of metal industry employees. *Pain, 53*(1), 89–94.

Linton, S. J., Nicholas, M. K., MacDonald, S., Boersma, K., Bergbom, S., Maher, C., et al. (2011). The role of depression and catastrophizing in musculoskeletal pain. *European Journal of Pain, 15*(4), 416–422.

Li, B., Piriz, J., Mirrione, M., Chung, C., Proulx, C. D., Schulz, D., et al. (2011). Synaptic potentiation onto habenula neurons in the learned helplessness model of depression. *Nature, 470*(7335), 535–539.

Lopez-Lopez, A., Gonzalez, J. L., Alonso-Fernandez, M., Cuidad, N., & Matias, B. (2014). Pain and symptoms of depression in older adults living in community and in nursing homes: the role of activity restriction as a potential mediator and moderator. *International Psychogeriatrics, 26*(10), 1679–1691.

Lopez-Martinez, A. E., Esteve-Zarazaga, R., & Ramirez-Maestre, C. (2008). Perceived social support and coping responses are independent variables explaining pain adjustment among chronic pain patients. *Journal of Pain, 9*(4), 373–379.

Lu, Q., Tsao, J. C., Myers, C. D., Kim, S. C., & Zeltzer, L. K. (2007). Coping predictors of children's laboratory-induced pain tolerance, intensity, and unpleasantness. *Journal of Pain, 8*(9), 708–717.

Magni, G., Caldieron, C., Rigatti-Luchini, S., & Merskey, H. (1990). Chronic musculo-skeletal pain and depressive symptoms in the general population. An analysis of the 1st National Health and Nutrition Examination Survey data. *Pain, 43*(3), 299–307.

Maxwell, T. D., Gatchel, R. J., & Mayer, T. G. (1998). Cognitive predictors of depression in chronic low back pain: toward an inclusive model. *Journal of Behavioural Medicine, 21*(2), 131–143.

McAllister, S. J., Vincent, A., Hassett, A. L., Whipple, M. O., Oh, T. H., Benzo, R. P., et al. (2015). Psychological resilience, affective mechanisms and symptom burden in a tertiary-care sample of patients with fibromyalgia. *Stress Health, 31*(4), 299–305.

McAuley, E., Konopack, J. F., Motl, R. W., Morris, K. S., Doerksen, S. E., & Rosengren, K. R. (2006). Physical activity and quality of life in older adults: influence of health status and self-efficacy. *Annals of Behavioural Medicine, 31*(1), 99–103.

McCracken, L. M., DaSilva, P., Skillicorn, B., & Doherty, R. (2014). The cognitive fusion questionnaire: a preliminary study of psychometric properties and prediction of func-tioning in chronic pain. *The Clinical Journal of Pain, 30*(10), 894–901.

McCracken, L. M., & Eccleston, C. (2003). Coping or acceptance: what to do about chronic pain? *Pain, 105*(1–2), 197–204.

McCracken, L. M., & Eccleston, C. (2005). A prospective study of acceptance of pain and patient functioning with chronic pain. *Pain, 118*(1–2), 164–169.

McCracken, L. M., & Vowles, K. E. (2008). A prospective analysis of acceptance of pain and values-based action in patients with chronic pain. *Health Psychology, 27*(2), 215–220.

McCracken, L. M., & Yang, S. Y. (2006). The role of values in a contextual cognitive-behavioral approach to chronic pain. *Pain, 123*(1–2), 137–145.

Miro, E., Martinez, M. P., Sanchez, A. I., Prados, G., & Medina, A. (2011). When is pain related to emotional distress and daily functioning in fibromyalgia syndrome? the mediating roles of self-efficacy and sleep quality. *British Journal of Health Psychology, 16*(4), 799–814.

Morasco, B. J., Lovejoy, T. I., Lu, M., Turk, D. C., Lewis, L., & Dobscha, S. K. (2013). The relationship between PTSD and chronic pain: mediating role of coping strategies and depression. *Pain, 154*(4), 609–616.

Niebuhr, R. (2014). *Reinhold niebuhr in Wikipedia.* Retrieved 10.03.14 from http://en. wikipedia.org/wiki/Psychology.

Okifuji, A., & Benham, B. (2011). Suicidal and self-harm behaviors in chronic pain patients. *Journal of Applied Biobehavioral Research, 16*(2), 57–77.

Okifuji, A., Turk, D. C., & Sherman, J. J. (2000). Evaluation of the relationship between depression and fibromyalgia syndrome: why aren't all patients depressed? *The Journal of Rheumatology, 27*(1), 212–219.

Onen, S. H., Onen, F., Courpron, P., & Dubray, C. (2005). How pain and analgesics disturb sleep. *The Clinical Journal of Pain, 21*(5), 422–431.

Ong, A. D., Bergeman, C. S., & Bisconti, T. L. (2004). The role of daily positive emotions during conjugal bereavement. *The Journal of Gerontology B Psychological Sciences and Social Sciences, 59*(4), P168–P176.

Osborne, T. L., Jensen, M. P., Ehde, D. M., Hanley, M. A., & Kraft, G. (2007). Psycho-social factors associated with pain intensity, pain-related interference, and psychological functioning in persons with multiple sclerosis and pain. *Pain, 127*(1–2), 52–62.

Overmier, J. B., & Seligman, M. E. (1967). Effects of inescapable shock upon subsequent escape and avoidance responding. *Journal of Comparitive and Physiological Psychology, 63*(1), 28–33.

Pakpour, A., Nikoobakht, M., & Campbell, P. (2014). Association of pain and depression in those with chronic low back pain: the mediation effect of patient sexual functioning. *The Clinical Journal of Pain, 31*(1), 44–51.

Palomino, R. A., Nicassio, P. M., Greenberg, M. A., & Medina, E. P., Jr. (2007). Helplessness and loss as mediators between pain and depressive symptoms in fibromyalgia. *Pain, 129*(1–2), 185–194.

Parmelee, P. A., Harralson, T. L., Smith, L. A., & Schumacher, H. R. (2007). Necessary and discretionary activities in knee osteoarthritis: do they mediate the pain-depression relationship? *Pain Medicine, 8*(5), 449–461.

Peng, D., Shi, F., Shen, T., Peng, Z., Zhang, C., Liu, X., et al. (2014). Altered brain network modules induce helplessness in major depressive disorder. *Journal of Affective Disorder, 168*, 21–29.

Peres, J. F., Foerster, B., Santana, L. G., Fereira, M. D., Nasello, A. G., Savoia, M., et al. (2011). Police officers under attack: resilience implications of an fMRI study. *Journal of Psychiatric Research, 45*(6), 727–734.

Pryce, C. R., Azzinnari, D., Spinelli, S., Seifritz, E., Tegethoff, M., & Meinlschmidt, G. (2011). Helplessness: a systematic translational review of theory and evidence for its relevance to understanding and treating depression. *Pharmacology and Therapeutics, 132*(3), 242–267.

Reitsma, M., Tranmer, J. E., Buchanan, D. M., & VanDenKerkhof, E. G. (2012). The epidemiology of chronic pain in Canadian men and women between 1994 and 2007: longitudinal results of the National Population Health Survey. *Pain Research and Managememnt, 17*(3), 166–172.

Richardson, E. J., Ness, T. J., Doleys, D. M., Banos, J. H., Cianfrini, L., & Richards, J. S. (2009). Depressive symptoms and pain evaluations among persons with chronic pain: catastrophizing, but not pain acceptance, shows significant effects. *Pain, 147*(1–3), 147–152.

Rudy, T. E., Kerns, R. D., & Turk, D. C. (1988). Chronic pain and depression: toward a cognitive-behavioral mediation model. *Pain, 35*(2), 129–140.

Sarda, J., Jr., Nicholas, M. K., Asghari, A., & Pimenta, C. A. (2009). The contribution of self-efficacy and depression to disability and work status in chronic pain patients: a comparison between Australian and Brazilian samples. *European Journal of Pain, 13*(2), 189–195.

Schwartz, L., Slater, M. A., Birchler, G. R., & Atkinson, J. H. (1991). Depression in spouses of chronic pain patients: the role of patient pain and anger, and marital satisfaction. *Pain, 44*(1), 61–67.

Shelby, R. A., Somers, T. J., Keefe, F. J., Silva, S. G., McKee, D. C., She, L., et al. (2009). Pain catastrophizing in patients with noncardiac chest pain: relationships with pain, anxiety, and disability. *Psychosomatic Medicine, 71*(8), 861–868.

Sherman, J. J., Turk, D. C., & Okifuji, A. (2000). Prevalence and impact of posttraumatic stress disorder-like symptoms on patients with fibromyalgia syndrome. *The Clinical Journal of Pain, 16*(2), 127–134.

Smith, M. T., Perlis, M. L., & Haythornthwaite, J. A. (2004). Suicidal ideation in outpatients with chronic musculoskeletal pain: an exploratory study of the role of sleep onset insomnia and pain intensity. *The Clinical Journal of Pain, 20*(2), 111–118.

Somers, T. J., Keefe, F. J., Carson, J. W., Pells, J. J., & Lacaille, L. (2008). Pain catastrophizing in borderline morbidly obese and morbidly obese individuals with osteoarthritic knee pain. *Pain Research Management, 13*(5), 401–406.

Somers, T. J., Keefe, F. J., Pells, J. J., Dixon, K. E., Waters, S. J., Riordan, P. A., et al. (2009). Pain catastrophizing and pain-related fear in osteoarthritis patients: relationships to pain and disability. *Journal of Pain and Symptom Management, 37*(5), 863–872.

Stahl, S. M. (2002). Does depression hurt? *Journal of Clinical Psychiatry, 63*(4), 273–274.

Sterling, M., Hodkinson, E., Pettiford, C., Souvlis, T., & Curatolo, M. (2008). Psychologic factors are related to some sensory pain thresholds but not nociceptive flexion reflex threshold in chronic whiplash. *The Clinical Journal of Pain, 24*(2), 124–130.

Sturgeon, J. A., Zautra, A. J., & Arewasikporn, A. (2014). A multilevel structural equation modeling analysis of vulnerabilities and resilience resources influencing affective adaptation to chronic pain. *Pain, 155*(2), 292–298.

Tinti, C., Schmidt, S., & Businaro, N. (2011). Pain and emotions reported after childbirth and recalled 6 months later: the role of controllability. *Journal of Psychosomatic Obstetrics Gynaecology, 32*(2), 98–103.

Tripp, D. A., VanDenKerkhof, E. G., & McAlister, M. (2006). Prevalence and determinants of pain and pain-related disability in urban and rural settings in southeastern Ontario. *Pain Research Management, 11*(4), 225–233.

Tsang, A., Von Korff, M., Lee, S., Alonso, J., Karam, E., Angermeyer, M. C., et al. (2008). Common chronic pain conditions in developed and developing countries: gender and age differences and comorbidity with depression-anxiety disorders. *Journal of Pain, 9*(10), 883–891.

Turk, D. (2000). Foreword. In K. B. Schmaling, & T. G. Sher (Eds.), *The psychology of couples and illness* (pp. xi–xiv). Washington, DC: American Psychological Association Press.

Turk, D., Kerns, R., & Rosenberg, R. (1992). Effects of marital interaction on chronic pain and disability: examining the down-side of social support. *Rehabilitation Psychology, 37*, 257–272.

Turk, D. C., Okifuji, A., & Scharff, L. (1995). Chronic pain and depression: role of perceived impact and perceived control in different age cohorts. *Pain, 61*(1), 93–101.

Turner, J. A., Jensen, M. P., & Romano, J. M. (2000). Do beliefs, coping, and catastrophizing independently predict functioning in patients with chronic pain? *Pain, 85*(1–2), 115–125.

Viane, I., Crombez, G., Eccleston, C., Poppe, C., Devulder, J., Van Houdenhove, B., et al. (2003). Acceptance of pain is an independent predictor of mental well-being in patients with chronic pain: empirical evidence and reappraisal. *Pain, 106*(1–2), 65–72.

Von Korff, M., Dworkin, S., LeResche, L., & Kruger, A. (1988). Epidemiology of temporomandibular disorders II. TMD pain compared to other common pain sites. In R. Dubner, G. Gebhart, & M. Bond (Eds.), *Proceedings of the 5th World Congress on Pain* (pp. 506–511). Amsterdam: Elsevier.

Wang, M., Perova, Z., Arenkiel, B. R., & Li, B. (2014). Synaptic modifications in the medial prefrontal cortex in susceptibility and resilience to stress. *Journal of Neuroscience, 34*(22), 7485–7492.

Weir, R., Browne, G. B., Tunks, E., Gafni, A., & Roberts, J. (1992). A profile of users of specialty pain clinic services: predictors of use and cost estimates. *Journal of Clinical Epidemiology, 45*(12), 1399–1415.

Wells-Federman, C., Arnstein, P., & Caudill, M. (2002). Nurse-led pain management program: effect on self-efficacy, pain intensity, pain-related disability, and depressive symptoms in chronic pain patients. *Pain Management Nursing, 3*(4), 131–140.

van der Werff, S. J., van den Berg, S. M., Pannekoek, J. N., Elzinga, B. M., & van der Wee, N. J. (2013). Neuroimaging resilience to stress: a review. *Frontier in Behavioural Neuroscience, 7*, 39.

Williamson, G. M. (2000). Extending the activity restriction model of depressed affect: evidence from a sample of breast cancer patients. *Health Psychology, 19*(4), 339–347.

Williamson, G. M., & Schulz, R. (1995). Activity restriction mediates the association between pain and depressed affect: a study of younger and older adult cancer patients. *Psychology and Aging, 10*(3), 369–378.

Wong, W. S., Chen, P. P., Yap, J., Mak, K. H., Tam, B. K., & Fielding, R. (2011). Assessing depression in patients with chronic pain: a comparison of three rating scales. *Journal of Affective Disorders, 133*(1–2), 179–187.

Wood, B. M., Nicholas, M. K., Blyth, F., Asghari, A., & Gibson, S. (2013). Catastrophizing mediates the relationship between pain intensity and depressed mood in older adults with persistent pain. *Journal of Pain, 14*(2), 149–157.

Youssef, N. A., Green, K. T., Beckham, J. C., & Elbogen, E. B. (2013). A 3-year longitudinal study examining the effect of resilience on suicidality in veterans. *Annals of Clinical Psychiatry, 25*(1), 59–66.

Zautra, A. J., Fasman, R., Reich, J. W., Harakas, P., Johnson, L. M., Olmsted, M. E., et al. (2005). Fibromyalgia: evidence for deficits in positive affect regulation. *Psychosomatic Medicine, 67*(1), 147–155.

CHAPTER 10

Addiction, Pain, and Stress Response

Motohiro Nakajima, Mustafa al'Absi
University of Minnesota Medical School, Minneapolis, Duluth, MN, USA

INTRODUCTION

Experience of stress and pain can be modified at multiple levels including genetic, biological, cognitive, behavioral, and social determinants. Substance use is a global phenomenon that poses threats to health, social, and economic welfare. Accumulating evidence indicates that acute and chronic administration of abused drugs induces various neurochemical changes in the brain and peripheral physiological systems that produce alterations in the stress response and pain sensitivity. This chapter is aimed at providing a general overview of how drug use and misuse are associated with pain and stress. We will briefly discuss findings from studies showing the mediating role of stress in the link between pain and addiction. Finally, we will discuss other factors such as sex differences and mental health problems that modify the associations between drug use, pain, and stress. We will conclude this chapter by discussing current limitations and future directions.

ADDICTION AND PAIN
Epidemiology of Drug Use

Substance use, including use of opioids, alcohol, tobacco, cannabis, amphetamine-type stimulants, and cocaine, continues to pose threats to health, social, and economic welfare locally and globally (SAMHSA, 2014; UNODC, 2012). It is estimated that between 26 and 36 million people across the globe consume opioids (UNODC, 2012). While the rate of use has been generally stable in illicit drugs (UNODC, 2012) or in high-income countries (Eriksen, Mackay, & Ross, 2012), the prevalence remains high in low- and middle-income countries, especially among the youth (Eriksen et al., 2012; UNODC, 2012). In the United States, approximately 136 million individuals who were 12 years or older were

The Neuroscience of Pain, Stress, and Emotion
http://dx.doi.org/10.1016/B978-0-12-800538-5.00010-8

current alcohol drinkers, 66 million individuals were current tobacco product users, and 24 million were current illicit drug users in 2013 (SAMHSA, 2014). The use of illicit drugs showed an increase over the past 15 years (SAMHSA, 2014). More than 21.5 million individuals at the age of 12 or older fall under the category of substance dependence or abuse as defined by the *Diagnostic and Statistical Manual of Mental Disorders*, fourth edition, although only about 10% of them received facility-based treatment (SAMHSA, 2014).

Substance Use and Pain

Substance use is a risk factor of pain-related morbidity (Ditre, Brandon, Zale, & Meagher, 2011; Garland, Froeliger, Zeidan, Partin, & Howard, 2013; Sehgal, Manchikanti, & Smith, 2012; Shi, Weingarten, Mantilla, Hooten, & Warner, 2010). Prescription opioids are commonly abused drugs (Wilson, 2007) and are a growing public health concern in many countries, including the United States (Garland et al., 2013; Maxwell, 2011). Various studies have shown positive associations of drug use, such as opioids (Edwards et al., 2011; Eriksen, Sjogren, Bruera, Ekholm, & Rasmussen, 2006; Fischer, Lusted, Roerecke, Taylor, & Rehm, 2012; Jamison, Link, & Marceau, 2009; Macey, Morasco, Duckart, & Dobscha, 2011; Rosenblum et al., 2003; Trafton, Oliva, Horst, Minkel, & Humphreys, 2004), tobacco (Andersson, Ejlertsson, & Leden, 1998; Brage & Bjerkedal, 1996; Ekholm, Gronbaek, Peuckmann, & Sjogren, 2009; Hagg, Fritzell, & Nordwall, 2002; Jakobsson, 2008; Jamison, Stetson, & Parris, 1991; Palmer, Syddall, Cooper, & Coggon, 2003; Pisinger et al., 2011; Scott, Goldberg, Mayo, Stock, & Poitras, 1999; Shiri, Karppinen, Leino-Arjas, Solovieva, & Viikari-Juntura, 2010; Zvolensky, McMillan, Gonzalez, & Asmundson, 2009), alcohol (Brennan, Schutte, & Moos, 2005; Riley & King, 2009; Tsui et al., 2014), and heroin (Tsui et al., 2013), with pain-related symptoms. Laboratory studies using experimental pain procedures to examine pain sensitivity among drug abusers also support this relationship. Individuals who are addicted to opioids or at high risk for opioid abuse have lower pain tolerance than healthy comparisons (Edwards et al., 2011; Pud, Cohen, Lawental, & Eisenberg, 2006; Ren, Shi, Epstein, Wang, & Lu, 2009). Alcoholic patients who were undergoing alcohol withdrawal showed lower tolerance to heat pain than control individuals matched by gender and age (Jochum, Boettger, Burkhardt, Juckel, & Bar, 2010). Chronic smokers during ad libitum smoking (al'Absi, Nakajima, & Grabowski, 2013) and an initial phase of a quit attempt (Nakajima & al'Absi, 2014) showed lower pain tolerance to cold pressor test (CPT) relative to nonsmokers. Smokers who were administered CPT as part of the laboratory session reported greater levels of smoking urges and had shorter time until taking up a cigarette after the pain task than those who did not receive the pain task (Ditre & Brandon, 2008). Greater precessation pain ratings in the CPT predicted early smoking relapse (Nakajima & al'Absi, 2011). There is initial evidence to suggest that withdrawal from drugs enhances sensitivity to pain, which further increases the likelihood of subsequent drug use (Ditre & Brandon, 2008; Jochum et al., 2010; Nakajima & al'Absi, 2014). Taken together, epidemiological and laboratory-based studies strongly suggest positive associations between drug use and pain sensitivity.

Mechanisms of drug effects on pain perception are likely to involve multiple pathways. For instance, opioids interact with mu, kappa, and delta opioid receptors that are widely distributed throughout the brain and the spinal cord. Activation of those receptors causes analgesic effects by stimulating amino acids and neuropeptides that inhibit neurophysiological pathways related to nociceptive signals (Garland et al., 2013; Ossipov et al., 2004). Nicotine binds to nicotinic cholinergic (nACh) receptors in central and peripheral nervous systems, causing the release of neurotransmitters such as dopamine, norepinephrine, acetylcholine, glutamate, serotonin, β-endorphin, and γ-aminobutyric acid (GABA), mediating antinociceptive properties of nicotine (Bannon et al., 1998; Becker, Gandhi, & Schweinhardt, 2012; Ditre et al., 2011; Shi et al., 2010; Wewers, Dhatt, Snively, & Tejwani, 1999). Alcohol stimulates N-methyl-D-aspartate, $GABA_A$, $5\text{-}HT_3$, and nACh receptors that are associated with enhanced dopaminergic activity (Egli, Koob, & Edwards, 2012; Vengeliene, Bilbao, Molander, & Spanagel, 2008) and secretion of β-endorphin from the hypothalamus.

Substance use in general activates mesolimbic pathways including the ventral tegmental area, the nucleus accumbens, and the prefrontal cortex that promote the secretion of dopamine (Benowitz, 2010; Egli et al., 2012), a known agent responsible for self-administration of addictive drugs and stress (al'Absi, 2007; Benowitz, 2010). The dopaminergic pathway is regulated by the endogenous opioid system (Chong, Uhart, & Wand, 2007) because mu, delta, and kappa receptors are located in the nucleus accumbens (Mansour, Khachaturian, Lewis, Akil, & Watson, 1988). Drug-induced activation of this system has been suggested as one mechanism of drug reinforcement (Chong et al., 2007). The hypothalamic–pituitary–adrenal (HPA) axis is also activated by several drugs of abuse and is likely to be involved in pain suppression and reinforcement of drug use (see below). In summary, drug effects on antinociception are mediated by complex neurobiological cascades including the endogenous opioid system and the dopaminergic pathway and stress–related response systems including the HPA axis.

While acute administration of drugs of abuse suppresses pain, repetitive intake develops tolerance to the drug that could influence drug-related analgesia. Tolerance is developed when effects obtained with the first dose are attenuated after repeated doses or increased doses are needed to reach the effects attained by the original dose (Benowitz, 1988). Furthermore, chronic drug use may lead to dysregulations in the central and peripheral pain-inhibitory mechanisms (Haghparast, Khani, Naderi, Alizadeh, & Motamedi, 2008; Zarrindast, Khoshayand, & Shafaghi, 1999) that alter the severity of withdrawal symptoms and sensitivity to pain. This has been supported in studies reporting positive associations between withdrawal symptoms, drug-induced negative affect, and pain sensitivity (al'Absi, Nakajima, et al., 2013; Ditre & Brandon, 2008; Jochum et al., 2010; Nakajima & al'Absi, 2014; Pud et al., 2006; Ren et al., 2009). It is possible that habitual drug users take drugs as a means of self-medication to alleviate side effects and distress (Khantzian, 1997; Riley & King, 2009). In fact, one study (Brennan et al., 2005) found that problem alcohol drinkers reported more severe pain, and using alcohol to manage pain, relative to those who did not have an alcohol drinking problem. Another study found that male smokers who cited reduction of craving as a motive to smoke were more likely to relapse (Nakajima & al'Absi, 2012).

THE ROLE OF STRESS IN THE LINK BETWEEN ADDICTION AND PAIN

Brief Overview of Stress

Stress is associated with both addiction and pain, and evidence indicates that stress mediates this link. Stress response occurs at biochemical, physiological, cognitive, and behavioral levels (see Chapter 2 for more details). While acute or short-lived stress response reflects the adaptive capacity of the organism to meet environmental challenges, chronic or frequent stress, due to environment or predispositional characteristic, could lead to prolonged activation of central and peripheral neurobiological mechanisms that have pathophysiological consequences (Lazarus & Folkman, 1984; Lovallo, 2004). Maladaptive physiological changes in response to stress cause wear and tear of the system (McEwen, 1998), which mediates medical conditions including chronic pain and unhealthy behaviors such as smoking and alcohol drinking (McEwen, 1998). In the next sections we will briefly review the associations of stress with addiction and pain.

Stress and Drug Use

Stress is a well-known risk factor for addiction (al'Absi, 2007; Sinha, 2008). The link between psychosocial stress and substance use has been consistently reported (al'Absi, 2006; Cohen & Lichtenstein, 1990; Shiffman, Paty, Gnys, Kassel, & Hickcox, 1996; Slopen et al., 2012; Webb & Carey, 2008). Studies have shown neurobiological mechanisms of stress and addictive behaviors (Koob & Le Moal, 1997; Kreek & Koob, 1998; Lovallo, 2006; Van Bockstaele, Reyes, & Valentino, 2010). Stress involves activation of the HPA axis, which sensitizes central neurophysiological pathways that are associated with drug reward (Rouge-Pont, Deroche, Le, & Piazza, 1998; Rouge-Pont, Marinelli, Le, Simon, & Piazza, 1995; Tidey & Miczek, 1997) that facilitates self-administration of the drug (Koob & Le Moal, 1997; Piazza & Le Moal, 1998). In fact, both drug use and stress are independently linked with dopaminergic activity. Animal studies have shown that the dopaminergic pathway can be activated by administration of addictive drugs and moderate levels of stress; however, the system tends to be inhibited during the absence of drug use and prolonged or unpredictable stress (Marinelli, 2007). The interplay between stress-related HPA response and the risk for drug abuse has also been found in human studies (al'Absi, 2006; Lovallo, 2006; Sinha, 2008; Uhart & Wand, 2009). Altered HPA stress response or basal activity was found in chronic smokers (al'Absi, Nakajima, et al., 2013; al'Absi, Wittmers, Erickson, Hatsukami, & Crouse, 2003; Kirschbaum, Strasburger, & Langkrar, 1993), alcoholic patients (Bernardy, King, Parsons, & Lovallo, 1996; Errico, Parsons, King, & Lovallo, 1993; Lovallo, Dickensheets, Myers, Thomas, & Nixon, 2000), individuals with family history of alcoholism (Croissant & Olbrich, 2004; Dawes et al., 1999; Sorocco, Lovallo, Vincent, & Collins, 2006; Uhart, Oswald, McCaul, Chong, & Wand, 2006; Zimmermann et al., 2004), those who were at risk of engaging in harmful drinking (Nakajima, Kumar, Wittmers, Scott, & al'Absi, 2013), amphetamine-type substance users (al'Absi, Khalil, et al., 2013), and opioid-dependent users (Fatseas et al., 2011; Zhang et al., 2008). Altered HPA response to stress was predictive of relapse to smoking (al'Absi, Hatsukami, & Davis, 2005; al'Absi, Nakajima, Allen, Lemieux, & Hatsukami, 2015) and cocaine use (Sinha, Garcia, Paliwal, Kreek,

& Rounsaville, 2006) as well as drug experimenting and drinking relapse in the future (Junghanns et al., 2003, 2005; Moss, Vanyukov, Yao, & Kirillova, 1999). These studies suggest the usefulness of the HPA stress response in identifying individuals who are at high risk of drug relapse. Other studies have shown dysregulations in cardiovascular (Roy, Steptoe, & Kirschbaum, 1994; Straneva, Hinderliter, Wells, Lenahan, & Girdler, 2000) responses to stress among habitual chronic smokers. These alterations have been proposed as a risk factor of enhanced pain sensitivity of this group (Girdler et al., 2005).

Stress and Pain

Acute stress suppresses pain perception (i.e., stress-induced analgesia (SIA); al'Absi & Petersen, 2003; Butler & Finn, 2009; Janssen, Spinhoven, & Brosschot, 2001; Rhudy & Meagher, 2000). While the exact mechanism of this association has yet to be determined, studies have found stress-related changes in cardiovascular activity (France & Stewart, 1995; Janssen et al., 2001), baroreceptor activity (France, 1999; Guasti et al., 2002; Sheps et al., 1989), the endogenous opioid system (al'Absi et al., 2004; al'Absi, Wittmers, Hatsukami, & Westra, 2008; Girdler et al., 2005; Randich & Maixner, 1984), and hypothalamic–autonomic activation (al'Absi, Nakajima, et al., 2013; France, 1999; Guasti et al., 2002; Nakajima & al'Absi, 2014) as potential mediators. For instance, elevated blood pressure is linked with reduction in pain (al'Absi, Buchanan, & Lovallo, 1996; al'Absi, Buchanan, Marrero, & Lovallo, 1999; al'Absi & Petersen, 2003; Ghione, 1996). The HPA system has also been shown to mediate pain perception (al'Absi, Petersen, & Wittmers, 2002; Lariviere & Melzack, 2000). While acute stress-related physiological activation attenuates pain, there is evidence that chronic stress is related to enhanced pain perception (Lundberg, 1999). This is indicated in prolonged conditions in which individuals suffer high levels of mental and physical distress. Impaired adrenocortical activity has been observed in patients with chronic neck pain (Shahidi, Sannes, Laudenslager, & Maluf, 2015), irritable bowel syndrome (Dinan et al., 2006; Fukudo, Nomura, & Hongo, 1998), chronic pelvic pain (Heim, Ehlert, Hanker, & Hellhammer, 1998; Wingenfeld et al., 2009), chronic migraine (Patacchioli et al., 2006), low back pain (Muhtz et al., 2013; Theorell, Hasselhorn, Vingrd, & Andersson, 2000), fibromyalgia (Geiss, Rohleder, & Anton, 2012; Wingenfeld et al., 2008; Wingenfeld, Nutzinger, Kauth, Hellhammer, & Lautenbacher, 2010), rheumatoid arthritis (Dekkers et al., 2001; Eijsbouts et al., 2005), chronic musculoskeletal pain (Generaal et al., 2014), and chronic fatigue syndrome (Nijhof et al., 2014; Roberts, Wessely, Chalder, Papadopoulos, & Cleare, 2004). Psychiatric disorders such as posttraumatic stress disorder (PTSD) (Gureje, 2008) and major depression (Bair, Robinson, Katon, & Kroenke, 2003; Gambassi, 2009) have been shown to exacerbate pain. It is possible that stress-related chronic activation of physiological systems may alter central mechanisms responsible for modulation of pain.

Taken together, numerous studies have reported that stress is associated with addiction and pain, respectively. However, to our best knowledge, very few studies have systematically examined the mediating role of psychobiological stress response in chronic substance use and pain sensitivity. In the next section, we will discuss data from our laboratory examining this hypothesis among nicotine-dependent men and women.

Stress as a Mediator of the Link between Addiction and Pain

We have examined the role of stress in the relationship between pain and nicotine addiction in two cross-sectional studies (al'Absi, Nakajima, et al., 2013; Nakajima & al'Absi, 2014). Part of a larger project, which investigated psychobiological determinants of smoking relapse (al'Absi et al., 2015), this project included chronic smokers and nonsmokers to directly compare influences of smoking on psychobiological responses to stress and SIA. The laboratory protocol included the following: (1) 45 min initial baseline; (2) 40 min pain assessment 1; (3) 20 min rest period; (4) 40 min pain assessment 2; (5) 20 min rest period. The pain assessment was included twice: one after rest (rest–pain) and one after stress (stress–pain). The order of pain assessment (rest–pain condition first or not) was counterbalanced across participants to minimize order effects. To assess psychobiological responses to stress, self-report measures of mood as well as blood and saliva samples for the measurement of stress-related hormones (adrenocorticotropic hormone (ACTH) and cortisol) were collected at the end of each period. In addition, cardiovascular measures including blood pressure (BP) and heart rate (HR) were collected multiple times during baseline, stress, and rest periods. Subjective craving and withdrawal symptoms were assessed from smokers. Public speaking and mental arithmetic tasks were used as stressors. These tasks have been found to reliably induce subjective and biological changes (al'Absi et al., 1997) that are similar to stress-related changes observed in the natural environment. The CPT and thermal heat pain induction tests were used. Pain threshold and tolerance and the short version of the McGill pain questionnaire (MPQ) (Melzack, 1975) were administered to evaluate pain.

The first study (al'Absi, Nakajima, et al., 2013) was conducted when smokers interested in quitting were smoking at their own pace. Non-smokers completed the same protocol. The results indicated that reported distress was higher and positive affect was lower in smokers than in non-smokers (p < 0.05). Craving and withdrawal symptoms increased in response to stress in smokers (p < 0.05). Smokers exhibited reduced cardiovascular (systolic and diastolic BP, HR) and salivary cortisol responses to stress relative to nonsmokers (p < 0.05). Pain tolerance to CPT was lower in smokers than in nonsmokers, pain tolerance to thermal heat was higher after stress than after rest regardless of smoking status, and women had lower pain tolerance than men regardless of smoking status (p <0.05). When the model was adjusted for confounding variables (e.g., demographics), we found smoking group × pain condition interactions (p < 0.05), reflecting greater heat pain threshold and tolerance poststress compared to postrest in nonsmokers but not in smokers. Additional correlational analysis further revealed that greater systolic BP (SBP) was associated with higher pain tolerance to CPT, and greater SBP and salivary cortisol levels were related to higher pain tolerance to thermal heat (p < 0.05). In general, reported distress and withdrawal symptoms (in smokers) were positively linked to MPQ measures after CPT and thermal heat procedures. These findings collectively indicate a lack of SIA among smokers. It also suggests dissociations between subjective and biological responses to stress in smokers. Smokers reported higher distress than nonsmokers but cardiovascular and hormonal stress responses were attenuated in smokers relative to nonsmokers. This blunted stress response profile may be a risk factor of enhanced pain perception in smokers. The finding of smoking group difference in SIA and inverse associations of physiological measures with pain perception support this hypothesis.

Participants then set a quit day and completed the same protocol again approximately 2 weeks after the previous laboratory session. This study (Nakajima & al'Absi, 2014) was completed 48 h after smokers quit smoking. Smoking status was verified biochemically. Nonsmokers were tested in the same time frame without any smoking component. Results of this study expanded the previous study. In addition to attenuated cardiovascular responses to stress, smokers showed lower pain tolerance to CPT than nonsmokers. Pain tolerance to CPT was greater after stress than after rest (pain condition effect: p < 0.05) and greater in men than in women (sex effect: $p < 0.05$). We also found moderating effects of smoking status on pain condition. That is, pain tolerance to CPT increased after stress in nonsmokers but not in smokers ($p < 0.05$). Also, MPQ scores in response to CPT tended to increase after stress in smokers but this was not found in nonsmokers ($p < 0.05$). Correlations of self-report and physiological measures with pain measures found in this study were very similar to those observed in the previous study.

These two studies collectively indicate the importance of the central and peripheral stress-regulatory mechanisms in the link between pain and addiction. First, cardiovascular and adrenocortical responses to stress were attenuated in smokers relative to nonsmokers. Second, these alterations were associated with enhanced pain perception. Third, nonsmokers showed evidence of SIA from the two studies, while this was not the case with smokers. Fourth, stress-induced craving and withdrawal symptoms were positively related to pain perception. Finally, although direct comparison is not available, our results suggest that the link between altered stress response and enhanced pain perception was pronounced during smoking withdrawal (initial stage of smoking cessation). Taken together, alterations in psycho-biological stress response may contribute to enhanced pain experience and lack of SIA in chronic smokers.

The underlying mechanism should be elucidated. Accumulating evidence indicates that acute administration of nicotine (Fertig, Pomerleau, & Sanders, 1986; Jamner, Girdler, Shapiro, & Jarvik, 1998; Kanarek & Carrington, 2004; Pomerleau, Turk, & Fertig, 1984) and acute stress (al'Absi et al., 1996; al'Absi, Petersen, & Wittmers, 2000; al'Absi et al., 2002) are linked with analgesia; however, chronic nicotine exposure may dysregulate this relationship (Ditre et al., 2011; Girdler et al., 2005; Shi et al., 2010). For instance, repeated drug exposure, including nicotine, is associated with β-endorphin deficit (Girdler et al., 2005; Scanlon, Lazar-Wesley, Grant, & Kunos, 1992). Animals repeatedly treated with nicotine show a lack of hypoalgesia in response to morphine (Zarrindast et al., 1999). Maladaptive cardiovascular and hormonal adjustments to acute stressors have been found in habitual smokers (al'Absi et al., 2003; Kirschbaum et al., 1993; Roy et al., 1994; Straneva et al., 2000). Taken together, our and other studies suggest that chronic smoking downregulates or desensitizes central and peripheral functions that are responsible for antinociceptive effects of nicotine (Nakajima & al'Absi, 2014). We further propose the blunted stress response as one key component of the enhanced pain sensitivity in smokers. Correlations between stress-related increase in craving and withdrawal symptoms and pain found in our studies support relevant literature (Anderson et al., 2004; Mousa, Aloyo, & Van Loon, 1988; Nesbitt, 1973; Silverstein, 1982), suggesting that chronic nicotine exposure develops tolerance to nicotine, and nicotine withdrawal contributes to heightened pain sensitivity, potentially leading to smoking relapse. While more research is clearly needed to elucidate the role of stress in the link between pain and addiction, attenuated stress response pattern has been found in other chronic substance use (Nakajima et al., 2013; Sinha et al., 2011).

Effects of Opioid Blockade on Addiction and Pain

Studies have been undertaken to examine the extent to which chronic smoking is associated with altered endogenous opioid mechanisms. This work is guided by preclinical studies showing that nicotine increases the release of endogenous opioids (Dhatt et al., 1995; Kishioka, Kiguchi, Kobayashi, & Saika, 2014) and that the endogenous opioid system regulates the HPA axis (Chong et al., 2007). In this study (al'Absi et al., 2008), chronic smokers and nonsmokers completed two laboratory sessions in which they received a placebo or 50 mg of naltrexone using a double-blind method. The laboratory sessions included pain assessments, CPT, and thermal heat pain. Self-report measures of mood, blood and saliva samples for hormonal measures, and cardiovascular measures were collected multiple times during the study to track changes in response to noxious stimuli. The protocol included: (1) 30 min initial baseline; (2) administration of a pill (placebo or drug); (3) 60-min rest; (4) pain assessments (the first pain (CPT or heat); (5) 20 min rest; (6) the second pain (CPT or heat)); (7) 60 min rest. The order of pain was counterbalanced across participants. The results indicated that ACTH and plasma and salivary cortisol increased during the postdrug periods. In addition, in plasma and salivary cortisol, the increase was pronounced in the naltrexone condition relative to the placebo condition ($p < 0.05$). Naltrexone-induced increase in ACTH and plasma cortisol levels were smaller in smokers than in nonsmokers ($p < 0.05$). As to pain measures, female nonsmokers reported greater pain to both CPT and thermal heat stimuli than male nonsmokers, while this sex difference was not found in smokers ($p < 0.01$). Collectively, these findings suggest that influences of the endogenous opioid system on the HPA function are altered among chronic smokers.

While the underlying mechanism responsible for altered opioid effects on the HPA axis among chronic smokers is not clear, multiple neurobiological systems are likely to be involved. Our finding of increased HPA-related hormonal levels after opioid blockade exposure is supported by animal studies showing the direct regulatory effects of β-endorphin on the HPA axis via inhibition of corticotropin-releasing hormone (CRH) neuronal activity (Wand, Mangold, El Deiry, McCaul, & Hoover, 1998). Another proposed mechanism is opioid's indirect effects on CRH through the locus coeruleus (LC). The LC is a pontine nucleus that synthesizes norepi-nephrine, which has been identified as a target in response to stress and opiates. Opioids inhibit LC, which decreases secretion of norepinephrine, resulting in regulation of the HPA axis activity (Van Bockstaele et al., 2010). Attenuation of opioid-related increase in HPA activity among smokers observed in our study suggests the influence of smoking on the opioid–HPA link. Nicotine modulates opioid receptors and produces opiate peptides (Dhatt et al., 1995; Kishioka et al., 2014). It is plausible that chronic use of nicotine overstimulates opioid receptors and induces struc-tural and/or functional changes in opioid receptors (al'Absi et al., 2008). This could in turn disrupt opioid neuronal activity in multiple brain regions such as the hypothalamus and LC. Our two studies described in the previous section indicate the link between chronic nicotine exposure and altered HPA axis. Taken together, we propose that enhanced pain sensitivity and emotional distress are mediated by dysfunctions of the endogenous opioid and HPA stress-regulating systems.

OTHER FACTORS
Sex Differences

Sex moderates the relationship between addiction, pain, and stress. First, sex differences have been reported in patterns of substance use (Grunberg, Winders, & Wewers, 1991), sensitivity to drugs (Perkins, Jacobs, Sanders, & Caggiula, 2002; Perkins & Scott, 2008), and psychosocial (Nakajima & al'Absi, 2012) and neurobiological (al'Absi, 2006; al'Absi et al., 2015) correlates of drug relapse. For instance, female smokers use smoking to cope with negative affect (Dicken, 1978; D'Angelo, Reid, Brown, & Pipe, 2001; File, Dinnis, Heard, & Irvine, 2002), report more distress after exposure to nonsmoking and smoking-specific stimuli (McKee, Maciejewski, Falba, & Mazure, 2003; Swan, Ward, Jack, & Javitz, 1993), and generally have more difficulty quitting (Ward, Klesges, Zbikowski, Bliss, & Garvey, 1997; Wetter et al., 1999) than male smokers. Changes in hormonal response to stress are predictive of early smoking relapse in men (al'Absi, 2006; al'Absi et al., 2015), while trait negative affect and self-report withdrawal symptoms are predictive of cessation failure in women (al'Absi, 2006; Nakajima & al'Absi, 2012). Menstrual cycle phase correlated with smoking behavior, craving, and relapse (Bobzean, DeNobrega, & Perrotti, 2014; Carpenter, Upadhyaya, LaRowe, Saladin, & Brady, 2006) as well as effects of opioid blockade (Roche & King, 2015). In addition, there is evidence showing a link of sex hormones, such as progesterone (Fox, Sofuoglu, Morgan, Tuit, & Sinha, 2013) and its metabolite allopregnanolone (Allen, al'Absi, Lando, & Allen, 2015; Anker & Carroll, 2010a, 2010b; Marx et al., 2006), with cocaine and nicotine dependence. Second, sex differences have been observed in pain perception, with lower pain tolerance in women than in men (Bartley & Fillingim, 2013). This may be moderated by substance use status and pain modality. One study (Girdler et al., 2005) found that smoking group differences (smokers vs nonsmokers) in ischemic pain sensitivity were found in women but not in men, whereas smoking group differences in CPT sensitivity were observed in men only. Another study (al'Absi, Nakajima, et al., 2013) found lower thermal heat pain tolerance in nonsmoking women than men; however, this sex difference was reduced (but still at a statistically significant level) among nicotine-dependent men and women. Interestingly, these findings were not observed in CPT (al'Absi, Nakajima, et al., 2013). In summary, neurobiological and psychosocial factors may account for sex differences in addiction and pain (Bartley & Fillingim, 2013; Fillingim & Gear, 2004).

Mental Health Comorbidity

Mental health problems have been shown to be associated with pain. Depression and anxiety disorders are very common among chronic pain sufferers (Jamison & Edwards, 2013; Lepine & Briley, 2004; McWilliams, Cox, & Enns, 2003). Some studies suggest altered pain sensitivity among individuals with PTSD (Macey et al., 2011; Mostoufi et al., 2014). A meta-analysis on epidemiological data showed greater risk of mental health problems and pain among individuals who have misused prescription opioids (Fischer et al., 2012). Accumulating evidence also indicates the link between mental health problems and drug addiction. Patients who have severe mental illness are 4 times more likely to be heavy alcohol users, 3.5 times more likely to be regular marijuana users, 4.6 times more likely to be habitual smokers, and 4.6 times more likely to use other drugs (Hartz et al., 2014). It is possible that comorbidity of mental illness and substance use disorders modifies pain sensitivity through alterations in central stress, emotion, and pain-modulating mechanisms, although this hypothesis has not been tested directly (Ditre et al., 2011).

In addition, individual differences including family history, socioeconomic and social status, depressive mood and anger, anxiety sensitivity and withdrawal tolerance, and pain catastrophizing have been shown to be linked with substance use (al'Absi, Carr, & Bongard, 2007; Brown, Lejuez, Kahler, Strong, & Zvolensky, 2005; Ditre et al., 2011; Helmerhorst, Vranceanu, Vrahas, Smith, & Ring, 2014; Kassel, Stroud, & Paronis, 2003; Lovallo, 2007; Zvolensky, Stewart, Vujanovic, Gavric, & Steeves, 2009). Polydrug use or concurrent use of two or more drugs is not uncommon (Agrawal, Budney, & Lynskey, 2012; Baggio, Studer, Mohler-Kuo, Daeppen, & Gmel, 2014; Ekholm et al., 2009; Peters, Budney, & Carroll, 2012; Weinberger, Pilver, Hoff, Mazure, & McKee, 2013; Weinberger & Sofuoglu, 2009) and there is initial evidence suggesting that concurrent drug use is associated with altered psychophysiological stress response and cognitive functions (al'Absi et al., 2014; Fox, Tuit, & Sinha, 2013; Lovallo et al., 2000; Weinberger & Sofuoglu, 2009). These could in turn alter endogenous pain mechanisms.

FUTURE DIRECTIONS AND CONCLUSIONS
Causal Directions

The current literature provides an overview to understand the complex association of addiction with pain and stress. In general, drugs of abuse such as opioids, alcohol, and nicotine both have antinociceptive properties and play an important role in worsening pain conditions (Ditre et al., 2011; Jochum et al., 2010; Shi et al., 2010). These drugs also stimulate the HPA axis and dopaminergic pathways that are associated with stress and reward. It is likely that acute analgesic effects of drugs would be diminished across time with chronic drug exposure via neuroadaptations in central and peripheral pain- and stress-regulating systems. These neurobiological alterations may increase sensitivity to the withdrawal experience and physical discomfort including pain. As a result, these vulnerable individuals may use drugs to alleviate these symptoms (see Figure 1).

Studies have shown enhanced pain perception and negative mood during absence of drug use (Jochum et al., 2010; Nakajima & al'Absi, 2014) and pain as a risk factor for subsequent substance use (Brennan et al., 2005; Ditre & Brandon, 2008) and drug relapse (Nakajima & al'Absi, 2011). While drug use may temporally relieve physical discomfort and negative

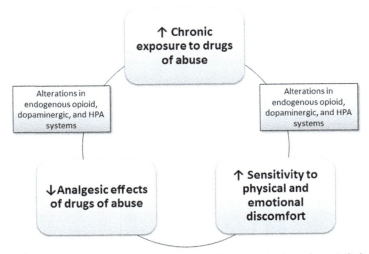

Figure 1 Proposed pathway of cycle through which chronic drug abuse is linked with decreased analgesic properties of the drug and increased sensitivity to physical and emotional discomfort, which leads to further drug abuse. The relationships are probably mediated by multiple central pain- and stress-regulating systems.

emotional states associated with pain, it facilitates the neuroadaptation process, enhancing sensitivity to pain and stress when drug use is terminated. This vicious cycle of addiction, pain, and stress has not been directly tested, and the majority of available data are based on cross-sectional studies. Thus, it is not clear whether chronic exposure to drugs disrupts the endogenous opioid system, dopaminergic pathways, and HPA axis, or if individuals who are predisposed to having heightened sensitivity to pain, drug-related reward, and stress initiate and maintain drug use and develop dependence. Longitudinal studies are warranted to examine the trajectory of substance use, stress vulnerability, and pain sensitivity. Such approach should also lead to an examination of the extent to which substance use and psychosocial stress, independently or interactively, affect psychobiological responses to acute pain as well as identifying those who are more likely to develop chronic pain conditions in the future.

Effects of Drug Withdrawal on Pain

While accumulating evidence indicates the associations between addiction, stress, and pain, more research is warranted to identify specific mechanisms. For instance, the effects of abstinence on stress and pain sensitivity have not been fully characterized. Cessation of drug use induces changes at multiple levels including the HPA axis, dopaminergic pathways, and the cardiovascular system. There is initial evidence to show changes in psychophysiological responses to stress during acute nicotine withdrawal (al'Absi et al., 2003; Nakajima & al'Absi, 2014). Opioid blockade effects on HPA axis activity are attenuated in patients who were in the early phase of alcohol withdrawal (Besirli, Esel, Ozsoy, & Turan, 2014). Alterations in HPA activity have also been reported in opioid withdrawal (Zhang et al., 2008). However, these studies used a cross-sectional design testing influences of withdrawal in between-subject comparisons. It would be fruitful to address this question using repeated assessment of the same individuals across different drug use conditions (e.g., ad libitum drug use, acute drug withdrawal). Such methods should provide better understanding of the subjective and physiological changes due to withdrawal. It is also important to have a rigorous control of drug withdrawal. Self-report and objective (e.g., biomarkers) verification of substance use are desirable to have adequate assessment of withdrawal manipulation. The definition of withdrawal should be carefully determined because it varies across drugs based on factors such as use pattern of the drug (e.g., accessibility) and metabolism. The duration of a laboratory session could potentially confound the results. For example, one study found that nicotine withdrawal symptoms could develop as soon as after 4 h of abstinence (Morrell, Cohen, & al'Absi, 2008).

Generalization of Laboratory Pain Procedures to Chronic Pain Model

The extent to which experimentally induced pain is generalizable to the chronic pain condition is not clear (Fillingim & Gear, 2004). Some studies have shown effects of pain modality on SIA (al'Absi, Nakajima, et al., 2013; Girdler et al., 2005; Nakajima & al'Absi, 2014). Future research should examine different pain stimuli (e.g., CPT, thermal heat pain, ischemic pain, and electrical pain) and assess the potential usefulness and applicability of these tests to chronic pain models. Also, as described above, the mediating or moderating roles of sex differences, mental health comorbidity, family history of substance abuse, psychosocial factors, and personality traits on addiction, stress vulnerability, and chronic pain are not well understood.

Research on Intervention Related to Addiction, Pain, and Stress

Finally, findings from laboratory studies need to be considered in informing the development of effective treatment strategies and programs. There are some indications that a combination of psychosocial and behavioral interventions and pharmacological treatments could be effective at reducing pain. However, there is very little research to elucidate specific components responsible for these outcomes. Subjective and biological measures that have been shown to be predictive of substance use, stress, and pain from laboratory models should be systematically tested in prevention and intervention programs. For example, one could examine patterns of change in substance use and stress- and pain-related psychobiological measures over the course of psychosocial and/or pharmacological interventions aimed at pain management. The intervention could be targeted at the reduction of stress and/or substance use because both are independently associated with pain symptoms. These models provide opportunities to assess not only the effects of intervention on pain sensitivity but also deterrents and protective factors associated with the intervention. Such models could also help elucidate the extent to which certain psychological or physiological systems normalize through the intervention and improve the outcomes. Results of these could also be helpful in refining models in the laboratory-based studies to inform future therapeutic developments.

In conclusion, drug addiction plays a role in shaping subjective and neurobiological regulation of stress and pain perception. Numerous animal and human studies have shown that chronic drug exposure modifies pain sensitivity through alterations in central circuits responsible for antinociception. These include the endogenous opioid system, HPA stress-regulatory system, and dopaminergic reward pathways. Research is needed to identify causal directions of these relationships. Also, mediators and moderators shown to be promising in laboratory studies should be incorporated to inform the development of prevention and intervention programs and to systematically evaluate their outcomes.

REFERENCES

al'Absi, M. (2006). Hypothalamic-pituitary-adrenocortical responses to psychological stress and risk for smoking relapse. *International Journal of Psychophysiology, 59*(3), 218–227. http://dx.doi.org/10.1016/j.ijpsycho.2005.10.010.

al'Absi, M. (2007). *Stress and addiction: Biological and psychological mechanisms.* London: Academic Press/Elsevier.

al'Absi, M., Bongard, S., Buchanan, T., Pincomb, G., Licinio, J., & Lovallo, W. R. (1997). Neuroendocrine and hemodynamic responses to extended mental and interpersonal stressors. *Psychophysiology, 34,* 266–275.

al'Absi, M., Buchanan, T., & Lovallo, W. R. (1996). Pain perception and cardiovascular responses in men with positive parental history for hypertension. *Psychophysiology, 33*(6), 655–661.

al'Absi, M., Buchanan, T. W., Marrero, A., & Lovallo, W. R. (1999). Sex differences in pain perception and cardiovascular responses in persons with parental history for hypertension. *Pain, 83*(2), 331–338.

al'Absi, M., Carr, S. B., & Bongard, S. (2007). Anger and psychobiological changes during smoking abstinence and in response to acute stress: prediction of smoking relapse. *International Journal of Psychophysiology*, *66*(2), 109–115. http://dx.doi.org/10.1016/j.ijpsycho.2007.03.016.

al'Absi, M., Hatsukami, D., & Davis, G. L. (2005). Attenuated adrenocorticotropic responses to psychological stress are associated with early smoking relapse. *Psychopharmacology (Berlin)*, *181*(1), 107–117. http://dx.doi.org/10.1007/s00213-005-2225-3.

al'Absi, M., Khalil, N. S., Al Habori, M., Hoffman, R., Fujiwara, K., & Wittmers, L. (2013). Effects of chronic khat use on cardiovascular, adrenocortical, and psychological responses to stress in men and women. *The American Journal on Addictions*, *22*(2), 99–107. http://dx.doi.org/10.1111/j.1521-0391.2013.00302.x.

al'Absi, M., Nakajima, M., Allen, S., Lemieux, A., & Hatsukami, D. (2015). Sex differences in hormonal responses to stress and smoking relapse: a prospective examination. *Nicotine & Tobacco Research*.

al'Absi, M., Nakajima, M., Dokam, A., Sameai, A., Alsoofi, M., Saem Khalil, N., et al. (2014). Concurrent tobacco and khat use is associated with blunted cardiovascular stress response and enhanced negative mood: a cross-sectional investigation. *Human Psychopharmacology*. http://dx.doi.org/10.1002/hup.2403.

al'Absi, M., Nakajima, M., & Grabowski, J. (2013). Stress response dysregulation and stress-induced analgesia in nicotine dependent men and women. *Biological Psychology*, *93*(1), 1–8. http://dx.doi.org/10.1016/j.biopsycho.2012.12.007.

al'Absi, M., & Petersen, K. L. (2003). Blood pressure but not cortisol mediates stress effects on subsequent pain perception in healthy men and women. *Pain*, *106*(3), 285–295.

al'Absi, M., Petersen, K. L., & Wittmers, L. E. (2000). Blood pressure but not parental history for hypertension predicts pain perception in women. *Pain*, *88*(1), 61–68.

al'Absi, M., Petersen, K. L., & Wittmers, L. E. (2002). Adrenocortical and hemodynamic predictors of pain perception in men and women. *Pain*, *96*(1–2), 197–204.

al'Absi, M., Wittmers, L. E., Ellestad, D., Nordehn, G., Kim, S. W., Kirschbaum, C., et al. (2004). Sex differences in pain and hypothalamic-pituitary-adrenocortical responses to opioid blockade. *Psychosomatic Medicine*, *66*(2), 198–206.

al'Absi, M., Wittmers, L. E., Erickson, J., Hatsukami, D., & Crouse, B. (2003). Attenuated adrenocortical and blood pressure responses to psychological stress in ad libitum and abstinent smokers. *Pharmacology Biochemistry & Behavior*, *74*(2), 401–410.

al'Absi, M., Wittmers, L. E., Hatsukami, D., & Westra, R. (2008). Blunted opiate modulation of hypothalamic-pituitary-adrenocortical activity in men and women who smoke. *Psychosomatic Medicine*, *70*(8), 928–935. http://dx.doi.org/10.1097/PSY.0b013e31818434ab.

Agrawal, A., Budney, A. J., & Lynskey, M. T. (2012). The co-occurring use and misuse of cannabis and tobacco: a review. *Addiction*, *107*(7), 1221–1233. http://dx.doi.org/10.1111/j.1360-0443.2012.03837.x.

Allen, A. M., al'Absi, M., Lando, H., & Allen, S. S. (2015). Allopregnanolone association with psychophysiological and cognitive functions during acute smoking abstinence in premenopausal women. *Experimental and Clinical Psychopharmacology*, *23*(1), 22–28. http://dx.doi.org/10.1037/a0038747.

Anderson, K. L., Pinkerton, K. E., Uyeminami, D., Simons, C. T., Carstens, M. I., & Carstens, E. (2004). Antinociception induced by chronic exposure of rats to cigarette smoke. *Neuroscience Letters*, *366*(1), 86–91.

Andersson, H., Ejlertsson, G., & Leden, I. (1998). Widespread musculoskeletal chronic pain associated with smoking. An epidemiological study in a general rural population. *Scandinavian Journal of Rehabilitation Medicine*, *30*(3), 185–191.

Anker, J. J., & Carroll, M. E. (2010a). Sex differences in the effects of allopregnanolone on yohimbine-induced reinstatement of cocaine seeking in rats. *Drug and Alcohol Dependence*, *107*(2–3), 264–267. http://dx.doi.org/10.1016/j.drugalcdep.2009.11.002.

Anker, J. J., & Carroll, M. E. (2010b). The role of progestins in the behavioral effects of cocaine and other drugs of abuse: human and animal research. *Neuroscience and Biobehavioral Reviews, 35*(2), 315–333. http://dx.doi.org/10.1016/j.neubiorev.2010.04.003.

Baggio, S., Studer, J., Mohler-Kuo, M., Daeppen, J. B., & Gmel, G. (2014). Concurrent and simultaneous polydrug use among young Swiss males: use patterns and associations of number of substances used with health issues. *International Journal of Adolescent Medicine and Health, 26*(2), 217–224. http://dx.doi.org/10.1515/ijamh-2013-0305.

Bair, M. J., Robinson, R. L., Katon, W., & Kroenke, K. (2003). Depression and pain comorbidity: a literature review. *Archives of Internal Medicine, 163*(20), 2433–2445. http://dx.doi.org/10.1001/archinte.163.20.2433.

Bannon, A. W., Decker, M. W., Holladay, M. W., Curzon, P., Donnelly-Roberts, D., Puttfarcken, P. S., et al. (1998). Broad-spectrum, non-opioid analgesic activity by selective modulation of neuronal nicotinic acetylcholine receptors. *Science, 279*(5347), 77–81.

Bartley, E. J., & Fillingim, R. B. (2013). Sex differences in pain: a brief review of clinical and experimental findings. *British Journal of Anaesthesia, 111*(1), 52–58. http://dx.doi.org/10.1093/bja/aet127.

Becker, S., Gandhi, W., & Schweinhardt, P. (2012). Cerebral interactions of pain and reward and their relevance for chronic pain. *Neuroscience Letters, 520*(2), 182–187. http://dx.doi.org/10.1016/j.neulet.2012.03.013.

Benowitz, N. L. (1988). Drug therapy. Pharmacologic aspects of cigarette smoking and nicotine addition. *The New England Journal of Medicine, 319*(20), 1318–1330.

Benowitz, N. L. (2010). Nicotine addiction. *The New England Journal of Medicine, 362*(24), 2295–2303.

Bernardy, N. C., King, A. C., Parsons, O. A., & Lovallo, W. R. (1996). Altered cortisol response in sober alcoholics: an examination of contributing factors. *Alcohol, 13*(5), 493–498.

Besirli, A., Esel, E., Ozsoy, S., & Turan, T. (2014). Hypothalamic-pituitary-adrenal axis response to oral naltrexone in alcoholics during early withdrawal. *Pharmacopsychiatry, 47*(4–5), 151–155. http://dx.doi.org/10.1055/s-0034-1381983.

Bobzean, S. A., DeNobrega, A. K., & Perrotti, L. I. (2014). Sex differences in the neurobiology of drug addiction. *Experimental Neurology, 259*, 64–74. http://dx.doi.org/10.1016/j.expneurol.2014.01.022.

Brage, S., & Bjerkedal, T. (1996). Musculoskeletal pain and smoking in Norway. *Journal of Epidemiology and Community Health, 50*(2), 166–169.

Brennan, P. L., Schutte, K. K., & Moos, R. H. (2005). Pain and use of alcohol to manage pain: prevalence and 3-year outcomes among older problem and non-problem drinkers. *Addiction, 100*(6), 777–786. http://dx.doi.org/10.1111/j.1360-0443.2005.01074.x.

Brown, R. A., Lejuez, C. W., Kahler, C. W., Strong, D. R., & Zvolensky, M. J. (2005). Distress tolerance and early smoking lapse. *Clinical Psychology Review, 25*(6), 713–733.

Butler, R. K., & Finn, D. P. (2009). Stress-induced analgesia. *Progress in Neurobiology, 88*(3), 184–202.

Carpenter, M. J., Upadhyaya, H. P., LaRowe, S. D., Saladin, M. E., & Brady, K. T. (2006). Menstrual cycle phase effects on nicotine withdrawal and cigarette craving: a review. *Nicotine & Tobacco Research, 8*, 627–638. England.

Chong, R. Y., Uhart, M., & Wand, G. S. (2007). Endogenous opiates, addiction, and stress response. In M. al'Absi (Ed.), *Stress and addiction: Biological and psychological mechanisms* (pp. 85–104). London: Academic Press/Elsevier.

Cohen, S., & Lichtenstein, E. (1990). Perceived stress, quitting smoking, and smoking relapse. *Health Psychology, 9*(4), 466–478.

Croissant, B., & Olbrich, R. (2004). Stress response dampening indexed by cortisol in subjects at risk for alcoholism. *Journal of Studies on Alcohol, 65*(6), 701–707.

Dawes, M. A., Dorn, L. D., Moss, H. B., Yao, J. K., Kirisci, L., Ammerman, R. T., et al. (1999). Hormonal and behavioral homeostasis in boys at risk for substance abuse. *Drug and Alcohol Dependence, 55*(1–2), 165–176.

Dekkers, J. C., Geenen, R., Godaert, G. L., Glaudemans, K. A., Lafeber, F. P., van Doornen, L. J., et al. (2001). Experimentally challenged reactivity of the hypothalamic pituitary adrenal axis in patients with recently diagnosed rheumatoid arthritis. *The Journal of Rheumatology, 28*(7), 1496–1504.

Dhatt, R. K., Gudehithlu, K. P., Wemlinger, T. A., Tejwani, G. A., Neff, N. H., & Hadjiconstantinou, M. (1995). Preproenkephalin mRNA and methionine-enkephalin content are increased in mouse striatum after treatment with nicotine. *Journal of Neurochemistry, 64*(4), 1878–1883.

Dicken, C. (1978). Sex roles, smoking, and smoking cessation. *Journal of Health and Social Behavior, 19*(3), 324–334.

Dinan, T. G., Quigley, E. M., Ahmed, S. M., Scully, P., O'Brien, S., O'Mahony, L., et al. (2006). Hypothalamic-pituitary-gut axis dysregulation in irritable bowel syndrome: plasma cytokines as a potential biomarker? *Gastroenterology, 130*(2), 304–311. http://dx.doi.org/10.1053/j.gastro.2005.11.033.

Ditre, J. W., & Brandon, T. H. (2008). Pain as a motivator of smoking: effects of pain induction on smoking urge and behavior. *Journal of Abnormal Psychology, 117*(2), 467–472.

Ditre, J. W., Brandon, T. H., Zale, E. L., & Meagher, M. M. (2011). Pain, nicotine, and smoking: research findings and mechanistic considerations. *Psychological Bulletin, 137*(6), 1065–1093.

D'Angelo, M. E., Reid, R. D., Brown, K. S., & Pipe, A. L. (2001). Gender differences in predictors for long-term smoking cessation following physician advice and nicotine replacement therapy. *Canadian Journal of Public Health, 92*(6), 418–422.

Edwards, R. R., Wasan, A. D., Michna, E., Greenbaum, S., Ross, E., & Jamison, R. N. (2011). Elevated pain sensitivity in chronic pain patients at risk for opioid misuse. *The Journal of Pain, 12*(9), 953–963. http://dx.doi.org/10.1016/j.jpain.2011.02.357.

Egli, M., Koob, G. F., & Edwards, S. (2012). Alcohol dependence as a chronic pain disorder. *Neuroscience & Biobehavioral Reviews, 36*(10), 2179–2192. http://dx.doi.org/10.1016/j.neubiorev.2012.07.010.

Eijsbouts, A. M., van den Hoogen, F. H., Laan, R. F., Hermus, A. R., Sweep, C. G., & van de Putte, L. B. (2005). Hypothalamic-pituitary-adrenal axis activity in patients with rheumatoid arthritis. *Clinical and Experimental Rheumatology, 23*(5), 658–664.

Ekholm, O., Gronbaek, M., Peuckmann, V., & Sjogren, P. (2009). Alcohol and smoking behavior in chronic pain patients: the role of opioids. *European Journal of Pain, 13*(6), 606–612. http://dx.doi.org/10.1016/j.ejpain.2008.07.006.

Eriksen, M., Mackay, J., & Ross, H. (2012). *The tobacco atlas* (4th ed.). Atlanta, GA: American Cancer Society, and New York, NY: World Lung Foundation.

Eriksen, J., Sjogren, P., Bruera, E., Ekholm, O., & Rasmussen, N. K. (2006). Critical issues on opioids in chronic non-cancer pain: an epidemiological study. *Pain, 125*(1–2), 172–179. http://dx.doi.org/10.1016/j.pain.2006.06.009.

Errico, A. L., Parsons, O. A., King, A. C., & Lovallo, W. R. (1993). Attenuated cortisol response to biobehavioral stressors in sober alcoholics. *Journal of Studies on Alcohol, 54*(4), 393–398.

Fatseas, M., Denis, C., Massida, Z., Verger, M., Franques-Reneric, P., & Auriacombe, M. (2011). Cue-induced reactivity, cortisol response and substance use outcome in treated heroin dependent individuals. *Biological Psychiatry, 70*(8), 720–727. http://dx.doi.org/10.1016/j.biopsych.2011.05.015.

Fertig, J. B., Pomerleau, O. F., & Sanders, B. (1986). Nicotine-produced antinociception in minimally deprived smokers and ex-smokers. *Addictive Behaviors, 11*(3), 239–248.

File, S. E., Dinnis, A. K., Heard, J. E., & Irvine, E. E. (2002). Mood differences between male and female light smokers and nonsmokers. *Pharmacology Biochemistry & Behavior*, 72(3), 681–689.

Fillingim, R. B., & Gear, R. W. (2004). Sex differences in opioid analgesia: clinical and experimental findings. *European Journal of Pain*, 8(5), 413–425.

Fischer, B., Lusted, A., Roerecke, M., Taylor, B., & Rehm, J. (2012). The prevalence of mental health and pain symptoms in general population samples reporting nonmedical use of prescription opioids: a systematic review and meta-analysis. *The Journal of Pain*, 13(11), 1029–1044. http://dx.doi.org/10.1016/j.jpain.2012.07.013.

Fox, H. C., Sofuoglu, M., Morgan, P. T., Tuit, K. L., & Sinha, R. (2013). The effects of exogenous progesterone on drug craving and stress arousal in cocaine dependence: impact of gender and cue type. *Psychoneuroendocrinology*, 38(9), 1532–1544. http://dx.doi.org/10.1016/j.psyneuen.2012.12.022.

Fox, H. C., Tuit, K. L., & Sinha, R. (2013). Stress system changes associated with marijuana dependence may increase craving for alcohol and cocaine. *Human Psychopharmacology*, 28(1), 40–53. http://dx.doi.org/10.1002/hup.2280.

France, C. R. (1999). Decreased pain perception and risk for hypertension: considering a common physiological mechanism. *Psychophysiology*, 36(6), 683–692.

France, C. R., & Stewart, K. M. (1995). Parental history of hypertension and enhanced cardiovascular reactivity are associated with decreased pain ratings. *Psychophysiology*, 52, 571–578.

Fukudo, S., Nomura, T., & Hongo, M. (1998). Impact of corticotropin-releasing hormone on gastrointestinal motility and adrenocorticotropic hormone in normal controls and patients with irritable bowel syndrome. *Gut*, 42(6), 845–849.

Gambassi, G. (2009). Pain and depression: the egg and the chicken story revisited. *Archives of Gerontology and Geriatrics*, 49(Suppl. 1), 103–112. http://dx.doi.org/10.1016/j.archger.2009.09.018.

Garland, E. L., Froeliger, B., Zeidan, F., Partin, K., & Howard, M. O. (2013). The downward spiral of chronic pain, prescription opioid misuse, and addiction: cognitive, affective, and neuropsychopharmacologic pathways. *Neuroscience & Biobehavioral Reviews*, 37(10 Pt 2), 2597–2607. http://dx.doi.org/10.1016/j.neubiorev.2013.08.006.

Geiss, A., Rohleder, N., & Anton, F. (2012). Evidence for an association between an enhanced reactivity of interleukin-6 levels and reduced glucocorticoid sensitivity in patients with fibromyalgia. *Psychoneuroendocrinology*, 37(5), 671–684. http://dx.doi.org/10.1016/j.psyneuen.2011.07.021.

Generaal, E., Vogelzangs, N., Macfarlane, G. J., Geenen, R., Smit, J. H., Penninx, B. W., et al. (2014). Reduced hypothalamic-pituitary-adrenal axis activity in chronic multi-site musculoskeletal pain: partly masked by depressive and anxiety disorders. *BMC Musculoskeletal Disorders*, 15, 227. http://dx.doi.org/10.1186/1471-2474-15-227.

Ghione, S. (1996). Hypertension-associated hypalgesia. Evidence in experimental animals and humans, pathophysiological mechanisms, and potential clinical consequences. *Hypertension*, 28(3), 494–504.

Girdler, S. S., Maixner, W., Naftel, H. A., Stewart, P. W., Moretz, R. L., & Light, K. C. (2005). Cigarette smoking, stress-induced analgesia and pain perception in men and women. *Pain*, 114(3), 372–385. http://dx.doi.org/10.1016/j.pain.2004.12.035.

Grunberg, N. E., Winders, S. E., & Wewers, M. E. (1991). Gender differences in tobacco use. *Health Psychology*, 10(2), 143–153.

Guasti, L., Zanotta, D., Mainardi, L. T., Petrozzino, M. R., Grimoldi, P., Garganico, D., et al. (2002). Hypertension-related hypoalgesia, autonomic function and spontaneous baroreflex sensitivity. *Autonomic Neuroscience*, 99(2), 127–133.

Gureje, O. (2008). Comorbidity of pain and anxiety disorders. *Current Psychiatry Reports*, 10(4), 318–322.

Hagg, O., Fritzell, P., & Nordwall, A. (2002). Characteristics of patients with chronic low back pain selected for surgery: a comparison with the general population reported from the Swedish lumbar spine study. *Spine (Phila Pa 1976), 27*(11), 1223–1231.

Haghparast, A., Khani, A., Naderi, N., Alizadeh, A. M., & Motamedi, F. (2008). Repeated administration of nicotine attenuates the development of morphine tolerance and dependence in mice. *Pharmacology Biochemistry & Behavior, 88*(4), 385–392. http://dx.doi.org/10.1016/j.pbb.2007.09.010.

Hartz, S. M., Pato, C. N., Medeiros, H., Cavazos-Rehg, P., Sobell, J. L., Knowles, J. A., et al. (2014). Comorbidity of severe psychotic disorders with measures of substance use. *JAMA Psychiatry, 71*(3), 248–254. http://dx.doi.org/10.1001/jamapsychiatry.2013.3726.

Heim, C., Ehlert, U., Hanker, J. P., & Hellhammer, D. H. (1998). Abuse-related post-traumatic stress disorder and alterations of the hypothalamic-pituitary-adrenal axis in women with chronic pelvic pain. *Psychosomatic Medicine, 60*(3), 309–318.

Helmerhorst, G. T., Vranceanu, A. M., Vrahas, M., Smith, M., & Ring, D. (2014). Risk factors for continued opioid use one to two months after surgery for musculoskeletal trauma. *The Journal of Bone and Joint Surgery, 96*(6), 495–499. http://dx.doi.org/10.2106/jbjs.l.01406.

Jakobsson, U. (2008). Tobacco use in relation to chronic pain: results from a Swedish population survey. *Pain Medicine, 9*(8), 1091–1097. http://dx.doi.org/10.1111/j.1526-4637.2008.00473.x.

Jamison, R. N., & Edwards, R. R. (2013). Risk factor assessment for problematic use of opioids for chronic pain. *The Clinical Neuropsychologist, 27*(1), 60–80. http://dx.doi.org/10.1080/13854046.2012.715204.

Jamison, R. N., Link, C. L., & Marceau, L. D. (2009). Do pain patients at high risk for substance misuse experience more pain? A longitudinal outcomes study. *Pain Medicine, 10*(6), 1084–1094. http://dx.doi.org/10.1111/j.1526-4637.2009.00679.x.

Jamison, R. N., Stetson, B. A., & Parris, W. C. (1991). The relationship between cigarette smoking and chronic low back pain. *Addictive Behaviors, 16*(3–4), 103–110.

Jamner, L. D., Girdler, S. S., Shapiro, D., & Jarvik, M. E. (1998). Pain inhibition, nicotine, and gender. *Experimental and Clinical Psychopharmacology, 6*(1), 96–106.

Janssen, S. A., Spinhoven, P., & Brosschot, J. F. (2001). Experimentally induced anger, cardiovascular reactivity, and pain sensitivity. *Journal of Psychosomatic Research, 51*(3), 479–485.

Jochum, T., Boettger, M. K., Burkhardt, C., Juckel, G., & Bar, K. J. (2010). Increased pain sensitivity in alcohol withdrawal syndrome. *European Journal of Pain, 14*(7), 713–718. http://dx.doi.org/10.1016/j.ejpain.2009.11.008.

Junghanns, K., Backhaus, J., Tietz, U., Lange, W., Bernzen, J., Wetterling, T., et al. (2003). Impaired serum cortisol stress response is a predictor of early relapse. *Alcohol and Alcoholism, 38*(2), 189–193.

Junghanns, K., Tietz, U., Dibbelt, L., Kuether, M., Jurth, R., Ehrenthal, D., et al. (2005). Attenuated salivary cortisol secretion under cue exposure is associated with early relapse. *Alcohol and Alcoholism, 40*(1), 80–85.

Kanarek, R. B., & Carrington, C. (2004). Sucrose consumption enhances the analgesic effects of cigarette smoking in male and female smokers. *Psychopharmacology (Berlin), 173*(1–2), 57–63.

Kassel, J. D., Stroud, L. R., & Paronis, C. A. (2003). Smoking, stress, and negative affect: correlation, causation, and context across stages of smoking. *Psychological Bulletin, 129*(2), 270–304.

Khantzian, E. J. (1997). The self-medication hypothesis of substance use disorders: a reconsideration and recent applications. *Harvard Review of Psychiatry, 4*(5), 231–244. http://dx.doi.org/10.3109/10673229709030550.

Kirschbaum, C., Strasburger, C. J., & Langkrar, J. (1993). Attenuated cortisol response to psychological stress but not to CRH or ergometry in young habitual smokers. *Pharmacology Biochemistry & Behavior, 44*(3), 527–531.

Kishioka, S., Kiguchi, N., Kobayashi, Y., & Saika, F. (2014). Nicotine effects and the endogenous opioid system. *Journal of Pharmacological Sciences, 125*(2), 117–124.

Koob, G. F., & Le Moal, M. (1997). Drug abuse: hedonic homeostatic dysregulation. *Science, 278*(5335), 52–58.

Kreek, M. J., & Koob, G. F. (1998). Drug dependence: stress and dysregulation of brain reward pathways. *Drug and Alcohol Dependence, 51*(1–2), 23–47.

Lariviere, W. R., & Melzack, R. (2000). The role of corticotropin-releasing factor in pain and analgesia. *Pain, 84*(1), 1–12.

Lazarus, R. S., & Folkman, S. (1984). *Stress, appraisal, and coping.* New York: Springer Publishing Company.

Lepine, J. P., & Briley, M. (2004). The epidemiology of pain in depression. *Human Psychopharmacology, 19*(Suppl. 1), S3–S7. http://dx.doi.org/10.1002/hup.618.

Lovallo, W. R. (2004). *Stress & health : Biological and psychological interactions.* Thousand Oaks, CA.

Lovallo, W. R. (2006). Cortisol secretion patterns in addiction and addiction risk. *The International Journal of Psychophysiology, 59*(3), 195–202.

Lovallo, W. (2007). Individual differences in response to stress and risk for addiction. In M. al'Absi (Ed.), *Stress and addiction: Biological and psychological mechanisms* (pp. 265–284). London: Academic Press/Elsevier.

Lovallo, W. R., Dickensheets, S. L., Myers, D. A., Thomas, T. L., & Nixon, S. J. (2000). Blunted stress cortisol response in abstinent alcoholic and polysubstance-abusing men. *Alcoholism: Clinical and Experimental Research, 24*(5), 651–658.

Lundberg, U. (1999). Stress responses in low-status jobs and their relationship to health risks: musculoskeletal disorders. *Annals of the New York Academy of Sciences, 896*, 162–172.

Macey, T. A., Morasco, B. J., Duckart, J. P., & Dobscha, S. K. (2011). Patterns and correlates of prescription opioid use in OEF/OIF veterans with chronic noncancer pain. *Pain Medicine, 12*(10), 1502–1509. http://dx.doi.org/10.1111/j.1526-4637.2011.01226.x.

Mansour, A., Khachaturian, H., Lewis, M. E., Akil, H., & Watson, S. J. (1988). Anatomy of CNS opioid receptors. *Trends in Neurosciences, 11*, 308–314.

Marinelli, M. (2007). Dopaminergic reward pathways and effects of stress. In M. al'Absi (Ed.), *Stress and addiction: Biological and psychological mechanisms* (pp. 41–83). London: Academic Press/Elsevier.

Marx, C. E., Trost, W. T., Shampine, L., Behm, F. M., Giordano, L. A., Massing, M. W., et al. (2006). Neuroactive steroids, negative affect, and nicotine dependence severity in male smokers. *Psychopharmacology (Berlin), 186*(3), 462–472. http://dx.doi.org/10.1007/s00213-005-0226-x.

Maxwell, J. C. (2011). The prescription drug epidemic in the United States: a perfect storm. *Drug and Alcohol Review, 30*(3), 264–270. http://dx.doi.org/10.1111/j.1465-3362.2011.00291.x.

McEwen, B. S. (1998). Protective and damaging effects of stress mediators. *The New England Journal of Medicine, 338*, 171–179.

McKee, S. A., Maciejewski, P. K., Falba, T., & Mazure, C. M. (2003). Sex differences in the effects of stressful life events on changes in smoking status. *Addiction, 98*(6), 847–855.

McWilliams, L. A., Cox, B. J., & Enns, M. W. (2003). Mood and anxiety disorders associated with chronic pain: an examination in a nationally representative sample. *Pain, 106*(1–2), 127–133.

Melzack, R. (1975). The McGill pain questionnaire: major properties and scoring methods. *Pain, 1*, 277–299.

Morrell, H. E., Cohen, L. M., & al'Absi, M. (2008). Physiological and psychological symptoms and predictors in early nicotine withdrawal. *Pharmacology Biochemistry & Behavior, 89*(3), 272–278. http://dx.doi.org/10.1016/j.pbb.2007.12.020.

Moss, H. B., Vanyukov, M., Yao, J. K., & Kirillova, G. P. (1999). Salivary cortisol responses in prepubertal boys: the effects of parental substance abuse and association with drug use behavior during adolescence. *Biological Psychiatry, 45*(10), 1293–1299.

Mostoufi, S., Godfrey, K. M., Ahumada, S. M., Hossain, N., Song, T., Wright, L. J., et al. (2014). Pain sensitivity in posttraumatic stress disorder and other anxiety disorders: a preliminary case control study. *Annals of General Psychiatry, 13*(1), 31. http://dx.doi.org/10.1186/s12991-014-0031-1.

Mousa, S. A., Aloyo, V. J., & Van Loon, G. R. (1988). Tolerance to tobacco smoke- and nicotine-induced analgesia in rats. *Pharmacology Biochemistry & Behavior, 31*(2), 265–268.

Muhtz, C., Rodriguez-Raecke, R., Hinkelmann, K., Moeller-Bertram, T., Kiefer, F., Wiedemann, K., et al. (2013). Cortisol response to experimental pain in patients with chronic low back pain and patients with major depression. *Pain Medicine, 14*(4), 498–503. http://dx.doi.org/10.1111/j.1526-4637.2012.01514.x.

Nakajima, M., & al'Absi, M. (2011). Enhanced pain perception prior to smoking cessation is associated with early relapse. *Biological Psychology, 88*(1), 141–146. http://dx.doi.org/10.1016/j.biopsycho.2011.07.006.

Nakajima, M., & al'Absi, M. (2012). Predictors of risk for smoking relapse in men and women: a prospective examination. *Psychology of Addictive Behaviors, 26*(3), 633–637. http://dx.doi.org/10.1037/a0027280.

Nakajima, M., & al'Absi, M. (2014). Nicotine withdrawal and stress-induced changes in pain sensitivity: a cross-sectional investigation between abstinent smokers and non-smokers. *Psychophysiology, 51*(10), 1015–1022. http://dx.doi.org/10.1111/psyp.12241.

Nakajima, M., Kumar, S., Wittmers, L., Scott, M. S., & al'Absi, M. (2013). Psychophysiological responses to stress following alcohol intake in social drinkers who are at risk of hazardous drinking. *Biological Psychology, 93*(1), 9–16. http://dx.doi.org/10.1016/j.biopsycho.2012.12.009.

Nesbitt, P. D. (1973). Smoking, physiological arousal, and emotional response. *Journal of Personality and Social Psychology, 25*(1), 137–144.

Nijhof, S. L., Rutten, J. M., Uiterwaal, C. S., Bleijenberg, G., Kimpen, J. L., & Putte, E. M. (2014). The role of hypocortisolism in chronic fatigue syndrome. *Psychoneuroendocrinology, 42*, 199–206. http://dx.doi.org/10.1016/j.psyneuen.2014.01.017.

Ossipov, M. H., Lai, J., King, T., Vanderah, T. W., Malan, T. P., Jr., Hruby, V. J., et al. (2004). Antinociceptive and nociceptive actions of opioids. *Journal of Neurobiology, 61*(1), 126–148. http://dx.doi.org/10.1002/neu.20091.

Palmer, K. T., Syddall, H., Cooper, C., & Coggon, D. (2003). Smoking and musculoskeletal disorders: findings from a British national survey. *Annals of the Rheumatic Diseases, 62*(1), 33–36.

Patacchioli, F. R., Monnazzi, P., Simeoni, S., De Filippis, S., Salvatori, E., Coloprisco, G., et al. (2006). Salivary cortisol, dehydroepiandrosterone-sulphate (DHEA-S) and testosterone in women with chronic migraine. *The Journal of Headache and Pain, 7*(2), 90–94. http://dx.doi.org/10.1007/s10194-006-0274-6.

Perkins, K. A., Jacobs, L., Sanders, M., & Caggiula, A. R. (2002). Sex differences in the subjective and reinforcing effects of cigarette nicotine dose. *Psychopharmacology (Berlin), 163*(2), 194–201. http://dx.doi.org/10.1007/s00213-002-1168-1.

Perkins, K. A., & Scott, J. (2008). Sex differences in long-term smoking cessation rates due to nicotine patch. *Nicotine & Tobacco Research, 10*(7), 1245–1250.

Peters, E. N., Budney, A. J., & Carroll, K. M. (2012). Clinical correlates of co-occurring cannabis and tobacco use: a systematic review. *Addiction, 107*(8), 1404–1417. http://dx.doi.org/10.1111/j.1360-0443.2012.03843.x.

Piazza, P. V., & Le Moal, M. (1998). The role of stress in drug self-administration. *Trends in Pharmacological Sciences, 19*(2), 67–74.

Pisinger, C., Aadahl, M., Toft, U., Birke, H., Zytphen-Adeler, J., & Jorgensen, T. (2011). The association between active and passive smoking and frequent pain in a general population. *European Journal of Pain*, *15*(1), 77–83. http://dx.doi.org/10.1016/j.ejpain.2010.05.004.

Pomerleau, O. F., Turk, D. C., & Fertig, J. B. (1984). The effects of cigarette smoking on pain and anxiety. *Addictive Behaviors*, *9*(3), 265–271.

Pud, D., Cohen, D., Lawental, E., & Eisenberg, E. (2006). Opioids and abnormal pain perception: new evidence from a study of chronic opioid addicts and healthy subjects. *Drug and Alcohol Dependence*, *82*(3), 218–223. http://dx.doi.org/10.1016/j.drugalcdep.2005.09.007.

Randich, A., & Maixner, W. (1984). [D-Ala2]-methionine enkephalinamide reflexively induces antinociception by activating vagal afferents. *Pharmacology Biochemistry & Behavior*, *21*(3), 441–448.

Ren, Z. Y., Shi, J., Epstein, D. H., Wang, J., & Lu, L. (2009). Abnormal pain response in pain-sensitive opiate addicts after prolonged abstinence predicts increased drug craving. *Psychopharmacology (Berlin)*, *204*(3), 423–429. http://dx.doi.org/10.1007/s00213-009-1472-0.

Rhudy, J. L., & Meagher, M. W. (2000). Fear and anxiety: divergent effects on human pain thresholds. *Pain*, *84*(1), 65–75.

Riley, J. L., 3rd, & King, C. (2009). Self-report of alcohol use for pain in a multi-ethnic community sample. *The Journal of Pain*, *10*(9), 944–952. http://dx.doi.org/10.1016/j.jpain.2009.03.005.

Roberts, A. D., Wessely, S., Chalder, T., Papadopoulos, A., & Cleare, A. J. (2004). Salivary cortisol response to awakening in chronic fatigue syndrome. *The British Journal of Psychiatry*, *184*, 136–141.

Roche, D. J., & King, A. C. (2015). Sex differences in acute hormonal and subjective response to naltrexone: the impact of menstrual cycle phase. *Psychoneuroendocrinology*, *52*, 59–71. http://dx.doi.org/10.1016/j.psyneuen.2014.10.013.

Rosenblum, A., Joseph, H., Fong, C., Kipnis, S., Cleland, C., & Portenoy, R. K. (2003). Prevalence and characteristics of chronic pain among chemically dependent patients in methadone maintenance and residential treatment facilities. *JAMA*, *289*(18), 2370–2378. http://dx.doi.org/10.1001/jama.289.18.2370.

Rouge-Pont, F., Deroche, V., Le, M. M., & Piazza, P. V. (1998). Individual differences in stress-induced dopamine release in the nucleus accumbens are influenced by corticosterone. *European Journal of Neuroscience*, *10*(12), 3903–3907.

Rouge-Pont, F., Marinelli, M., Le, M. M., Simon, H., & Piazza, P. V. (1995). Stress-induced sensitization and glucocorticoids. II. Sensitization of the increase in extracellular dopamine induced by cocaine depends on stress-induced corticosterone secretion. *Journal of Neuroscience*, *15*(11), 7189–7195.

Roy, M. P., Steptoe, A., & Kirschbaum, C. (1994). Association between smoking status and cardiovascular and cortisol stress responsivity in healthy young men. *International Journal of Behavioral Medicine*, *1*(3), 264–283.

SAMHSA. (2014). *Results from the 2013 national survey on drug use and health: Summary of national findings (Vol. NSDUH series H-48, HHS)*. Rockville, MD: Substance Abuse and Mental Health Services Administration.

Scanlon, M. N., Lazar-Wesley, E., Grant, K. A., & Kunos, G. (1992). Proopiomelanocortin messenger RNA is decreased in the mediobasal hypothalamus of rats made dependent on ethanol. *Alcoholism: Clinical and Experimental Research*, *16*(6), 1147–1151.

Scott, S. C., Goldberg, M. S., Mayo, N. E., Stock, S. R., & Poitras, B. (1999). The association between cigarette smoking and back pain in adults. *Spine (Phila Pa 1976)*, *24*(11), 1090–1098.

Sehgal, N., Manchikanti, L., & Smith, H. S. (2012). Prescription opioid abuse in chronic pain: a review of opioid abuse predictors and strategies to curb opioid abuse. *Pain Physician, 15*(Suppl. 3), Es67–92.

Shahidi, B., Sannes, T., Laudenslager, M., & Maluf, K. (2015). Cardiovascular responses to an acute psychological stressor are associated with the cortisol awakening response in individuals with chronic neck pain. *Physiology & Behavior.* http://dx.doi.org/10.1016/j.physbeh.2015.02.010.

Sheps, D. S., Maixner, W., Hinderliter, A. L., Herbst, M. C., Bragdon, E. E., Herdt, J., et al. (1989). Relationship between systolic blood pressure, ventricular volume and ischemic pain perception in patients with angina pectoris: a potential role for baroreceptors. *Israel Journal of Medical Sciences, 25*(9), 482–487.

Shiffman, S., Paty, J. A., Gnys, M., Kassel, J. A., & Hickcox, M. (1996). First lapses to smoking: within-subjects analysis of real-time reports. *Journal of Consulting and Clinical Psychology, 64*(2), 366–379.

Shiri, R., Karppinen, J., Leino-Arjas, P., Solovieva, S., & Viikari-Juntura, E. (2010). The association between smoking and low back pain: a meta-analysis. *The American Journal of Medicine, 123*(1), 87.e7–87.e35. http://dx.doi.org/10.1016/j.amjmed.2009.05.028.

Shi, Y., Weingarten, T. N., Mantilla, C. B., Hooten, W. M., & Warner, D. O. (2010). Smoking and pain: pathophysiology and clinical implications. *Anesthesiology, 113*(4), 977–992.

Silverstein, B. (1982). Cigarette smoking, nicotine addiction, and relaxation. *Journal of Personality and Social Psychology, 42*(5), 946–950.

Sinha, R. (2008). Chronic stress, drug use, and vulnerability to addiction. *Annals of the New York Academy of Sciences, 1141*, 105–130.

Sinha, R., Fox, H. C., Hong, K. I., Hansen, J., Tuit, K., & Kreek, M. J. (2011). Effects of adrenal sensitivity, stress- and cue-induced craving, and anxiety on subsequent alcohol relapse and treatment outcomes. *Archives of General Psychiatry, 68*(9), 942–952. http://dx.doi.org/10.1001/archgenpsychiatry.2011.49.

Sinha, R., Garcia, M., Paliwal, P., Kreek, M. J., & Rounsaville, B. J. (2006). Stress-induced cocaine craving and hypothalamic-pituitary-adrenal responses are predictive of cocaine relapse outcomes. *Archives of General Psychiatry, 63*(3), 324–331. http://dx.doi.org/10.1001/archpsyc.63.3.324.

Slopen, N., Dutra, L. M., Williams, D. R., Mujahid, M. S., Lewis, T. T., Bennett, G. G., et al. (2012). Psychosocial stressors and cigarette smoking among African American adults in midlife. *Nicotine & Tobacco Research, 14*(10), 1161–1169. http://dx.doi.org/10.1093/ntr/nts011.

Sorocco, K. H., Lovallo, W. R., Vincent, A. S., & Collins, F. L. (2006). Blunted hypothalamic-pituitary-adrenocortical axis responsivity to stress in persons with a family history of alcoholism. *The International Journal of Psychophysiology, 59*(3), 210–217.

Straneva, P., Hinderliter, A., Wells, E., Lenahan, H., & Girdler, S. (2000). Smoking, oral contraceptives, and cardiovascular reactivity to stress. *Obstetrics & Gynecology, 95*(1), 78–83.

Swan, G. E., Ward, M. M., Jack, L. M., & Javitz, H. S. (1993). Cardiovascular reactivity as a predictor of relapse in male and female smokers. *Health Psychology, 12*(6), 451–458.

Theorell, T., Hasselhorn, H. M., Vingrd, E., & Andersson, B. (2000). Interleukin 6 and cortisol in acute musculoskeletal disorders: results from a case-referent study in Sweden. *Stress Medicine, 16*, 27–35.

Tidey, J. W., & Miczek, K. A. (1997). Acquisition of cocaine self-administration after social stress: role of accumbens dopamine. *Psychopharmacology (Berlin), 130*(3), 203–212.

Trafton, J. A., Oliva, E. M., Horst, D. A., Minkel, J. D., & Humphreys, K. (2004). Treatment needs associated with pain in substance use disorder patients: implications for concurrent treatment. *Drug and Alcohol Dependence, 73*(1), 23–31.

Tsui, J. I., Cheng, D. M., Coleman, S. M., Blokhina, E., Bridden, C., Krupitsky, E., et al. (2013). Pain is associated with heroin use over time in HIV-infected Russian drinkers. *Addiction, 108*(10), 1779–1787. http://dx.doi.org/10.1111/add.12274.

Tsui, J. I., Cheng, D. M., Coleman, S. M., Lira, M. C., Blokhina, E., Bridden, C., et al. (2014). Pain is associated with risky drinking over time among HIV-infected persons in St. Petersburg, Russia. *Drug and Alcohol Dependence, 144*, 87–92. http://dx.doi.org/10.1016/j.drugalcdep.2014.08.013.

Uhart, M., Oswald, L., McCaul, M. E., Chong, R., & Wand, G. S. (2006). Hormonal responses to psychological stress and family history of alcoholism. *Neuropsychopharmacology, 31*(10), 2255–2263.

Uhart, M., & Wand, G. S. (2009). Stress, alcohol and drug interaction: an update of human research. *Addiction Biology, 14*(1), 43–64.

UNODC. (2012). *World drug report 2012: United Nations publication, sales No. E.12.XI.1.*

Van Bockstaele, E. J., Reyes, B. A., & Valentino, R. J. (2010). The locus coeruleus: a key nucleus where stress and opioids intersect to mediate vulnerability to opiate abuse. *Brain Research, 1314*, 162–174. http://dx.doi.org/10.1016/j.brainres.2009.09.036.

Vengeliene, V., Bilbao, A., Molander, A., & Spanagel, R. (2008). Neuropharmacology of alcohol addiction. *British Journal of Pharmacology, 154*(2), 299–315. http://dx.doi.org/10.1038/bjp.2008.30.

Wand, G. S., Mangold, D., El Deiry, S., McCaul, M. E., & Hoover, D. (1998). Family history of alcoholism and hypothalamic opioidergic activity. *Archives of General Psychiatry, 55*(12), 1114–1119.

Ward, K. D., Klesges, R. C., Zbikowski, S. M., Bliss, R. E., & Garvey, A. J. (1997). Gender differences in the outcome of an unaided smoking cessation attempt. *Addictive Behaviors, 22*(4), 521–533.

Webb, M. S., & Carey, M. P. (2008). Tobacco smoking among low-income Black women: demographic and psychosocial correlates in a community sample. *Nicotine & Tobacco Research, 10*(1), 219–229. http://dx.doi.org/10.1080/14622200701767845.

Weinberger, A. H., Pilver, C. E., Hoff, R. A., Mazure, C. M., & McKee, S. A. (2013). Changes in smoking for adults with and without alcohol and drug use disorders: longitudinal evaluation in the US population. *The American Journal of Drug and Alcohol Abuse, 39*(3), 186–193. http://dx.doi.org/10.3109/00952990.2013.785557.

Weinberger, A. H., & Sofuoglu, M. (2009). The impact of cigarette smoking on stimulant addiction. *The American Journal of Drug and Alcohol Abuse, 35*(1), 12–17. http://dx.doi.org/10.1080/00952990802326280.

Wetter, D. W., Kenford, S. L., Smith, S. S., Fiore, M. C., Jorenby, D. E., & Baker, T. B. (1999). Gender differences in smoking cessation. *Journal of Consulting and Clinical Psychology, 67*(4), 555–562.

Wewers, M. E., Dhatt, R. K., Snively, T. A., & Tejwani, G. A. (1999). The effect of chronic administration of nicotine on antinociception, opioid receptor binding and met-enkephalin levels in rats. *Brain Research, 822*(1–2), 107–113.

Wilson, J. F. (2007). Strategies to stop abuse of prescribed opioid drugs. *Annals of Internal Medicine, 146*(12), 897–900.

Wingenfeld, K., Heim, C., Schmidt, I., Wagner, D., Meinlschmidt, G., & Hellhammer, D. H. (2008). HPA axis reactivity and lymphocyte glucocorticoid sensitivity in fibromyalgia syndrome and chronic pelvic pain. *Psychosomatic Medicine, 70*(1), 65–72. http://dx.doi.org/10.1097/PSY.0b013e31815ff3ce.

Wingenfeld, K., Hellhammer, D. H., Schmidt, I., Wagner, D., Meinlschmidt, G., & Heim, C. (2009). HPA axis reactivity in chronic pelvic pain: association with depression. *Journal of Psychosomatic Obstetrics and Gynaecology, 30*(4), 282–286. http://dx.doi.org/10.3109/01674820903254732.

Wingenfeld, K., Nutzinger, D., Kauth, J., Hellhammer, D. H., & Lautenbacher, S. (2010). Salivary cortisol release and hypothalamic pituitary adrenal axis feedback sensitivity in fibromyalgia is associated with depression but not with pain. *The Journal of Pain, 11*(11), 1195–1202. http://dx.doi.org/10.1016/j.jpain.2010.02.011.

Zarrindast, M. R., Khoshayand, M. R., & Shafaghi, B. (1999). The development of cross-tolerance between morphine and nicotine in mice. *European Neuropsychopharmacology, 9*(3), 227–233.

Zhang, G. F., Ren, Y. P., Sheng, L. X., Chi, Y., Du, W. J., Guo, S., et al. (2008). Dysfunction of the hypothalamic-pituitary-adrenal axis in opioid dependent subjects: effects of acute and protracted abstinence. *The American Journal of Drug and Alcohol Abuse, 34*(6), 760–768. http://dx.doi.org/10.1080/00952990802385781.

Zimmermann, U., Spring, K., Kunz-Ebrecht, S. R., Uhr, M., Wittchen, H. U., & Holsboer, F. (2004). Effect of ethanol on hypothalamic-pituitary-adrenal system response to psychosocial stress in sons of alcohol-dependent fathers. *Neuropsychopharmacology, 29*(6), 1156–1165.

Zvolensky, M. J., McMillan, K., Gonzalez, A., & Asmundson, G. J. (2009). Chronic pain and cigarette smoking and nicotine dependence among a representative sample of adults. *Nicotine & Tobacco Research, 11*(12), 1407–1414. http://dx.doi.org/10.1093/ntr/ntp153.

Zvolensky, M. J., Stewart, S. H., Vujanovic, A. A., Gavric, D., & Steeves, D. (2009). Anxiety sensitivity and anxiety and depressive symptoms in the prediction of early smoking lapse and relapse during smoking cessation treatment. *Nicotine & Tobacco Research, 11*(3), 323–331.

CHAPTER 11

Pain, Blood Pressure, and Hypertension

Blaine Ditto[1], Kristin Horsley[1], Tavis S. Campbell[2]
[1]Department of Psychology, McGill University, Montreal, QC, Canada; [2]Department of Psychology, University of Calgary, Calgary, AB, Canada

INTRODUCTION

Some of the most fascinating and potentially clinically important interactions related to pain, stress, and emotion involve blood pressure. In large measure, this is due to the bidirectional nature of the pathways. For example, building on the rationale and surgical procedures for pacemakers, there is growing interest in the use of implantable vagus nerve stimulators to reduce demand on the heart in people with heart failure (De Ferrari et al., 2011). At the same time, the cuff electrodes used by these devices stimulate afferent as well as efferent vagal activity. Inhibitory effects on a number of aspects of central nervous system (CNS) function have been observed, and implantable vagus nerve stimulators are now approved for difficult-to-control epilepsy and depression, and a number of other applications are under investigation, including the treatment of chronic pain (Goadsby, Grosberg, Mauskop, Cady, & Simmons, 2014; Multon & Schoenen, 2005). Similarly, blood pressure can be increased by both painful and nonpainful stimuli, and blood pressure elevation due to pain, emotion, or a purely nonemotional physical stimulus can reduce pain in many individuals. This review will address empirical and theoretical aspects of this area including a brief discussion of potential clinical implications such as silent myocardial ischemia (SI) and the development of chronic pain.

HISTORICAL OVERVIEW

Current understanding of the relationships between blood pressure and pain can be traced to innovative experiments in two laboratories in the 1970s. Noting previous anatomical and pharmacological findings suggesting an overlap in brain centers involved in blood pressure regulation and pain,

The Neuroscience of Pain, Stress, and Emotion
http://dx.doi.org/10.1016/B978-0-12-800538-5.00011-X

231

Zamir studied the effects of experimentally induced hypertension in rats (induced by a renal artery clip; restriction of blood flow to a kidney can produce hypertension by activation of the renin–angiotensin–aldosterone system) on responses to a hot plate (Zamir & Segal, 1979). Rats with experimental hypertension displayed significantly delayed paw licking compared to those in two control groups. This hypoalgesia was reduced by administration of the opioid antagonist naloxone and subsequent surgical removal of the stenotic kidney. Zamir also extended this research to humans, finding that unmedicated hypertensive individuals had higher pain threshold levels during electrical stimulation of dental pulp than individuals with normal blood pressure levels (Zamir & Shuber, 1980).

A second line of early research in the area focused more explicitly on feedback of information about systemic blood pressure, building on long-standing speculation about the ability of peripheral blood pressure receptors to influence aspects of CNS function beyond those involved in cardiovascular control (Dworkin, Filewich, Miller, Craigmyle, & Pickering, 1979). Rats with intact or denervated baroreceptors received either a placebo or a blood pressure-elevating drug (phenylephrine) and were placed in a situation in which wheel running could reduce the probability of receiving an electric shock. Phenylephrine significantly reduced wheel running but only in rats with intact baroreceptors. The limitation to rats with intact baroreceptors eliminated some alternative explanations (e.g., drug-induced fatigue) and indicated the importance of baroreflex activity in blood pressure-related modulation of CNS activity. Although the researchers were not specifically interested in the phenomenon of pain (e.g., the effect of blood pressure on wheel running may have been more related to decreased anxiety than pain), they raised the fascinating idea that high blood pressure might be learned response.

These experiments set the stage for many others using similar methods (e.g., animal research using different procedures to produce acute or sustained increases in blood pressure) and issues (e.g., the possible involvement of the baroreflex and endogenous opioid mechanisms). Following its publication in *Science*, the Dworkin (1979) paper was especially influential. On the other hand, it is important to note that this area of study falls within a broader context of interest in the inhibition of psychological function by cardiovascular activity that extends back in time much longer—indeed, for millennia. For example, there are anthropological reports of the use of carotid massage (a sort of early vagus nerve stimulation) for the treatment of insomnia (Schlager & Meier, 1947). Relatedly, in 350 BCE (approximately), Aristotle discussed relationships among variables such as blood flow, body size, alcohol consumption, and sleep (Aristotle, 350 BCE). Anticipating much later research on the impact of blood pressure-related baroreflex stimulation on CNS function, he noted that "persons who have the blood vessels in the neck compressed become insensible." Admittedly, the meaning of the translated word "insensible" is open to interpretation, and even though the topic of the discussion is sleep it could be argued that this was the simple observation that physical disruption of blood flow to the brain can produce unconsciousness (vs a more functional effect). However, he continues "persons whose veins are inconspicuous … are addicted to sleep … (in contrast) those whose veins are large are, thanks to the easy flow through the veins, not addicted to sleep." In describing the results of early experimental evaluations of the carotid baroreflex, Waller (1862) supports this view, stating "It is easily ascertained that the symptoms above described are not owing to compression of the carotid artery, as they may be produced without obliterating the calibre of the artery." Thus, people have been aware of associations among vasoconstriction, increased blood pressure, baroreceptor and vagal stimulation, and CNS inhibition for a very long time.

Many years later, modern psychophysiology was essentially invented in the 1960s, when John Lacey observed that responses to reaction time stimuli varied depending on when the stimulus was administered within the cardiac cycle (Lacey & Lacey, 1978). In particular, he found that participants responded less quickly when the stimulus was presented during the period of maximal baroreceptor stimulation, the systolic phase, as opposed to the diastolic phase. Lacey had the insight to suspect that this curious association reflected an important psychophysiological relationship.

THE BAROREFLEX

While not all of the findings on blood pressure–pain interactions can be explained by the baroreflex, it is important to understand the basics of this key homeostatic reflex. That said, one useful thing to note at the outset is that although this is typically referred to in the singular ("the" baroreflex), pressure-sensitive cells (baroreceptors) are embedded in the walls of arteries in several areas of the body and compensatory responses can be elicited by changes in flow in any area. Indeed, though a common expression, it is even somewhat inaccurate to refer to baroreceptors as pressure-sensitive cells as they do not measure blood pressure per se. Rather, baroreceptors are a subset of mechanoreceptors sensitive to stretch that can be found in many areas outside as well as within the cardiovascular system. However, given the crucial importance of ensuring proper blood flow to the brain, the primary baroreflex circuit begins with baroreceptors located in the aortic arch and carotid sinus (Figure 1).

Information about blood flow in these areas is conveyed to the nucleus of the solitary tract in the medulla by afferents in the vagus and glosso-pharyngeal nerves. If an adjustment to heart rate is required, outgoing vagal activity is adjusted by intermediary centers in the nucleus ambiguus and dorsal motor nucleus. For example, standing up leads to a decrease in baroreceptor stretch and a reduction in outgoing vagal activity to the heart, promoting a compensatory increase in heart rate. Outgoing sympathetic nervous system activity to the heart and blood vessels is also increased. This negative feedback system can dampen sympathetic activity in response to an increase in blood pressure. Of crucial importance in the present context, the inhibition of CNS activity extends beyond processes involved in cardiovascular control. For example, other connections include a number

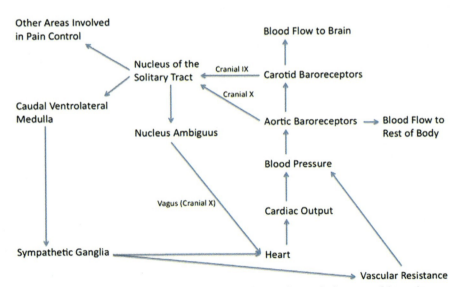

Figure 1 Schematic diagram of the sinoaortic baroreflex including possible pathways to pain control areas. See text for more details.

of areas involved in sensation and pain such as the nucleus raphe magnus, locus coeruleus, and caudal ventrolateral medulla (Randich & Gebhart, 1992).

Highlighting the fact that baroreceptors are "simple" stretch receptors that can have widespread effects on CNS function, it is interesting to note that the system can be misled by an external stimulus into responding as though blood pressure has decreased or increased. For example, though less common in today's culture, "necktie fainting" was not unusual at one time and remains an exclusionary criterion in the clinical evaluation of syncope. That is, external pressure over the carotid sinus can distort blood vessels. Even without an increase in systemic blood pressure, the combination of normal pressure and mechanical distortion can open cation channels and depolarize baroreceptors, triggering "compensatory" heart rate deceleration and vasodilation that may lead to dizziness and perhaps fainting. As will be discussed in more detail later, researchers have taken advantage of the ability to stretch baroreceptors with different pharmacological and physical manipulations.

ANIMAL RESEARCH ON BLOOD PRESSURE-RELATED HYPOALGESIA

Zamir and Dworkin's studies were soon followed by a number of interesting and largely consistent experiments on blood pressure-related hypoalgesia in animals. In addition to acute elevation of blood pressure by phenylephrine (Dworkin et al., 1979) and sustained elevation of blood pressure by attachment of a renal clip (Zamir & Segal, 1979), other models of hypertension produced reduced pain. For example, expansion of blood volume using Ficoll (Maixner & Randich, 1984), deoxycorticosterone acetate (Zamir, Simantov, & Segal, 1980), and dietary sodium loading (Afolabi, Mudashiru, Abdullateef, & Alagbonsi, 2013) decreased sensitivity to several pain stimuli, though some did not observe this effect (Sitsen & de Jong, 1984b) and others found it limited primarily to animals with a genetic predisposition to hypertension (Friedman, Murphy, Persons, & McCaughran, 1984; Randich, 1986).

Research implicating the baroreflex accumulated. For example, Randich and Hartunian (1983) extended Dworkin's findings in several respects. Blood pressure elevation by phenylephrine reduced sensitivity to a more classical pain test (tail flick to radiant heat). The magnitude of the effect was correlated with degree of heart rate deceleration and, once again, eliminated by denervation of the baroreceptors. Comparable results were reported by Maixner and Randich (1984). Electrical stimulation of the nucleus of the solitary tract was found to reduce pain (Aicher & Randich, 1990; Lewis, Baldrighi, & Akil, 1987), and the involvement of descending pain modulation was indicated by the ability of a spinal cold block to eliminate the reduction in pain produced by a surgical procedure (occlusion of the abdominal aorta) that increased blood pressure and baroreflex activity (Thurston & Randich, 1990). Similarly, renal clip hypertension leads to reduced spinal transmission of pain information as indicated by the number of Fos-immunoreactive cells (Lima, Albino-Teixeira, & Tavares, 2002). Lima and colleagues suggest that blood pressure-related hypoalgesia may be due to a circuit involving the nucleus of the solitary tract, the caudal ventrolateral medullary reticular formation, and descending inhibition of spinal pain transmission.

Comparable results were obtained in a large number of studies using a genetic model of hypertension, the spontaneously hypertensive (SHR) rat (Hoffmann, Plesan, & Wiesenfeld-Hallin, 1998; Maixner, Touw, Brody, Gebhart, & Long, 1982; Saavedra, 1981; Sitsen & de Jong, 1984a; Taylor, Roderick, St Lezin, & Basbaum, 2001; Wendel & Bennett, 1981; Zamir et al., 1980). Similar to rats with experimental hypertension, the hypoalgesia of SHR rats appears to depend on having intact baroreceptor connections to the nucleus of the solitary tract (Maixner et al., 1982) and subsequent inhibition of spinal transmission of pain information (Randich & Robertson, 1994).

Perhaps more important, this has been observed *across the age span*, including young, prepubertal SHR rats (Maixner et al., 1982; Saavedra, 1981; Sitsen & de Jong, 1984a; Wendel & Bennett, 1981). While, at first glance, the observation of lower sensitivity to pain in young SHR rats may seem noncontroversial and supportive of the overall picture, it raises what is probably the key theoretical and clinical puzzle in the area, since these rats *do not yet display high blood pressure.*

Thus, the question becomes: does this research area indicate a relationship between blood pressure and pain, a relationship between risk for hypertension and pain, a relationship between cardiovascular control mechanisms and pain, or all of the above? A relationship between risk for hypertension and pain in currently normotensive individuals (as is discussed below, similar results have been obtained in humans) does not preclude the involvement of the baroreflex as part of the process but requires elaboration of the idea.

Another ongoing puzzle is the involvement of endogenous opioids. Hypoalgesia in SHR rats has often been found to be naloxone or naltrexone reversible (e.g., Maixner et al., 1982; Saavedra, 1981; Wendel & Bennett, 1981; Zamir et al., 1980), and other interactions involving opioid activity have been observed. For example, Hoffman et al. (1998) found that SHR rats were more sensitive to the pain–reducing effects of morphine than a comparison group of Wistar-Kyoto rats. Although it is possible that this was due to some peripheral effect of morphine, administration of an opioid blocker that does not cross the blood–brain barrier (N-methylnaloxone) did not reduce hypoalgesia of SHR rats (Sitsen & de Jong, 1984b). In addition, hypoalgesia produced by experimental elevation of blood pressure (Zamir & Segal, 1979; Zamir et al., 1980) and electrical stimulation of the nucleus of the solitary tract (Lewis et al., 1987) has been found to be naloxone reversible. Thus, descending inhibition appears to be at least partly mediated by endogenous opioid activity, though there may be other opioid and nonopioid mechanisms. Previous reviews of this topic cover various aspects of the animal literature (Bruehl & Chung, 2004; Bruehl, McCubbin, & Harden, 1999; France & Ditto, 1996; France, 1999; Ghione, 1996; Koltyn & Umeda, 2006; Maixner, 1991; Randich & Maixner, 1984; Saccò et al., 2013; Zamir & Maixner, 1986).

HUMAN RESEARCH ON BLOOD PRESSURE-RELATED HYPOALGESIA

As noted above, Zamir and Shuber (1980) found that unmedicated hypertensive individuals were significantly less sensitive to electrical stimulation of dental pulp compared to normotensive individuals. Comparable results have been obtained in a number of other studies, though the literature involving human participants is smaller owing to ethical and methodological constraints including individual needs and differences in antihypertensive treatment.

Ghione, Rosa, Mezzasalma and Panattoni (1988) used electrical stimulation of dental pulp to measure pain in 42 individuals with established hypertension, 34 with borderline hypertension, 43 outpatients with problems other than hypertension, 18 medical staff members, and 19 medical students. On the one hand, the diversity of the sample is useful, though, on the other hand, it complicates interpretation of the results. Not surprisingly, hypertensive patients were generally older than the control participants. However, no significant correlations between age and reported pain were observed and the significant group differences between hypertensive (both established and borderline) patients and controls were maintained following statistical control of potential confounds. Guasti et al. (1995) studied a less diverse but tighter sample of 67 drug-free men ages 30–50 who were referred for assessment of ambulatory blood pressure. Men who were subsequently determined to have hypertension had higher pulpar shock pain threshold and tolerance values than similarly aged normotensive men. Although, obviously, there are no direct analog to animal pain tests such as the hot plate test, the results of other studies indicate that these trends are not limited to verbal behavior. For example, Rosa, Vignocchi, Panattoni, Rossi, and Ghione (1994) found that hypertensive individuals required stronger shocks to elicit a defensive eyeblink response, suggesting that this phenomenon does not reflect simply willingness to report pain. Lower ratings and higher pain thresholds and tolerance levels have been observed among hypertensives in a number of other studies involving shock (Ghione et al., 1985; Rosa, Ghione, Panattoni, Mezzasalma, & Giuliano, 1986), heat (Ditto, Lewkowski, Rainville, & Duncan, 2009; Rau et al., 1994; Sheps et al., 1992), and mechanically induced pain (Schobel et al., 1996, 1998).

While the need for clinical intervention varies among hypertensives and the literature examining the effects of antihypertensive medications on pain sensitivity in hypertensives is small, it is interesting to note that several studies have found that treatment can lead to an *increase* in sensitivity to pain (Guasti et al., 1998, 2002; Rosa & Ghione, 1990), though one did not (Ghione et al., 1988).

Similar to the animal research, there is also clear evidence that risk for hypertension in humans is associated with a diminished sensitivity to pain. These studies focus on having a normative elevation of blood pressure (Al'Absi, Petersen, & Wittmers, 2000; Bruehl, Carlson, & McCubbin, 1992; Bruehl, Chung, Ward, Johnson, & McCubbin, 2002; Fillingim & Maixner, 1996; Frew & Drummond, 2009; Lewkowski, Young, Ghosh, & Ditto, 2008; Myers, Robinson, Riley, & Sheffield, 2001) and/or a family history of the disorder.

In an important early study of the effects of family history, France, Adler, France and Ditto (1994) found that inexperienced female blood donors with a confirmed parental history of hypertension reported significantly less pain during the procedure than women without a parental history of hypertension. This study anticipated application of this research to the area of clinical and chronic pain. Since the effect was limited to more anxious, inexperienced blood donors, it also raised the possible involvement of acute cardiovascular reactions in the phenomenon.

More controlled (but possibly more artificial) laboratory studies observed similar associations between family history and reduced pain due to electric shock, the cold pressor test, and several stimuli that produce local ischemia (Al'Absi et al., 2005; Al'Absi, Buchanan, & Lovallo, 1996; Bragdon, Light, Girdler, & Maixner, 1997; Campbell & Ditto, 2002; Cook, Jackson, O'Connor, & Dishman, 2004; D'Antono, Ditto, Rios, & Moskowitz, 1999; Ditto, France, & France, 1997; France, Ditto, & Adler, 1991; France & Stewart, 1995), though effects have not been observed by all (Al'Absi et al., 2000; Ghione et al., 1988; Guasti et al., 1999).

France and colleagues used the shock–induced nociceptive flexion reflex (NFR) in this context. In general, offspring of hypertensives required stronger shocks to elicit a reflex withdrawal response of the biceps femoris muscle as detected by electromyography (France, Froese, & Stewart, 2002; France & Suchowiecki, 2001; Page & France, 1997). In addition to providing objective evidence of a reduced sensitivity to pain in offspring of hypertensives, these differences in a relatively simple spinally mediated withdrawal reflex, which were not observed with elicitation of a non–pain–related reflex (France et al., 2002), further support the notion that hypoalgesia is at least partly due to descending inhibition of spinal pain transmission. Nevertheless, additional research is required as the effect was not observed in two studies (Al'Absi et al., 2005; Edwards et al., 2007), though in both cases NFR assessment was embedded in a complex protocol including other manipulations that may have obscured effects.

Although most of these studies employed young adult or middle–aged participants, several studies have observed effects among children. Ditto, Seguin, Boulerice, Pihl and Tremblay (1998) studied the joint effects of parental history of hypertension and normative elevation of systolic blood pressure on the response of 14–year–old boys to mechanical finger pressure. In analyses limited to those with a confirmed medical history, boys who had a parental history of hypertension and above average blood pressure had significantly lower average and maximum pain ratings than boys at lower risk for eventual hypertension. In a larger group that included participants whose blood pressure was measured but medical history could not be confirmed, boys with above average systolic blood pressure were also found to tolerate finger pressure longer than boys with lower blood pressure.

While the results differ somewhat for boys and girls and different pain stimuli, similar cross-sectional findings were obtained by Haas, Lu, Evans, Tsao, and Zeltzer (2011) and Drouin and McGrath (2013). Even more intriguing was the observation of an association between family history of hypertension and reduced crying in neonates who received a vitamin injection after birth (France, Taddio, Shah, Pagé, & Katz, 2009). It is not clear if this (1) is unrelated to the larger literature on blood pressure-related hypoalgesia, (2) reflects a genetic effect that is manifest at birth, or (3) indicates that a new perspective on blood pressure-related hypo-algesia may be required. Although speculative, McCubbin (2009) suggests that it may be the last and that blood pressure-related hypoalgesia could be the result of intrauterine influences. Indeed, this is a plausible explanation for the results of France et al. (2009), since reduced crying was observed only among babies whose *mothers* had a parental history of hypertension (owing to the low prevalence of hypertension in the mothers and fathers of the children, family history of hypertension was operationalized in terms of the babies' grandparents) as opposed to those whose fathers had a parental history of hypertension. Thus, they may have developed in a more "stressed" environment than babies whose fathers had a parental history of hypertension and the results may fall into the general context of research indicating that early exposure to stress and stress hormones can have an impact on pain modulation. For example, returning briefly to the animal literature, an interesting study found that neonatal rats who received a one-time injection of pain-inducing carrageenan subsequently developed hypoalgesia and higher blood pressure (Chu et al., 2012). Though this may seem inconsistent with the idea that baroreflex stimu-lation is involved in the process, Chu et al. (2012) suggest that hypoalgesia may have been the result of a postcarrageenan predisposition to exag-gerated blood pressure reactivity that eventually led to sustained high blood pressure.

Indeed, some studies in humans have found that individual differences among children in sensitivity to pain are prospectively associated with blood pressure. In two projects, Campbell and colleagues reassessed participants in the study of Ditto et al. (1998), examining laboratory blood pressure at age 19 (Campbell et al., 2002) and ambulatory blood pressure at age 22 (Campbell, Ditto, Seguin, Sinray, & Tremblay, 2003). In both cases, lower pain sensitivity at age 14 was found to predict greater increase in blood pressure above and beyond what would be predicted based on age 14 blood pressure alone, suggesting that hypoalgesia is associated with some dysregulation of blood pressure control mechanisms. These findings were replicated and extended by Drouin and McGrath (2013), who administered a different pain stimulus (finger prick for a blood draw) to a larger sample including both boys and girls.

In sum, though the human literature is smaller than the animal literature, especially in terms of research with youth, and the causal arrows seem complex and multidirectional, the overall pattern of results is fairly consistent. For example, the previously discussed results from children and young adults are consistent with those from young SHR rats, who display a reduced sensitivity to pain before the onset of sustained high blood pressure (Maixner et al., 1982; Saavedra, 1981; Sitsen & de Jong, 1984a; Wendel & Bennett, 1981).

That said, one feature of the human literature is less clear. Somewhat surprisingly, despite fairly consistent results indicating the involvement of endogenous opioids in experimental animals, most human studies that administered either naloxone or naltrexone to participants have *not* observed an impact on blood pressure-related hypoalgesia (Al'Absi, France, Harju, France, & Wittmers, 2006; Bruehl et al., 2002; Edwards, Ring, France, McIntyre, & Martin, 2008; France et al., 2005; McCubbin & Bruehl, 1994; Ring, France, et al., 2008; Schobel et al., 1998), though more positive evidence was obtained in several blocking studies (Bruehl et al., 2010; Frew & Drummond, 2009; Lewkowski et al., 2008; McCubbin, Helfer, Switzer, Galloway, & Griffith, 2006) as well as related research. For example, similar to research suggesting greater sensitivity to the pain-reducing effects of morphine in SHR rats (Hoffmann et al., 1998), a form of transcutaneous electrical nerve stimulation (TENS) thought work by engaging endogenous opioid activity (low-frequency TENS) was found to produce greater pain reduction in normotensive individuals at risk for hypertension compared to those at lower risk (Campbell & Ditto, 2002). Based on the collective results of studies with humans and experimental animals, most reviewers have reached the somewhat unsatisfying but probably correct conclusion that both opioid and nonopioid mechanisms are involved in blood pressure-related hypoalgesia (Bruehl & Chung, 2004; Bruehl et al., 1999; France & Ditto, 1996; France, 1999; Ghione, 1996; Koltyn & Umeda, 2006; Maixner, 1991; Randich & Maixner, 1984; Saccò et al., 2013; Zamir & Maixner, 1986), operating in the brain, spinal cord, and perhaps periphery, for example, involving vascular sympathetic activity or subclinical neuropathy (Edwards, Ring, McIntyre, Winer, & Martin, 2008).

CLINICAL IMPLICATIONS

While many researchers remain interested in theoretical issues related to the association between blood pressure and pain, this is largely an elaboration of earlier animal work (Marques-Lopes et al., 2012), and recent research has tended to focus more on clinical implications. For example, does blood pressure influence clinical pain? In general, this seems to be the case. As noted earlier, risk for hypertension was associated with decreased sensitivity to needle-related pain during blood donation (France et al., 1994) and injections (France et al., 2009), as well as reduced postsurgical pain (France & Katz, 1999). Beyond pain induced by medical procedures, several studies have found inverse relationships between hypertension or risk for hypertension and nonclinical daily aches and pains (D'Antono et al., 1999; Hagen et al., 2005; Stewart, France, & Sheffield, 2003; Stovner & Hagen, 2009).

In fact, perhaps the most important application of this area has been to the study of serious chronic pain. However, among individuals with chronic pain the blood pressure–pain relationship is usually reversed, that is, higher blood pressure is associated with greater pain. Bruehl and colleagues (Bruehl & Chung, 2004; Bruehl et al., 1999) discuss a number of studies that indicate this is due to a reversal of the typical negative association between blood pressure and pain rather than the elevation of blood pressure by pain, arguing that this is due to exhaustion of pain control mechanisms. For example, baroreflex sensitivity may be reduced owing to repeated engagement of the system.

One interesting study that supports this idea used the technique of phase-related external suction (PRES). PRES is focused suction over the carotid sinus that stretches baroreceptors. It can be applied in brief bursts such as during the systolic or diastolic phase of the cardiac cycle. In addition to maximizing stretch when administered during the systolic phase, suction during the diastolic phase is a useful "placebo control" since it is impossible for participants to distinguish the point in the cardiac cycle at which suction is applied. Normally, PRES during the systolic phase decreases response to an acute pain stimulus relative to PRES during the diastolic phase (Dworkin et al., 1994; Rau et al., 1994). However, this was reversed in a group of chronic low back pain patients (Brody et al., 1997).

Several studies suggest that baroreflex sensitivity is reduced in certain types of chronic pain (Chung et al., 2008; Maixner et al., 2011; Reyes del Paso, Garrido, Pulgar, & Duschek, 2011). Ironically, given the importance of the baroreflex in blood pressure control, this may set the stage for the development of hypertension, and one study found that the prevalence of hypertension in chronic pain patients was almost twice the rate observed in a control group (Bruehl, Chung, Jirjis, & Biridepalli, 2005)! This may point to the importance of blood pressure control among individuals with chronic pain.

Another potentially important clinical implication of blood pressure-related hypoalgesia is SI. Although painful angina is clearly unpleasant, it serves an important warning of the need for medical care. Inverse relationships between blood pressure and degree of experimentally induced pain have been observed in cardiac patients (Falcone, Auguadro, Sconocchia, & Angoli, 1997; Sheffield et al., 1997). More important, independent of the severity of coronary atherosclerosis, higher blood pressure has been found to be associated with reduced angina even in the very controlled context of exercise stress testing. Interestingly, both patients with higher resting blood pressure (Ditto et al., 2010; Falcone et al., 1997; Krittayaphong & Sheps, 1996) and those who experienced large but temporary increases in blood pressure during exercise (Bacon et al., 2006; Ditto, D'Antono, Dupuis, & Burelle, 2007; Go, Sheffield, Krittayaphong, Maixner, & Sheps, 1997) experienced less pain. As a result, higher blood pressure may increase the risk of SI. While there are certainly other risk factors for SI, blood pressure-related hypoalgesia may be especially relevant given the strong association between blood pressure and risk for atherosclerosis.

CONCLUDING THOUGHTS

Research on the links between blood pressure and pain has yielded important insights concerning the regulation of cardiovascular activity, pain, and emotion and clinical phenomena such as chronic pain and SI (Figure 2), despite a number of ongoing questions such as the role of endogenous opioid activity. The relationship between the risk for hypertension and hypoalgesia is also unclear, though accumulating research suggests this is due to acute blood pressure reactivity. As noted at the outset, acute pharmacologically induced elevation of blood pressure can reduce pain (Dworkin et al., 1979; Randich & Hartunian, 1983). There is even some buffering of pain by short-term cardiac cycle effects (Edwards, Inui, et al., 2008; Edwards, McIntyre, Carroll, Ring, & Martin, 2002). In addition to studies indicating a relationship between pain and the degree of change in blood pressure produced by exercise, a number have observed inverse

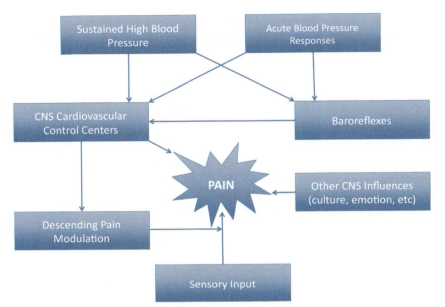

Figure 2 Simplified diagram of possible connections between cardiovascular activity and pain. For clarity, not all connections are noted, for example, part of the impact of emotion on pain may be mediated by blood pressure response.

relationships between pain and degree of short-term cardiovascular response to the pain protocol (Bragdon et al., 1997; Campbell, Holder, & France, 2006; Ditto et al., 1997; France & Stewart, 1995; Vassend & Knardahl, 2004). This may explain some of the variation in findings concerning the impact of parental history of hypertension and pain. As noted earlier, most but not all studies point to a relationship. This may depend on the degree to which those with a family history display an exaggerated blood pressure response (e.g., France & Stewart, 1995). In sum, while some studies do not support this conclusion (e.g., Schobel et al., 1996) and all of these phenomena do not require a common explanation, it seems parsimonious to suggest that hypoalgesia among nonhypertensives can be produced by a short-term increase in blood pressure that also stimulates the baroreflex.

One final interesting topic is the sociobiological origin of this relationship. Blood pressure-related hypoalgesia is often discussed in the context of stress-induced analgesia and there are many empirical and theoretical connections. However, this begs an important question. Simply put, why would the brain require information about peripheral blood pressure to let it know the organism is in a stressful situation? It is possible that blood pressure-related hypoalgesia is one of several redundant mechanisms to ensure an adaptive stress-related decrease in pain. Alternatively, it is interesting to consider the fact that this relationship is probably very old from an evolutionary perspective. For example, variations of the baroreflex are present in fish, lizards, and snakes. Although research is limited, a 2006 review linked exercise-related analgesia to blood pressure-related hypoalgesia, noting inverse relationships between blood pressure response to exercise and sensitivity to experimental pain stimuli (Koltyn & Umeda, 2006). This is supported by a more recent study (Ring, Edwards, & Kavussanu, 2008) and the research discussed above linking angina to magnitude of blood pressure response to exercise stress testing. Thus, while speculative, blood pressure-related hypoalgesia may be an early mechanism of stress-induced analgesia once triggered primarily by vigorous reflexive withdrawal responses that influence blood pressure. Regardless, there are fascinating relationships among pain, blood pressure, hypertension, and cardiovascular control mechanisms with important theoretical and clinical implications.

REFERENCES

Afolabi, A. O., Mudashiru, S. K., Abdullateef, I., & Alagbonsi, I. A. (2013). Effects of salt-loading hypertension on nociception in rats. *Journal of Pain Research, 6,* 387–392.

Aicher, S. A., & Randich, A. (1990). Antinociception and cardiovascular responses produced by electrical stimulation in the nucleus tractus solitarius, nucleus reticularis ventralis, and the caudal medulla. *Pain, 42,* 103–119.

Al'Absi, M., Buchanan, T., & Lovallo, W. R. (1996). Pain perception and cardiovascular responses in men with positive parental history for hypertension. *Psychophysiology, 33,* 655–661.

Al'Absi, M., France, C. R., Harju, A., France, J., & Wittmers, L. (2006). Adrenocortical and nociceptive responses to opioid blockade in hypertension-prone men and women. *Psychosomatic Medicine, 68,* 292–298.

Al'Absi, M., France, C. R., Ring, C., France, J., Harju, A., McIntyre, D., et al. (2005). Nociception and baroreceptor stimulation in hypertension-prone men and women. *Psychophysiology, 42,* 83–91.

Al'Absi, M., Petersen, K. L., & Wittmers, L. E. (2000). Blood pressure but not parental history for hypertension predicts pain perception in women. *Pain, 88,* 61–68.

Aristotle (350BCE). On sleep and sleeplessness. J. Beare (Ed.). Adelaide, Australia: eBooks@Adelaide.

Bacon, S. L., Lavoie, K. L., Campbell, T. S., Fleet, R., Arsenault, A., & Ditto, B. (2006). The role of ischaemia and pain in the blood pressure response to exercise stress testing in patients with coronary heart disease. *Journal of Human Hypertension, 20,* 672–678.

Bragdon, E. E., Light, K. C., Girdler, S. S., & Maixner, W. (1997). Blood pressure, gender, and parental hypertension are factors in baseline and poststress pain sensitivity in normotensive adults. *International Journal of Behavioral Medicine, 4,* 17–38.

Brody, S., Angrilli, A., Weiss, U., Birbaumer, N., Mini, A., Veit, R., et al. (1997). Somatosensory evoked potentials during baroreceptor stimulation in chronic low back pain patients and normal controls. *International Journal of Psychophysiology, 25*, 201–210.

Bruehl, S., Burns, J. W., Chung, O. Y., Magid, E., Chont, M., Gilliam, W., et al. (2010). Hypoalgesia associated with elevated resting blood pressure: evidence for endogenous opioid involvement. *Journal of Behavioral Medicine, 33*, 168–176.

Bruehl, S., Carlson, C. R., & McCubbin, J. A. (1992). The relationship between pain sensitivity and blood pressure in normotensives. *Pain, 48*, 463–467.

Bruehl, S., & Chung, O. Y. (2004). Interactions between the cardiovascular and pain regulatory systems: an updated review of mechanisms and possible alterations in chronic pain. *Neuroscience and Biobehavioral Reviews, 28*, 395–414.

Bruehl, S., Chung, O. Y., Jirjis, J. N., & Biridepalli, S. (2005). Prevalence of clinical hypertension in patients with chronic pain compared to nonpain general medical patients. *The Clinical Journal of Pain, 21*, 147–153.

Bruehl, S., Chung, O. Y., Ward, P., Johnson, B., & McCubbin, J. A. (2002). The relationship between resting blood pressure and acute pain sensitivity in healthy normotensives and chronic back pain sufferers: the effects of opioid blockade. *Pain, 100*, 191–201.

Bruehl, S., McCubbin, J. A., & Harden, R. N. (1999). Theoretical review: altered pain regulatory systems in chronic pain. *Neuroscience and Biobehavioral Reviews, 23*, 877–890.

Campbell, T. S., & Ditto, B. (2002). Exaggeration of blood pressure-related hypoalgesia and reduction of blood pressure with low frequency transcutaneous electrical nerve stimulation. *Psychophysiology, 39*, 473–481.

Campbell, T. S., Ditto, B., Seguin, J. R., Assaad, J. M., Pihl, R. O., Nagin, D., et al. (2002). A longitudinal study of pain sensitivity and blood pressure in adolescent boys: results from a 5-year follow-up. *Health Psychology, 21*, 594–600.

Campbell, T. S., Ditto, B., Seguin, J. R., Sinray, S., & Tremblay, R. E. (2003). Adolescent pain sensitivity is associated with cardiac autonomic function and blood pressure over 8 years. *Hypertension, 41*, 1228–1233.

Campbell, T. S., Holder, M. D., & France, C. R. (2006). The effects of experimenter status and cardiovascular reactivity on pain reports. *Pain, 125*, 264–269.

Chung, O. Y., Bruehl, S., Diedrich, L., Diedrich, A., Chont, M., & Robertson, D. (2008). Baroreflex sensitivity associated hypoalgesia in healthy states is altered by chronic pain. *Pain, 138*, 87–97.

Chu, Y.-C., Yang, C. C. H., Lin, H.-T., Chen, P.-T., Chang, K.-Y., Yang, S.-C., et al. (2012). Neonatal nociception elevated baseline blood pressure and attenuated cardiovascular responsiveness to noxious stress in adult rats. *International Journal of Developmental Neuroscience, 30*, 421–426.

Cook, D. B., Jackson, E. M., O'Connor, P., & Dishman, R. K. (2004). Muscle pain during exercise in normotensive AfricanAmerican women: effect of parental hypertension history. *The Journal of Pain: Official Journal of the American Pain Society, 5*, 111–118.

De Ferrari, G. M., Crijns, H. J. G. M., Borggrefe, M., Milasinovic, G., Smid, J., Zabel, M., et al. (2011). Chronic vagus nerve stimulation: a new and promising therapeutic approach for chronic heart failure. *European Heart Journal, 32*, 847–855.

Ditto, B., D'Antono, B., Dupuis, G., & Burelle, D. (2007). Chest pain is inversely associated with blood pressure during exercise among individuals being assessed for coronary heart disease. *Psychophysiology, 44*, 183–188.

Ditto, B., France, J., & France, C. R. (1997). Risk for hypertension and pain sensitivity in women. *International Journal of Behavioral Medicine, 4*, 117–130.

Ditto, B., Lavoie, K. L., Campbell, T. S., Gordon, J., Arsenault, A., & Bacon, S. L. (2010). Negative association between resting blood pressure and chest pain in people undergoing exercise stress testing for coronary artery disease. *Pain, 149,* 501–505.

Ditto, B., Lewkowski, M. D., Rainville, P., & Duncan, G. H. (2009). Effects of cardiopulmonary baroreceptor activation on pain may be moderated by risk for hypertension. *Biological Psychology, 82,* 211–213.

Ditto, B., Seguin, J. R., Boulerice, B., Pihl, R. O., & Tremblay, R. E. (1998). Risk for hypertension and pain sensitivity in adolescent boys. *Health Psychology, 17,* 249–254.

Drouin, S., & McGrath, J. J. (2013). Blood pressure and pain sensitivity in children and adolescents. *Psychophysiology, 50,* 513–520.

Dworkin, B. R., Elbert, T., Rau, H., Birbaumer, N., Pauli, P., Droste, C., et al. (1994). Central effects of baroreceptor activation in humans: attenuation of skeletal reflexes and pain perception. *Proceedings of the National Academy of Sciences, 91,* 6329–6333.

Dworkin, B. R., Filewich, R. J., Miller, N. E., Craigmyle, N., & Pickering, T. G. (1979). Baroreceptor activation reduces reactivity to noxious stimulation: implications for hypertension. *Science (New York, N.Y.), 205,* 1299–1301.

D'Antono, B., Ditto, B., Rios, N., & Moskowitz, D. S. (1999). Risk for hypertension and diminished pain sensitivity in women: autonomic and daily correlates. *International Journal of Psychophysiology, 31,* 175–187.

Edwards, L., Inui, K., Ring, C., Wang, X., & Kakigi, R. (2008a). Pain-related evoked potentials are modulated across the cardiac cycle. *Pain, 137,* 488–494.

Edwards, L., McIntyre, D., Carroll, D., Ring, C., & Martin, U. (2002). The human nociceptive flexion reflex threshold is higher during systole than diastole. *Psychophysiology, 39,* 678–681.

Edwards, L., Ring, C., France, C. R., Al'Absi, M., McIntyre, D., Carroll, D., et al. (2007). Nociceptive flexion reflex thresholds and pain during rest and computer game play in patients with hypertension and individuals at risk for hypertension. *Biological Psychology, 76,* 72–82.

Edwards, L., Ring, C., France, C. R., McIntyre, D., & Martin, U. (2008b). Effects of opioid blockade on nociceptive flexion reflex thresholds and nociceptive responding in hypertensive and normotensive individuals. *International Journal of Psychophysiology, 69,* 96–100.

Edwards, L., Ring, C., McIntyre, D., Winer, J. B., & Martin, U. (2008c). Cutaneous sensibility and peripheral nerve function in patients with unmediated essential hypertension. *Psychophysiology, 45,* 141–147.

Falcone, C., Auguadro, C., Sconocchia, R., & Angoli, L. (1997). Susceptibility to pain in hypertensive and normotensive patients with coronary artery disease: response to dental pulp stimulation. *Hypertension, 30,* 1279–1283.

Fillingim, R. B., & Maixner, W. (1996). The influence of resting blood pressure and gender on pain responses. *Psychosomatic Medicine, 58,* 326–332.

France, C. R. (1999). Decreased pain perception and risk for hypertension: considering a common physiological mechanism. *Psychophysiology, 36,* 683–692.

France, C. R., Adler, P. S., France, J., & Ditto, B. (1994). Family history of hypertension and pain during blood donation. *Psychosomatic Medicine, 56,* 52–60.

France, C. R., Al'absi, M., Ring, C., France, J. L., Brose, J., Spaeth, D., et al. (2005). Assessment of opiate modulation of pain and nociceptive responding in young adults with a parental history of hypertension. *Biological Psychology, 70,* 168–174.

France, C. R., & Ditto, B. (1996). Risk for high blood pressure and decreased pain perception. *Current Directions in Psychological Science, 5,* 120–125.

France, C. R., Ditto, B., & Adler, P. (1991). Pain sensitivity in offspring of hypertensives at rest and during baroreflex stimulation. *Journal of Behavioral Medicine, 14,* 513–525.

France, C. R., Froese, S. A., & Stewart, J. C. (2002). Altered central nervous system pro-cessing of noxious stimuli contributes to decreased nociceptive responding in individuals at risk for hypertension. *Pain, 98*, 101–108.

France, C. R., & Katz, J. (1999). Post surgical pain is attenuated in men with elevated presurgical systolic blood pressure. *Pain Research and Management, 4*, 100–103.

France, C. R., & Stewart, K. M. (1995). Parental history of hypertension and enhanced cardiovascular reactivity are associated with decreased pain ratings. *Psychophysiology, 32*, 571–578.

France, C. R., & Suchowiecki, S. (2001). Assessing supraspinal modulation of pain perception in individuals at risk for hypertension. *Psychophysiology, 38*, 107–113.

France, C. R., Taddio, A., Shah, V. S., Pagé, M. G., & Katz, J. (2009). Maternal family history of hypertension attenuates neonatal pain response. *Pain, 142*, 189–193.

Frew, A. K., & Drummond, P. D. (2009). Opposite effects of opioid blockade on the blood pressure-pain relationship in depressed and non-depressed participants. *Pain, 142*, 68–74.

Friedman, R., Murphy, D., Persons, W., & McCaughran, J. A. (1984). Genetic predispo-sition to hypertension, elevated blood pressure and pain sensitivity: a functional analysis. *Behavioural Brain Research, 12*, 75–79.

Ghione, S. (1996). Hypertension-associated hypalgesia: evidence in experimental animals and humans, pathophysiological mechanisms, and potential clinical consequences. *Hypertension, 28*, 494–504.

Ghione, S., Rosa, C., Mezzasalma, L., & Panattoni, E. (1988). Arterial hypertension is associated with hypalgesia in humans. *Hypertension, 12*, 491–497.

Ghione, S., Rosa, C., Panattoni, E., Nuti, M., Mezzasalma, L., & Giuliano, G. (1985). Comparison of sensory and pain threshold in tooth pulp stimulation in normotensive man and essential hypertension. *Journal of Hypertension, 3*, S113–S115.

Goadsby, P., Grosberg, B., Mauskop, A., Cady, R., & Simmons, K. (2014). Effect of noninvasive vagus nerve stimulation on acute migraine: an open-label pilot study. *Cephalalgia, 34*, 986–993.

Go, B. M., Sheffield, D., Krittayaphong, R., Maixner, W., & Sheps, D. S. (1997). Association of systolic blood pressure at time of myocardial ischemia with angina pectoris during exercise testing. *The American Journal of Cardiology, 79*, 954–956.

Guasti, L., Cattaneo, R., Rinaldi, O., Rossi, M. G., Bianchi, L., Gaudio, G., et al. (1995). Twenty-four-hour noninvasive blood pressure monitoring and pain perception. *Hypertension, 25*, 1301–1305.

Guasti, L., Gaudio, G., Zanotta, D., Grimoldi, P., Petrozzino, M. R., Tanzi, F., et al. (1999). Relationship between a genetic predisposition to hypertension, blood pressure levels and pain sensitivity. *Pain, 82*, 311–317.

Guasti, L., Grimoldi, P., Diolisi, A., Petrozzino, M. R., Gaudio, G., Grandi, A. M., et al. (1998). Treatment with enalapril modifies the pain perception pattern in hypertensive patients. *Hypertension, 31*, 1146–1150.

Guasti, L., Zanotta, D., Diolisi, A., Garganico, D., Simoni, C., Gaudio, G., et al. (2002). Changes in pain perception during treatment with angiotensin converting enzyme-inhibitors and angiotensin II type 1 receptor blockade. *Journal of Hypertension, 20*, 485–491.

Haas, K., Lu, Q., Evans, S., Tsao, J. C. I., & Zeltzer, L. K. (2011). Relationship between resting blood pressure and laboratory-induced pain among healthy children. *Gender Medicine, 8*, 388–398.

Hagen, K., Zwart, J. A., Holmen, J., Svebak, S., Bovim, G., & Stovner, L. J. (2005). Does hypertension protect against chronic musculoskeletal complaints? The Nord-Trondelag Health Study. *Archives of Internal Medicine, 165*, 916–922.

Hoffmann, O., Plesan, A., & Wiesenfeld-Hallin, Z. (1998). Genetic differences in morphine sensitivity, tolerance and withdrawal in rats. *Brain Research, 806*, 232–237.

Koltyn, K. F., & Umeda, M. (2006). Exercise, hypoalgesia and blood pressure. *Sports Medicine (Auckland, N.Z.), 36*, 207–214.

Krittayaphong, R., & Sheps, D. S. (1996). Relation between blood pressure at rest and perception of angina pectoris during exercise testing. *The American Journal of Cardiology, 77*, 1224–1226.

Lacey, B. C., & Lacey, J. I. (1978). Two-way communication between the heart and the brain. Significance of time within the cardiac cycle. *The American Psychologist, 33*, 99–113.

Lewis, J. W., Baldrighi, G., & Akil, H. (1987). A possible interface between autonomic function and pain control: opioid analgesia and the nucleus tractus solitarius. *Brain Research, 424*, 65–70.

Lewkowski, M. D., Young, S. N., Ghosh, S., & Ditto, B. (2008). Effects of opioid blockade on the modulation of pain and mood by sweet taste and blood pressure in young adults. *Pain, 135*, 75–81.

Lima, D., Albino-Teixeira, A., & Tavares, I. (2002). The caudal medullary ventrolateral reticular formation in nociceptive-cardiovascular integration. An experimental study in the rat. *Experimental Physiology, 87*, 267–274.

Maixner, W. (1991). Interactions between cardiovascular and pain modulatory systems: physiological and pathophysiological implications. *Journal of Cardiovascular Electrophysiology, 2*, s3–s12.

Maixner, W., Greenspan, J. D., Dubner, R., Bair, E., Mulkey, F., Miller, V., et al. (2011). Potential autonomic risk factors for chronic TMD: descriptive data and empirically identified domains from the OPPERA case-control study. *The Journal of Pain, 12*, T75–T91.

Maixner, W., & Randich, A. (1984). Role of the right vagal nerve trunk in antinociception. *Brain Research, 298*, 374–377.

Maixner, W., Touw, K. B., Brody, M. J., Gebhart, G. F., & Long, J. P. (1982). Factors influencing the altered pain perception in the spontaneously hypertensive rat. *Brain Research, 237*, 137–145.

Marques-Lopes, J., Martins, I., Pinho, D., Morato, M., Wilson, S. P., Albino-Teixeira, A., et al. (2012). Decrease in the expression of N-methyl-D-aspartate receptors in the nucleus tractus solitarii induces antinociception and increases blood pressure. *Journal of Neuroscience Research, 90*, 356–366.

McCubbin, J. A. (2009). Prenatal maternal stress hormones, risk for hypertension, and the neonatal pain response: Comment on France et al., "Maternal family history of hypertension attenuates neonatal pain response". *Pain, 142*, 173–174.

McCubbin, J. A., & Bruehl, S. (1994). Do endogenous opioids mediate the relationship between blood pressure and pain sensitivity in normotensives? *Pain, 57*, 63–67.

McCubbin, J. A., Helfer, S. G., Switzer, F. S., Galloway, C., & Griffith, W. V. (2006). Opioid analgesia in persons at risk for hypertension. *Psychosomatic Medicine, 68*, 116–120.

Multon, S., & Schoenen, J. (2005). Pain control by vagus nerve stimulation: from animal to man and back. *Acta Neurologica Belgica, 105*, 62–67.

Myers, C. D., Robinson, M. E., Riley, J. L., & Sheffield, D. (2001). Sex, gender, and blood pressure: contributions to experimental pain report. *Psychosomatic Medicine, 63*, 545–550.

Page, G. D., & France, C. R. (1997). Objective evidence of decreased pain perception in normotensives at risk for hypertension. *Pain, 73*, 173–180.

Randich, A. (1986). Volume loading hypoalgesia in SHR, WKY and F1 offspring of a SHR x WKY cross. *Brain Research, 363*, 178–182.

Randich, A., & Gebhart, G. F. (1992). Vagal afferent modulation of nociception. *Brain Research. Brain Research Reviews, 17*, 77–99.

Randich, A., & Hartunian, C. (1983). Activation of the sinoaortic baroreceptor reflex arc induces analgesia: interactions between cardiovascular and endogenous pain inhibition systems. *Physiological Psychology, 11*, 214–220.

Randich, A., & Maixner, W. (1984). Interactions between cardiovascular and pain regulatory systems. *Neuroscience and Biobehavioral Reviews, 8*, 343–367.

Randich, A., & Robertson, J. D. (1994). Spinal nociceptive transmission in the spontaneously hypertensive and Wistar-Kyoto normotensive rat. *Pain, 58*, 169–183.

Rau, H., Brody, S., Larbig, W., Pauli, P., Vohringer, M., Harsch, B., et al. (1994). Effects of PRES baroreceptor stimulation on thermal and mechanical pain threshold in borderline hypertensives and normotensives. *Psychophysiology, 31*, 480–485.

Reyes del Paso, G. A., Garrido, S., Pulgar, Á., & Duschek, S. (2011). Autonomic cardiovascular control and responses to experimental pain stimulation in fibromyalgia syndrome. *Journal of Psychosomatic Research, 70*, 125–134.

Ring, C., Edwards, L., & Kavussanu, M. (2008a). Effects of isometric exercise on pain are mediated by blood pressure. *Biological Psychology, 78*, 123–128.

Ring, C., France, C. R., Al'Absi, M., Edwards, L., McIntyre, D., Carroll, D., et al. (2008b). Effects of naltrexone on electrocutaneous pain in patients with hypertension compared to normotensive individuals. *Biological Psychology, 77*, 191–196.

Rosa, C., & Ghione, S. (1990). Effect of ketanserin on pain perception in arterial hypertension. *Cardiovascular Drugs and Therapy, 4*, 133–135.

Rosa, C., Ghione, S., Panattoni, E., Mezzasalma, L., & Giuliano, G. (1986). Comparison of pain perception in normotensives and borderline hypertensives by means of a tooth pulp-stimulation test. *Journal of Cardiovascular Pharmacology, 8*, S125–S127.

Rosa, C., Vignocchi, G., Panattoni, E., Rossi, B., & Ghione, S. (1994). Relationship between increased blood pressure and hypoalgesia: additional evidence for the existence of an abnormality of pain perception in arterial hypertension in humans. *Journal of Human Hypertension, 8*, 119–126.

Saavedra, J. M. (1981). Naloxone reversible decrease in pain sensitivity in young and adult spontaneously hypertensive rats. *Brain Research, 209*, 245–249.

Saccò, M., Meschi, M., Regolisti, G., Detrenis, S., Bianchi, L., Bertorelli, M., et al. (2013). The relationship between blood pressure and pain. *Journal of Clinical Hypertension, 15*, 600–605.

Schlager, E., & Meier, T. E. (1947). A strange Balinese method of inducing sleep. *Acta Tropica, 4*, 127–134.

Schobel, H. P., Handwerker, H. O., Schmieder, R. E., Heusser, K., Dominiak, P., & Luft, F. C. (1998). Effects of naloxone on hemodynamic and sympathetic nerve responses to pain in normotensive vs. borderline hypertensive men. *Journal of the Autonomic Nervous System, 69*, 49–55.

Schobel, H. P., Ringkamp, M., Behrmann, A., Forster, C., Schmieder, R. E., & Handwerker, H. O. (1996). Hemodynamic and sympathetic nerve responses to painful stimuli in normotensive and borderline hypertensive subjects. *Pain, 66*, 117–124.

Sheffield, D., Krittayaphong, R., Go, B. M., Christy, C. G., Biles, P. L., & Sheps, D. S. (1997). The relationship between resting systolic blood pressure and cutaneous pain perception in cardiac patients with angina pectoris and controls. *Pain, 71*, 249–255.

Sheps, D. S., Bragdon, E. E., Gray, T. F., Ballenger, M., Usedom, J. E., & Maixner, W. (1992). Relation between systemic hypertension and pain perception. *American Journal of Cardiology, 70*, 3F–5F.

Sitsen, J. M., & de Jong, W. (1984a). Hypoalgesia in genetically hypertensive rats (SHR) is absent in rats with experimental hypertension. *Hypertension, 5*, 185–190.

Sitsen, J. M., & de Jong, W. (1984b). Observations on pain perception and hypertension in spontaneously hypertensive rats. *Clinical and Experimental Hypertension. Part A, Theory and Practice, 6*, 1345–1356.

Stewart, J. C., France, C. R., & Sheffield, D. (2003). Hypertension awareness and pain reports: data from the NHANES III. *Annals of Behavioral Medicine, 26*, 8–14.

Stovner, L. J., & Hagen, K. (2009). Hypertension-associated hypalgesia: a clue to the co-morbidity of headache and other pain disorders. *Acta Neurologica Scandinavica. Supplementum, 189*, 46–50.

Taylor, B. K., Roderick, R. E., St Lezin, E., & Basbaum, A. I. (2001). Hypoalgesia and hyperalgesia with inherited hypertension in the rat. *American Journal of Physiology. Regulatory, Integrative and Comparative Physiology, 280*, R345–R354.

Thurston, C. L., & Randich, A. (1990). Acute increases in arterial blood pressure produced by occlusion of the abdominal aorta induces antinociception: peripheral and central substrates. *Brain Research, 519*, 12–22.

Vassend, O., & Knardahl, S. (2004). Cardiovascular responsiveness to brief cognitive challenges and pain sensitivity in women. *European Journal of Pain (London, England), 8*, 315–324.

Waller, A. (1862). Experimental researches on the functions of the vagus and the cervical sympathetic nerves in man. *Proceedings of the Royal Society of London, 11*, 302–303.

Wendel, O. T., & Bennett, B. (1981). The occurrence of analgesia in an animal model of hypertension. *Life Sciences, 29*, 515–521.

Zamir, N., & Maixner, W. (1986). The relationship between cardiovascular and pain regulatory systems. *Annals of the New York Academy of Sciences, 467*, 371–384.

Zamir, N., & Segal, M. (1979). Hypertension-induced analgesia: changes in pain sensitivity in experimental hypertensive rats. *Brain Research, 160*, 170–173.

Zamir, N., & Shuber, E. (1980). Altered pain perception in hypertensive humans. *Brain Research, 201*, 471–474.

Zamir, N., Simantov, R., & Segal, M. (1980). Pain sensitivity and opioid activity in genetically and experimentally hypertensive rats. *Brain Research, 184*, 299–310.

CHAPTER 12

Chronic Pain and Fatigue

Tore C. Stiles[1], Maria Hrozanova[2]

[1]Department of Psychology, Norwegian University of Science and Technology, Trondheim, Norway;
[2]Department of Neuroscience, Norwegian University of Science and Technology, Trondheim, Norway

INTRODUCTION

This chapter addresses two widespread and debilitating conditions that have troubled the lives of patients, researchers, and physicians for decades: chronic pain and chronic fatigue. Both of these syndromes are poorly understood by specialists, even though the symptoms are well described by patients. The consequences of this lack of understanding are alarming: people who suffer from chronic pain and chronic fatigue have to persistently cope with low quality of life, they lose their jobs owing to the inability to endure traditional hours at work, they suffer from depression and anxiety, and they often live isolated lives. Similarly, the health care system is faced with enormous expenses linked to the treatment of these patients, as they require prolonged attention of medical professionals and long-lasting stays in the hospital, followed by intensive rehabilitation. In addition, the efficacy of medication is often limited and can even lead to dependency.

Chronic pain and fatigue remind professionals that the human body is a fallible system, and therefore, much of the current research is trying to uncover the pathophysiology of these two conditions. Through the understanding of pathophysiology, treatment and diagnosis can improve on many levels: identification of new biomarkers can make the detection of the syndrome quicker, more reliable, and more effective, leading to more accurate diagnosis. Similarly, biomarkers can be employed to investigate the pharmacologic responses to therapeutic interventions, allowing valuable insight into the mechanisms of the syndromes. By using the correct biomarkers, the development of new, more helpful and disease-specific therapeutical methods can be enabled. When developing new treatment options, the aim is to achieve long-lasting effects while minimizing side effects and to encourage patients in their recovery through the setting of manageable, encouraging, short-term goals. Therefore, by understanding the pathology of chronic pain and fatigue, researchers will be able to identify useful biomarkers, which will allow for the development of

The Neuroscience of Pain, Stress, and Emotion
http://dx.doi.org/10.1016/B978-0-12-800538-5.00012-1

treatment options, both psychological and pharmacological, that will eventually make way for recovery.

CHRONIC FATIGUE

Background

Chronic fatigue is a condition that can be most commonly described as persistent and irrepressible tiredness that interferes with normal day-to-day functioning. It is often accompanied by diffuse migratory pain that manifests itself in the form of headaches, joint and muscle pain, or back pain, but it can be present elsewhere in the body, too. Common for chronic fatigue patients are also mental health issues such as depression and disruption in normal cognitive functioning. Short-term memory, problems with executive functioning, and impairments in concentration can be often seen. Even simple mental tasks for which the patient has to focus leaves him or her fatigued and discouraged. Other symptoms include lack of motivation, constant energy deficit, drowsiness, and apathy. The length of persistence of these symptoms is truly debilitating, as individual episodes of impaired well-being may last 6 months or longer. Such chronic fatigue can result in decades of wearing existence.

The symptoms present in chronic fatigue can be often linked to a wide range of other diseases, making it difficult for practitioners to diagnose correctly and to explore the causality of this syndrome. Often, chronic fatigue syndrome is misunderstood, misperceived, and thus goes untreated. The famous Canadian physician William Osler, also nicknamed the "Father of Modern Medicine," in 1889 said: "In all forms there is a striking lack of accordance between the symptoms of which the patients complain and the objective changes discoverable by the physician." This applies very accurately to chronic fatigue. However, the fact that the syndrome is difficult to diagnose and difficult to treat does not mean that it is not real. After decades of uncertainty and doubtfulness by the medical professionals, chronic fatigue is now accepted as a medical condition, giving patients the much needed validation and assurance.

Chronic fatigue is relatively widespread, and it has been estimated that as much as 10% of the world's population suffers from this condition at some point in their lifetime (Nordqvist, 2015). But, as a result of the lack of understanding of the syndrome's causes, only 15% of all chronic fatigue sufferers are thought to have been given the correct diagnosis. It is important to note that even when the diagnosis is correct, the prognosis of a recovery is rather slim—as of this writing, there is no efficient treatment that leads to reconvalescence.

The understanding of what causes the syndrome is actively evolving, and much research is now dedicated to uncovering the links between the symptoms and the pathophysiology. Currently, the most commonly considered possibilities of chronic fatigue causes are psychiatric disorders, metabolic disorders, certain types of medications, untreated infections, exposure to chemicals, cancer, weight, problematic lifestyle, and many more. Research lends a lot of support to the hypothesis that a wide variety of triggers can give rise to a series of events that cause hypothalamic–pituitary–adrenal (HPA) axis dysfunction.

In the upcoming sections, the possible pathophysiology of chronic fatigue is outlined. The main features of the neurological abnormalities in the syndrome, as well as the changes in the brain caused by white matter abnormalities, psychoneuroimmunological interactions, and neuroinflammation are defined. In addition, the available diagnostic procedures are described. Following is a description of the most widely used psychological treatment, namely cognitive behavioral therapy, and mindfulness-based therapy and graded exercise therapy. This account gives a fairly comprehensive picture of the current understanding of chronic fatigue.

PATHOPHYSIOLOGY
Neurological Abnormalities

Interestingly, research investigating endurance performance has shed light on the possible mechanisms underlying chronic fatigue. A link has been found between the patterns of neuronal processes and the level of muscle activity. The study showed that muscle nerve impulses have an inhibitory effect on the primary motor area of the brain during a task that requires great energy exertion. Therefore, when the body is under a lot of physical strain, the brain prompts inhibition of muscle performance, protecting the body from going beyond its physiological limits (Hilty, Langer, Pascual-Marqui, Boutellier, & Lutz, 2011). Furthermore, research employing functional magnetic resonance imaging (MRI) showed that it is the thalamus and the insular cortex that are involved in the halting of the ongoing high-energy activity to protect the organism (Hilty, Langer, Pascual-Marqui, Boutellier, & Lutz, 2011). These areas are normally both involved in the analysis of possible threat situations, such as pain or hunger.

However, the above findings can be generalized to chronic fatigue patients only with extreme caution. Even though it might seem straightforward to explain the tiredness of these patients by drawing a link to the processes at the level of muscle activity, the fact remains that chronic fatigue patients experience the debilitating tiredness even in the lack of exceptional exertion. Very simple chores, cognitive functioning, or short periods of physical movement leave the patients exhausted and unable to do anything else. Therefore, research has proposed to look further, beyond the motor system.

Assuming that the main perturbations of the chronic fatigue syndrome lie in the central nervous system, the functioning of the blood–brain barrier has been investigated in hopes of shining more light on the pathophysiology of this syndrome. It has been hypothesized that one of the main reasons for such debilitating symptoms in chronic fatigue patients is the dysfunctional permeability of the blood–brain barrier (Bested, Saunders, & Logan, 2001). The study showed that there are numerous elements of the central nervous system that can be detrimental to the normal permeability of the blood–brain barrier in chronic fatigue syndrome; namely viruses, cytokines, nitric oxide, stress, the lack of essential fatty acids, and more. The dysfunction of the blood–brain barrier functioning is thought to cause cellular dysfunction in the central nervous system, as well as abnormalities in neuronal transmission in patients with chronic fatigue. Therefore, research concluded that more resources should be dedicated to the study of the various elements of the central nervous system that show such detrimental effects in chronic fatigue patients.

Psychoneuroimmunological Interactions

The brain is greatly influenced by the immune system, and vice versa. In this interaction, the HPA axis and the sympathetic nervous system play crucial roles. Normal functioning of the immune system is actively hindered by stress exerted on mental well-being. This mechanism is mediated by certain hormones, such as cortisol. Cortisol is released upon the experience of stress. Prompted by abnormalities outside the brain, the release of cortisol gives rise the possible occurrence of neurological symptoms, mediated by neurotransmitter release in response to stress hormone activation. Furthermore, the presence of neuropsychiatric conditions in patients suffering from chronic fatigue syndrome was also linked to the abnormal cytokine synthesis by glial cells in the central nervous system.

HPA

The HPA axis has a very important role in the human body. It mediates the psychoneuroendocrine function of the stress response and immunity. The HPA axis synthesizes cortisol, a hormone closely linked to energy metabolism. This makes HPA disruptions crucial to chronic fatigue syndrome, and much research was devoted to investigating the relationship between the dysfunctional HPA axis and chronic fatigue syndrome. The link between a variety of markers of unstimulated salivary cortisol activity (markers included the cortisol awakening response, the circadian profiles of participants, and the diurnal cortisol slopes) in daily tasks of chronic fatigue patients, and the fatigue observed in healthy subjects, was investigated. The results revealed a gradual decrease in the effect of the cortisol awakening response increase in chronic fatigue patients relative to healthy subjects. Furthermore, the increase in cortisol awakening response and diurnal cortisol slopes were both linked to fatigue in both chronic fatigue patients and healthy subjects (Powell, Liossi, Moss-Morris, & Schlotz, 2013). Postexertional malaise has also been studied in reference to the cortisol awakening response, a marker of endocrine abnormalities linked to fatigue. Research found that having advanced stress management skills was linked to greater activity of the cortisol awakening response, which was linked to lesser experience of postexertional malaise in chronic fatigue patients (Hall et al., 2014). Clearly, these results further highlight the importance of understanding and maintaining the HPA axis functionally intact.

Neuroinflammation

Neuroinflammation is one among other possible causes of chronic fatigue syndrome. A greater amount of inflammatory markers in chronic fatigue patients with critical cognitive dysfunction is typical for regions of the brain such as the amygdala, thalamus, and midbrain. Furthermore, in chronic fatigue patients who suffered from greater amounts of pain, increased amounts of inflammatory markers were found in the thalamus and cingulate cortex. Chronic fatigue subjects suffering from depression had greater amounts of inflammatory markers in the hippocampus (Nakatomi et al., 2014). Such findings could potentially lead to the development of biologically based tests for the diagnosis of chronic fatigue, which would immensely help physicians in improving the patients' quality of life.

Directly linked to the fact that the brain experiences greater neuro-inflammation in conditions such as chronic fatigue is the fact that the brain also exhibits greater amounts of inflammatory cell-signaling proteins, cytokines. Cytokine levels are significantly correlated with the amounts of leptin. Leptin, found in the blood, has been found to be important in terms of the daily fluctuations of fatigue—it is directly linked to the self-reported changes in tiredness in chronic fatigue patients, further underlying the importance of cytokines in neuroinflammation (Brent et al., 2012; Stringer et al., 2013).

Along with the chronically activated immune system, another possible role in the development of chronic fatigue is played by oxidative and nitrosative stress. Research found that when the immune-inflammatory pathways as well as oxidative and nitrosative stress are persistently active, such activation results in a variety of self-preserving and self-intensifying pathological processes that are linked to the development of chronic fatigue syndrome. The cause of such persistent activation of oxidative and nitrosative stress, as well as the immune-inflammatory pathways, lies in chronic, sporadic, and opportunistic infections; bacterial translocations; autoimmune feedback; and abnormalities in mitochondrial functioning, as well as the inhibition of antioxidant functioning. Such instances then result in neuroinflammation, brain hypometabolism/hypoperfusion, toxic effects of nitric oxide and peroxynitrite, lipid peroxidation and oxidative damage to DNA, secondary autoimmune responses aimed against abnormal lipid membrane components and proteins, mitochondrial abnormalities with a dysfunction of energy metabolism (e.g., compromised ATP production), and abnormal intracellular signaling pathways. All of these variables then contribute to self-intensifying feed-forward loops, leading to persistent activation of oxidative and nitrosative stress and autoimmune pathways, which act to maintain and worsen the symptoms of chronic fatigue (Morris & Maes, 2014).

White Matter Abnormalities

A 2014 study, employing modern imaging methods, investigated whether the central nervous systems of chronic fatigue sufferers bears any differences from the brains of healthy subjects. This study was conducted with the aim of discovering a biomarker unique to chronic fatigue, which would make the diagnosis of this syndrome easier. The results found three important differences in the brains of the two subject groups. First, using MRI, the study showed that, overall, the white matter of chronic fatigue syndrome patients is significantly reduced in volume compared to the white matter of healthy subjects. This result was perhaps unsurprising, as chronic fatigue syndrome has been previously linked to neuroinflammation, which is known to negatively influence the structure and density of white matter structures. Second, using diffusion-tensor imaging, the study discovered uniform disruptions in a certain nerve tract of the right hemisphere of patients suffering from chronic fatigue—the right arcuate fasciculus. The right arcuate fasciculus is an area that connects the frontal and temporal lobes of the brain. In addition, the degree of disruption in the right arcuate fasciculus was correlated to the acuteness of the syndrome. Third, researchers observed consistent thickening of gray matter at the frontal and temporal lobes, connected with the deteriorated right arcuate fasciculus (Zeineh et al., 2014). These exciting results give ground to further research that may allow the exploration of changes in the chronic fatigue patients' brains.

Infectious Causes

It seems that in some portion of chronic fatigue patients, there is an infectious insult preceding the development of the debilitating syndrome. Research has focused on the investigation of various infectious agents to determine whether it is these that are responsible for the symptomatology seen in chronic fatigue patients. Some of the investigated infections include infectious mononucleosis/glandular fever (caused by the Epstein–Barr virus) (Hickie et al., 2006; Katz, Shiraishi, Mears, Binns, & Taylor, 2009; Montoya et al., 2013), Q fever (caused by the *Coxiella burnetii* pathogen), and infections caused by the Ross River virus (Hickie et al., 2006), as well as human herpesvirus 6 infections (Montoya et al., 2013).

In a study with 253 participants, glandular fever, Q fever, and infections caused by the Ross River virus were investigated. Six groups of symptoms were identified and thereafter measured in patients with the aforementioned infections. The symptom groups included, first, "acute sickness," which described the immediate pains of headaches and fevers. Second, "irritability" outlined the mental well-being of patients and the changes in their moods. Third, "fatigue" measured the exhaustion either after physical exertion or after rest; "musculoskeletal pain" described the pain in limbs and joints; "mood disturbance" reported the depressive state of the patients. Last, "neurocognitive disturbance" detailed the cognitive disruptions experienced by these patients. Not surprisingly, it was the "fatigue" symptom group that correlated most strongly and consistently with functional abnormalities experienced by these patients. The results of the study suggested that the fatigue experienced by these patients after they had been diagnosed with the infection decreased with time. At 6 weeks, the fatigue was experienced by 35% of all participants, but this number gradually dropped to 12% at 6 months, which is the time requirement for a diagnosis of chronic fatigue. In 12 months, the incidence decreased to 9%. Thus, the study's results suggest that the chronic fatigue experienced by some of the patients who have dealt with a glandular fever, Q fever, or infections caused by the Ross River virus is caused by the response of the host organism to the infection. These troublesome symptoms, in some cases, persisted as long as 12 months. These data show that chronic fatigue is a relatively common sequela for patients who have contracted the aforementioned infections, and the syndrome is often long-lasting. In this way, such patients create a subgroup of all chronic fatigue patients, distinguishable by the evidence of causality of their symptoms (Hickie et al., 2006). The goal of future research is to develop biomarkers that could effectively pinpoint those infectious patients likely to develop full-blown chronic fatigue syndrome and to develop efficacious interventions for alleviation of symptoms and improvement of the quality of life.

In the case of infectious mononucleosis, a study was designed with 1- and 2-year follow-ups to investigate whether some of the patients experience postinfection chronic fatigue syndrome. Fatigue is a common symptom among infectious mononucleosis patients, and thus the study included only those who experienced persistent fatigue 6 months after recovery. Three hundred one (13% of the original sample) such patients were identified. At 12-month follow-up, 7% of patients experienced chronic fatigue, while at 24-month follow-up, this included 4% of patients. From these results, the authors concluded that patients with infectious mononucleosis, or glandular fever, are at a risk of developing chronic fatigue syndrome. Reportedly, women and those having greater fatigue are at a greater risk of developing a persistent chronic fatigue syndrome that persists 6 months or longer. In this manner, infectious mononucleosis patients form another subgroup of patients that are at risk of developing chronic fatigue (Katz et al., 2009). In future research, this subgroup should be carefully investigated and other risk factors, demographical or psychological, should be assessed.

The risk of chronic fatigue syndrome in patients with human herpesvirus 6 infections and glandular fever has been investigated. A sample of 30 patients suffering from chronic fatigue was selected. These patients also exhibited elevated levels of IgG antibody titers against human herpesvirus 6 and the virus causing glandular fever—Epstein–Barr virus. A double-blind, placebo-controlled trial was carried out in which a portion of patients received placebo and a portion received valganciclovir, an antiviral medication effective in the treatment of infections caused by herpesviruses. Valganciclovir is often used to treat infections like glandular fever or other human herpesvirus 6-caused infections. Levels of mental as well as physical fatigue were recorded, along with assessments of cognitive functioning. Monocytes, neutrophil counts, and cytokine levels were the chosen markers of disease progression. A range of symptoms in patients administered valganciclovir improved significantly more than the symptoms in placebo patients, at 9 months after baseline. These symptoms included mental fatigue, cognitive function, and fatigue severity, and these improvements were evident as early as 3 months after treatment. Monocyte and cytokine levels also responded to the antiviral treatment. Therefore, the authors of this study concluded that treatment with valganciclovir in a group of patients with human herpesvirus 6 infections and glandular fever is clinically beneficial to cognitive and physical functioning, independent of a placebo effect. These improvements are thought to be brought about by immunomodulatory and/or antiviral effects. In the future, research in a larger patient sample with longer treatment duration and longer follow-up has been proposed to be designed (Montoya et al., 2013).

The above findings clearly point to the possibility that in some chronic fatigue patients, an infection may have caused the dramatic physiological and mental changes. Whether the cause of chronic fatigue syndrome lies in the infectious agent per se or rather in the powerful immune response to that agent remains unclear. If it were the case that the syndrome was caused by the infectious agent, then it would be important to investigate whether it might be possible to treat these patients with the correct long-term antimicrobial medication. Infectious causes seem to be a crucial avenue for future research, in the hope to elucidate the mechanisms of chronic fatigue syndrome.

As evident from the aforementioned research, there seems to be a plethora of possible causes of the chronic fatigue syndrome. Neurological changes, white matter abnormalities, infectious causes, neuroinflammation, and interactions with the immune and endocrine systems all offer some limited insight into the mechanisms of the syndrome. It is important to note that because the possible causes are so numerous, and because the research is so far very inconclusive, it might be the case that chronic fatigue syndrome is actually evolving. In addition, it is important to consider that a different cause altogether may be in control of the development of the syndrome in different patients. Therefore, it seems that rather than treating chronic fatigue patients as one homogeneous group, research would benefit from creating subclasses of patients whose syndrome is underlined by varying causalities.

DIAGNOSIS

Because tiredness is such a widespread symptom of not only diseases but also syndromes, lifestyles, and states, it is especially hard to diagnose chronic fatigue. Currently, physicians are restricted to the diagnosis through patients' self-reports, as no lab tests for the diagnosis of chronic fatigue are available. Because there are no tests for the diagnosis of chronic fatigue by itself, the usual strategy in the diagnosis of this condition is to employ diagnostic tests to either rule out or confirm any possible disorders or conditions that could be causing the symptoms secondarily. If a condition is confirmed, for example, if the patient is found to suffer from anemia, then it is the anemia that has to be treated for the fatigue symptoms to diminish. However, such method of diagnosis is often "hit or miss," as it can be virtually impossible to test for all the possible causes of chronic fatigue. Therefore, many patients suffering from this condition often go undiagnosed, which in turn halts the hope for treatment and recovery.

Primary evaluation of chronic fatigue syndrome is so far possible only through a careful evaluation of the patient's medical history. Any fatigue that is persistent and unexplainable by extraordinary exertion or lack of rest has to be clinically considered. Moreover, chronic fatigue should always be considered if the patient also experiences other classes of symptoms that prevent with the patient's daily functioning at work, personal life, and concentration, such as mental fog and cognitive dysfunction.

There is a lot of emphasis on developing diagnostic tools that would allow for the detection of chronic fatigue syndrome. Scientists have discovered protein biomarkers in the spinal fluid of chronic fatigue patients that are drastically distinct from the proteins found in the spinal fluid of healthy individuals. Such findings indicate that the malfunction of central nervous system proteins is crucial in chronic fatigue. According to the results of this study, patients suffering from chronic fatigue carry 738 proteins unique to this syndrome. Future research aims to identify the biomarker proteins that, after running diagnostic tests, would offer conclusive results as to whether the patient suffers from chronic fatigue. If such protein biomarkers are identified, it would then be possible to introduce specific treatments that would aim to attend to the specific protein biomarker pathway. Such approach could result in highly efficient treatments that would treat chronic pain where it originates (Schutzer et al., 2011).

TREATMENT
Cognitive Behavioral Therapy

Cognitive behavioral therapy, or CBT, is a therapeutical method aimed at establishing the most effective ways of symptom management. Through identifying problematic cognitions and behaviors, CBT aims to relieve the symptoms (affective, physical, social, etc.) of chronic fatigue, thus improving the patient's quality of life. CBT approaches chronic fatigue in one of the following two ways. The main goal of therapy is either (a) to change the patients' cognitions about the syndrome, thus shifting their perception toward a healthier perspective, or (b) to improve the patients' quality of life by helping them achieve a better understanding of their syndrome and teaching them how to manage their physical disability without straining them unnecessarily. Thus, this approach addresses the practicalities associated with the syndrome, instead of directly attempting to ameliorate the patients' physical or mental capacity (Price, Mitchell, Tidy, & Hunot, 2008).

Generally, CBT aims to achieve the following outcomes: get a better understanding of the fluctuating energy levels by monitoring the patients' daily activities, and consequently developing a plan of daily tasks at the right times, to minimize strain and exhaustion; maximize the efficacy of the daily activity plan by creating a routine sleeping pattern; establish varied targets of therapy, to keep the patient motivated; learn skills to gain control of various emotions and cognitions regarding the symptomatology of the syndrome, eliminating catastrophic thoughts; work on the patients' self-esteem by identifying their strengths and consequently utilizing them to maximize the outcome of therapy.

Various review studies found that CBT is an effective tool in managing chronic fatigue symptoms. According to one study, patients who undergo CBT suffer from less severe fatigue, in comparison with patients who do not receive treatment or who receive only the usual care from a physician. Specifically, 40% of patients who attended CBT saw clinical improvement, while 26% patients in usual care experienced alleviation of chronic fatigue symptoms. This review also addressed the longevity of the beneficial CBT effects. At follow-up (1–7 months after completion of CBT program, depending on the study), the patients who had successfully finished the CBT treatment showed that the improvements they gained through therapy persisted also long term. The most significant improvement was seen in decreased fatigability. This review also contrasted CBT with other types of therapy used to treat chronic fatigue: relaxation methods, counseling and support, and other types of psychological interventions. This comparison found that CBT patients, upon successful completion of treatment, suffered from less severe fatigability, experienced more effective physical functioning, and saw improvements in depression and anxiety. These results were not very consistent at follow-up, however, highlighting possible drawbacks of CBT (Price et al., 2008). Another review found similar results regarding the improvements in fatigue, physical functioning, and other common symptoms, adding that patients who received CBT were also more likely to maintain consistent school attendance. However, this review concluded that even after such improvements, patients were unlikely to return to work (Chambers, Bagnall, Hempel, & Forbes, 2006).

A large trial was carried out in the United Kingdom to assess the effectiveness of group CBT. This study compared group CBT with counseling and support and with usual medical care. The main outcome measure in this study was the Short Form-36 survey, investigating the mental and physical health of the participants. Further outcome measures included a specific fatigue scale and a scale investigating anxiety and depression, as well as an overall health and well-being measure. Measures of physical health and cognitive functions were included too. Data were collected at baseline and at 6- and 12-month follow-up after the initial evaluation. The results showed that group CBT was more effective than the other interventions, but its improvements were limited. Specifically, the patients who attended group CBT saw no significant improvements in their quality of life, cognitive function, work status, or health care utility measures. This is an interesting outcome, because the majority of the said variables were found to be improved when patients attended individual CBT. However, group CBT did improve the patients' mood and strength, and it also decreased overall tiredness, outcomes that are also reliably seen in individual CBT. The fact that patients experienced improvements in strength (in terms of both energy and endurance) is of crucial importance, as this allowed them to normalize their daily activities substantially (O'Dowd, Gladwell, Rogers, Hollinghurst, & Gregory, 2006).

Research has been carried out to investigate the usefulness of family-based CBT, focusing mostly on the efficiency of treatment in terms of improving school attendance and work ethic. Compared with psycho-education, it was found that in terms of school attendance and recovery rates, both treatment groups benefited from the given intervention. This improvement was maintained at the 24-month follow-up for both groups. Family-based CBT yielded important significant improvements in emotional and behavioral adaptation in the long term, whereas the effects seen in patients who received psycho-education treatment suggested deterioration in these measures (Lloyd, Chalder, & Rimes, 2012).

Apart from the type of CBT received by patients suffering from chronic fatigue, research found that the therapy relationship is of crucial importance to the outcomes, too. The outcome expectations and the trust between the therapist and the patient, as well as the perception of posttreatment malaise, are important variables. Research found that to effectively assist in the alleviation of fatigue-perpetuating factors, the efficiency of CBT depends on all previously mentioned variables. Therefore, not only should stress be put on choosing the right type of CBT for the patient, but importance should also be given to creating and managing a positive therapy relationship, preferably from the very beginning of CBT (Heins, Knoop, & Bleijenberg, 2013).

Mindfulness-Based Therapy

Mindfulness-based therapy aims to shift the attention of the patient away from the ever-persistent fatigue in a very specific way—toward the patient's purpose in the current moment. Mindfulness offers a nonjudgmental space for learning to accept the syndrome and the symptoms that come with it and to in turn make these cognitions peaceful. Through the development of such awareness, detrimental beliefs held against the self and the syndrome can be recognized, and other, more adaptive, positive and accepting schemes can be cultivated.

One of the main symptoms of chronic fatigue is stress. Patients may feel stressed because of their limited functioning, but simultaneously, stress might be the cause of their problems, too. It is often found that patients who suffer from chronic fatigue have adrenal exhaustion—characterized by over-production of the stress hormones adrenalin and noradrenalin. These hormones are secreted in stressful, so-called fight-or-flight situations, making the body highly alert. Chronic fatigue patients are thought to have long-lasting and intense activation of their adrenal system, leading to abnormalities and malfunction. Anything can be a potential stressor—family, employment, relationships, or physical activity with inadequate recovery time.

In such instances, when patients recognize that the stressors in their life are worsening their condition, mindfulness-based therapy can be very helpful. A number of programs aimed at chronic fatigue patients have been developed, primarily addressing the said stressors, as well as sources of anxiety, fatigue, and depression. One such approach that has proved efficient is so-called mindfulness-based cognitive therapy. This approach integrates mindfulness techniques with some aspects of CBT, to maximize the prevention of depressive relapse and change the perception of both internal and external stressors. Mindfulness-based cognitive therapy was found to improve the patients' quality of life and fatigability symptoms. The results were comparable to the results obtained from CBT studies; however, the improvement in symptoms was more rapid when patients practiced mindfulness (Fjorback et al., 2013).

Research addressing the shortcomings of CBT investigated the use of mindfulness-based cognitive therapy administered after the completion of a CBT program in patients who did not reach recovery and alleviation of symptoms. The study found that patients were satisfied with the accessibility, engagement, and helpfulness of the mindfulness-based program. The outcome showed that the patients who participated and completed mindfulness-based cognitive therapy saw improvements in fatigability, whereas the symptoms of patients who did not participate in this program remained unchanged and severe. In addition, the follow-up measures found that the improvements gained through mindfulness-based cognitive therapy were maintained up to 6 months after the completion of treatment. Furthermore, patients who engaged in mindfulness experienced improvements in their mood, catastrophic thinking, unhelpful cognitions about fatigue-related emotions, and self-compassion (Rimes & Wingrove, 2013).

Graded Exercise Therapy

Graded exercise therapy is a form of intervention that employs physical activity as its main method of treatment for chronic fatigue. The physical activity is introduced gradually, often in the form of gentle stretching, with duration of as little as 5 min per day for individuals who have been physically inactive owing to chronic fatigue. As the patient gains strength, the intensity of physical exertion is increased over time. This form of therapy is highly controlled, and to be done correctly, it has to be followed according to a strict, balanced exercise plan, which includes mandatory periods of rest, too. The main aim is not to overexercise and not to push the body to its limits, which would be detrimental to the patient's health. If the physician and the patient manage to develop a suitable plan of physical activity, this can be efficient in alleviating the burdens of disturbed sleep, low mood, pain, and other symptoms related to chronic fatigue, allowing the patient to improve the quality of life (Edmonds, McGuire, & Price, 2004).

Research evaluating the efficacy of graded exercise therapy in alleviating the symptoms of chronic fatigue found that after the completion of treatment, patients felt significant improvements in fatigue and energy levels. The mechanism of this improvement was thought to be a reduction in concentration on symptoms through the focus on physical activity, rather than the increase in fitness (Moss-Morris, Sharon, Tobin, & Baldi, 2005). Another study suggests combining CBT with graded exercise therapy to make patients aware of their body and its limits, recognizing the signals when their body has had enough exercise. In this way, the prevention of relapse depends on the principles of self-management, self-awareness, and respect for one's own mental and physical limitations (Nijs, Paul, & Wallman, 2008).

The same study also recognizes, however, that graded exercise therapy, especially when the patient's boundaries are not respected, can be severely detrimental to both the patient's mental and his or her physical health. Graded exercise therapy has been known to worsen the chronic fatigue symptoms through promotion of immune dysfunction and through the exertion of inappropriate strain on the body and mind (Nijs et al., 2008). Similarly, a large-scale Norwegian study found that as many as 79% of patients who underwent graded exercise therapy actually perceived that their symptoms had worsened as a result (Bjørkum, Wang, & Waterloo, 2009). Therefore, the effectiveness of graded exercise therapy must be treated with caution. Extra focus should be put on the cognitive factors during this type of therapy, to prevent relapse and exacerbation of symptoms.

CHRONIC PAIN

Background

Pain is a symptom of a vast variety of injuries and disorders, but it can sometimes be the cause of a disorder itself. Pain is fully produced by the nervous system, and therefore, anything that has an impact on the nervous system potentially bears the capacity to disrupt pain signaling, too. Chronic pain is a syndrome characterized by persistent, ongoing pain that lasts for 3 months or more. It troubles more people than one would expect—outcomes of several epidemiological studies, gathering data from different countries in the world, showed that prevalence of chronic pain in the general population can range anywhere from 12 to 80% (Abu-Saad, 2010). In Norway, approximately 30% of adults have experienced chronic pain, a number high enough to make chronic pain the main reason for long-term sick leave and physical disability affecting employment (Nielsen, Steingrímsdóttir, Berg, & Hånes, 2011).

Chronic pain has a debilitating impact on the patients' quality of life, taking a toll on their physical and emotional state, resulting in the loss of fitness needed for work motivation and affecting their employability, financial security, and self-esteem. The effects of chronic pain are also very detrimental on the economy—chronic pain patients require longer hospital stays, frequent rehabilitations, more frequent outpatient visits, and a range of necessary therapeutical interventions, resulting in enormous health care costs.

Chronic pain is not directly caused by tissue damage, although it may precede the development of chronic pain. Therefore, the focus of chronic pain research is not on the structural changes in the body, but rather, the focal point is the sensitivity of the nervous system. One's choices of lifestyle, diet, and physical activity all have an impact on sensitizing the nervous system to an extent of dysfunction. Therefore, chronic pain is more than "just" pain—it is influenced by many factors, some of these being social, psychological, biological, cultural, environmental. Currently, there is no single, fully efficient treatment for chronic pain. Therefore, clinicians have to choose a broad approach of evaluating each patient. Psychological therapy, seconded by medication, is necessary for alleviating the symptoms and coming to an understanding of the events that preceded the development of chronic pain. Physical therapy is useful for restoring the body's tissue. In this section, the mechanisms of pain will be outlined, and pathophysiology and available treatment will be defined. A variety of suggestions for future research will be identified, aiming to give an accurate description of the aspects of chronic pain that the scientific community has been focusing on.

MECHANISMS OF PAIN

When the body encounters a painful stimulus, nociceptive receptors start firing. As the nociceptors fire, powerful chemicals are released by the injured cells. These are identified by other nerves, which then intensify the pain signal. This whole process is called nociception, and it leads to the subjective perception of a painful stimulus by an individual. This perception depends on a myriad of factors, such as the unique and distinctive tolerance to pain of each person, the person's emotional and physical well-being, his or her attitude toward pain, and the context in which the painful stimulus occurs. This makes the perception of pain a highly individual experience, making it difficult for researchers to develop a better understanding of the condition.

Chronic pain, unlike acute pain, which signals immediate danger and the need to be careful, is persistent and continuous. Nociceptors, the pain receptors, fire constantly in the nervous system, making the pain a continuous sensation. At the beginning, there might be a trigger for the nociceptive receptors to start firing—the stimuli can be of thermal, mechanical, or chemical character, such as an injured back or untreated infection. However, the cause might be ongoing, caused by conditions such as arthritis or cancer. Acute pain recedes once the tissue has recovered. In the case of chronic pain, however, the nociceptors keep firing despite tissue recovery. Individuals suffering from chronic pain experience one or more of these conditions—spontaneous pain, with no obvious cause; hyperpathia, characterized by firing of nociceptive receptors that exceeds the expectation after injury; hyperalgesia, exacerbated intensity of pain with no further experience of a painful event; secondary hyperalgesia, in which the sensitivity to pain extends to intact, uninjured tissue; and allodynia, characterized by the experience of pain from a stimulus that does not normally activate nociceptors. The resulting chronic pain often manifests in the form of migraines, back pain, arthritis pain, neck pain, neurogenic pain, and so on. Back pain is the most common form of chronic pain. It has been reported that patients suffering from chronic back pain have lowered quality of life, mainly affecting their physical and mental health. Of these patients, 28% experience reduced physical ability.

Chronic pain sufferers are also three times more likely to be in fair or bad health and four times more likely to have mental health problems than adults with no chronic pain condition (US Department of Health & Human Services, 2006).

To gain a better understanding of chronic pain, it is important to explore the characteristics of the different nociceptive receptors. Nociceptors can be either stimulus specific, and thus respond to chemical, thermal, or mechanical injury of the body, or polymodal, meaning they respond to any of the said types of stimuli. These types of receptors are usually located in the periphery and can be sensitized over a prolonged period of time by recurrent application of the stimuli. These polymodal nociceptors, which play an important role in the peripheral sensitization of receptors, are thought to mediate the development and permanency of chronic pain.

From the polymodal receptors, the noxious information travels up the spinal cord and terminates in the brain. The axons in the central nervous system differ in terms of myelination—the greater the myelination, the faster the stimulus transmission. The myelination of axons is sensitive to injury-related changes in transmission. The more myelinated axons in the central nervous system are considered to have greater sensitivity to the changes in myelination as a result of injury. Therefore, if injury causes abnormalities in myelination (and thus the myelin cannot perform its protective and nourishing function), the mechanisms that convey action potentials along the axons can become dysfunctional. With such abnormalities in action potential mechanisms, we can often see excessive electrical activity within the nerves themselves, which in turn causes an increase in the nociceptors' firing rate, resulting in more severe perception of the noxious stimulus.

PATHOPHYSIOLOGY

Dysfunction at the Molecular Level

The cell bodies of nociceptors can be found in the dorsal root ganglia of the spinal cord. It is here, in the dorsal root ganglia, that the nociceptors have their intricate genetic infrastructure and metabolic apparatus. The genetic infrastructure is thought to be especially important in terms of the various pain states. In terms of chronic pain, the following intracellular factors have been known to occur. First, it has been noted that in chronic pain, even the neurons that are typically not designed to transmit pain information start synthesizing a chemical that is normally present when noxious stimulus is transferred through nociceptors—substance P. If a neuron starts synthesizing substance P, the resulting activity may be perceived as pain, even in the lack of injury.

Similarly, the perception of pain can be affected by the presence and expression of sodium channels. Sodium channels are present in every neuron that is capable of generating action potentials, mediating the passage of sodium ions through the cell membrane. Past research showed that a unique mutation of sodium channels plays an important role in a rare genetic disorder, which is characterized by the inability to feel pain (Fertleman et al., 2006). Often, genetic mutations in sodium channels do not disable their functionality completely, but merely change it. That is the case in another disorder, erythromelalgia, a rare genetic disorder with very painful symptoms (Drenth et al., 2005), and other illnesses with painful symptomatologies (Fertleman & Ferrie, 2006). Therefore, it is obvious that the genetic infrastructure of a cell that mediates the function of sodium channels may induce the perception of chronic pain even in the absence of a painful event.

Chemical Factors

Apart from the aforementioned substance P, there are also other compounds that are synthesized and released in the presence of noxious stimuli. These compounds modulate nerve excitability and thus the perception of pain, and include the amino acids gamma-aminobutyric acid and glycine, various peptides, and the nucleoside adenosine, whose function is to dampen the signal transmitted by nociceptors. Any damage or abnormalities of these compounds, in terms of their molecular foundation and changes to the intensity of synaptic input, have the capacity to cause long-term or even indefinite changes in the nociceptors. Such indefinite changes in nociceptor functioning may in turn be responsible for certain aspects of chronic pain.

Peripheral Nervous System Abnormalities

Certain abnormalities in the spinal cord have been thought to contribute to the perception of chronic pain. These abnormalities include phenomena such as central sensitization, wind-up, and microglial activation. Central sensitization refers to a situation in which the nociceptive receptors in the dorsal horns of the spinal cord become sensitized by prolonged presence of noxious stimuli in the periphery, caused by, for example, tissue damage or inflammation. Wind-up refers to the perceived intensification of the intensity of pain. This occurs over time, when a certain nonnoxious stimulus is applied recurrently above a critical rate. Such recurrent stimulation of group C peripheral nerve fibers then consequently causes gradual increases in electrical response in the corresponding spinal cord neurons. Last, but not least, microglia are located within the spinal cord and their major role is to mediate inflammatory processes. There is clear evidence showing that microglia have a role in the direct induction of peripheral injury-induced pain, as well as the maintenance of chronic pain (Hains & Waxman, 1994; Tsuda, Inoue, & Salter, 2005).

White Matter Abnormalities

A number of studies have found structural abnormalities in the brains of chronic pain patients, relative to the brains of healthy individuals. A 2013 study investigated two groups of patients. Upon recruitment to the study, each patient group had experienced pain for at least 3 months. At 12-month follow-up, the population of patients was split into two groups—those who still experienced pain and those in whom the pain had ceased. Diffusion tensor imaging was employed to study the white matter structure of these patients. The picture that emerged clearly indicated that the structure of the white matter in patients with persistent chronic pain differed from the white matter structures in patients who had recovered. Namely, it was the white matter structures connecting the medial prefrontal cortex and the nucleus accumbens, both known for their implication in pain, that showed abnormalities. Neuroimaging data were also collected at baseline, and the results showed an extraordinary degree of consistency—in most cases, those patients in which white matter abnormalities were seen at baseline had persistent chronic pain and the white matter structures remained abnormal at the 12-month follow-up. The same applies to the other sample of subjects—those who did not develop chronic pain showed intact white matter structures, both at baseline and at follow-up. The authors of this study suggested that abnormalities in these structures can in the future be used as a biomarker to distinguish the patients who will develop chronic pain from those who will not. Such ability to pinpoint the predisposition to chronic pain would be greatly beneficial in reducing the longevity of this burdensome syndrome and would offer a degree of insight yet unprecedented in chronic pain syndrome (Mansour et al., 2013).

Psychoneuroimmunological Factors

The nonneuronal contributors that play important roles in the development and sustainment of chronic pain include immune cells, neuroinflammation, cytokines, cortisol, the HPA axis, and others. Another important factor in chronic pain is the observed decrease in gray matter volume in the brain, which results in changes in thickness of the cortex (Baliki, Schnitzer, Bauer, & Apkarian, 2011). Another important factor is the reorganization of the networks in the brain that process pain-associated information, with much of the research focusing on the hippocampus (Baliki et al., 2011).

Furthermore, patients suffering from chronic pain often have an abnormally functioning HPA axis, manifesting the principal adaptation inflicted by the noxious stimulus, which is also thought to influence the structure and function of the hippocampus (McEwen & Kalia, 2010). The abnormal functioning of the HPA axis, which in turn influences the structure and function of the hippocampal network, is thought to be caused by the allostatic load and its sensitivity to the detrimental effects of continuously elevated levels of glucocorticoids (Mirescu & Gould, 2006). Such changes are crucial when the body tries to adjust its functioning in accordance with the chronic pain, as the unpredictability about the upcoming pain, the intensification of pain by premediated anxiety, and negative emotions are thought to activate the hippocampal network relevant to the processing of pain (Vachon-Presseau et al., 2013). Further research found that chronic pain may amount to an allostatic load in patients who are more prone to stress, causing permanent plastic changes in the brain that induce the worsening of the patient's condition (Vachon-Presseau et al., 2013).

The research investigating the pathophysiology of chronic pain has also focused on the role of the adaptive immune system, by the study of cytokines. Cytokines are small secreted proteins whose main function relates to interactions and communication between cells. There are two functional types of cytokines: pro- and anti-inflammatory. Research showed that certain types of cytokines are implicated in both the induction and the longevity of chronic pain by directly activating nociceptors. Specific inflammatory cytokines are also believed to play a role in inflammation- or nerve injury-caused central sensitization, thereby prompting the development of conditions such as hyperalgesia or allodynia (Sherman & Loomis, 1994; Zhang & An, 2007).

Chronic pain is also thought to depend on plastic changes in the body's stress network (Gatchel, Peng, Peters, Fuchs, & Turk, 2007), in which the hormone cortisol is a key factor. The stress network is mediated by elevated levels of cortisol. When the body is under long-lasting, unknown, and unmanageable threat, it adapts its functioning of metabolic activity to match the environmental demands. Such adaptation may ultimately cause abnormal responses of the stress system, prompting pathophysiological strain as a result (McEwen, 1998). This state of pathophysiological strain is also termed allostatic load, and it is instrumental in the persistence and intensifying of the perception of pain (Borsook, Maleki, Becerra, & McEwen, 2012).

TREATMENT

CBT

Patients with chronic pain looking for psychological therapy are most often advised to participate in CBT. CBT is now a widely used tool for the management of pain. With the help of a therapist's guidance, the patient who experiences chronic pain learns how to shift his or her attention from the pain toward the aspiration for recovery. CBT teaches that it is the person him- or herself who holds the key to the recovery gate. It teaches that individuals themselves are responsible for their own experiences and attitudes. This approach can be applied to many of the cognitions held by chronic pain patients. The patient learns to pinpoint and understand negative patterns in thoughts and behavior that are linked to the syndrome. Once these are identified, the patient then goes on to establish the skills needed to change the negative behavioral and mental patterns. Once these skills are successfully put into practice, chronic pain-related symptoms are expected do decrease, while the quality of life is expected to increase.

CBT is also efficient for becoming in control of stress. In stressful situations, the brain releases noradrenaline and serotonin, which affect pain control. In chronic pain patients, stressful situations can especially exacerbate the perception of pain. By learning and applying the CBT techniques, the arousal that has an influence on the release of noradrenaline and serotonin is reduced. In this manner, the body can gradually normalize its response to pain, and it can also increase the efficacy of its innate pain relief response.

Patients who completed CBT, in comparison to those who received no treatment, saw a small, but statistically significant, improvement in pain and the resulting disability, as well as average improvements in mood and the tendency for catastrophism. Greater improvements at follow-up were seen in mood (Williams, Eccleston, & Morley, 2012). In addition, CBT has been shown to help patients with their illness perception; as a result of therapy, they were able to identify, manage, and replace the troubling perception of their condition (Siemonsma et al., 2013).

When addressing specific types of chronic pain, reviews showed the following. Patients who received CBT for chronic back pain saw improvements in pain, engagement in physical activities, quality of life associated with health, and depression (Hoffman, Papas, Chatkoff, & Kerns, 2007). In terms of chronic headaches, patients who completed CBT experienced 30–60% alleviation of symptoms. These effects were long-lasting, and in some patients, the symptoms never returned (Andrasik, 2007). Patients suffering from chronic orofacial pain who completed a course of CBT experienced long-lasting improvements in the intensity of pain, depression, and engagement in physical activity that was previously impossible because of pain (Aggarwal et al., 2011). CBT is also known to be effective for other pain-related disorders, such as fibromyalgia and arthritis.

The advantages of CBT lay in its tailoring to different age groups—it is effective in both adults and children. Furthermore, a wide range of innovative CBT delivery formats has been developed, and it is now possible to hold CBT online, or on the phone; without having to compromise on efficiency.

Mindfulness

Mindfulness in chronic pain syndrome focuses on shifting the focus of the patient away from the pain. Rather, the attention is turned to the process of observing the patient's thought patterns, feelings, sensations in the body. Mindfulness aims to do this in a fully nonjudgmental way—without placing pressure on the patients and without subjecting them to criticism for how much pain they are experiencing. By exploring mindfulness, chronic pain patients learn how to respond to pain thoughtfully rather than adversely react to it.

One of the main symptoms seen in chronic pain patients is catastrophizing. Patients often engage in these harmful cognitions, whereby they exacerbate the perception of pain by ruminating about all its adverse impacts on daily functioning. The lack of efficacious treatment is another aspect of the syndrome that the patients often catastrophize about, persuading themselves that they will never be healthy because there is not one drug that could make them feel better. In this way, patients feel the pain much more deeply and persistently. Catastrophizing is often accompanied by stress, anxiety, and depression, all of which make the goal of recovery harder to reach.

Through mindfulness, chronic pain patients learn to adopt a fresh outlook, to take recovery step by step and set small goals. Any expectations should ideally be dropped. Such approach makes the patient's journey to health filled with acceptance. Patients learn to acknowledge their pain without fear and anger. There is a set of strategies the patients are encouraged to employ. First, a "brain scan" refers to the mental exercise of concentrating the focus to individual body parts and thus working against the brain, which wishes to minimize the pain and the awareness of it. This approach encourages acceptance and awareness of the whole body. Furthermore, breathing exercises are a vital part of mindfulness. They, too, aim to work against the brain. When the body feels pain, the brain reacts instantaneously, increasing the heart rate, inducing negative thoughts, and making breathing difficult. By employing the breathing exercises in mindfulness, the patient learns how to slow his or her breathing and calm his or her thoughts. This is a form of a grounding exercise. All attention is focused on making the body more relaxed, and the breathing more effortless. Last but not least, distractions are another powerful aspect of mindfulness. When pain is present, the patient is encouraged to spend some time engaging in a healthy, distracting activity of his or her choice. This may be listening to music, reading a magazine, or enjoying a cup of coffee. In this manner, the patient spends his or her energy in a much more positive way than when focusing on the pain (Gardner-Nix & Costin-Hall, 2009).

Research has shown that chronic pain patients can benefit from mindfulness in many ways. These include alleviation of bodily pain and negative mental symptoms, such as depression (Esmer, Blum, Rulf, & Pier, 2010) and catastrophizing, and decreased distress and disability (McCracken & Thompson). Mindfulness is most probably not more effective than CBT, but it is still a good therapy option, teaching patients patience, acceptance, and self-awareness, which can be utilized to alleviate some of the debilitating symptoms of chronic pain.

Acceptance-Commitment Therapy

Acceptance-commitment therapy (ACT) is another therapeutical intervention used for the treatment of chronic pain. It possesses certain characteristics similar to those of CBT and mindfulness: it teaches patients to reduce the avoidance strategies they have created for themselves as a way of keeping away from pain. In addition, through cognitive techniques, patients learn to disengage their harmful, negative thoughts that are linked to their actions. Coming closer to the desired goals and values in life is one of the main facets of ACT. Through these approaches, the patients gradually work to accept their situation and learn to refocus their energy away from the efforts of symptoms management and pain reduction. The main idea is to put as much as possible of the patient's attention at the desired private experiences (emotions, thoughts, and symptoms including pain) that are routinely avoided when struggling with chronic pain syndrome.

Through ACT, patients are intensely present-focused. They learn to step away from their emotions connected to pain. They are encouraged to develop their psychological flexibility and courage to experience pain. This can be achieved by paying close attention to their thoughts, feelings, and perceptions just they way they are—patients are encouraged not to change them. This acceptance enables them to act in a compatible manner with their therapy goals and way of life. ACT aims to help the patient understand that when the patient perceives pain in his or her body, it is the struggle he or she wages with pain that makes his or her hardship. The perception of the noxious stimulus is barely a reflex necessary for survival, functioning to alert us to danger. Therefore, the principles of commitment and acceptance are especially helpful when attempts to medicate the pain have failed and when the causes and sustaining factors of chronic pain are unknown.

Research has shown that ACT has proven beneficial in re-introducing previously enjoyable activities with friends and family, involvement in work, and the self-satisfaction that follows (McCracken & Eccleston, 2004). In addition, ACT has been shown to significantly decrease the perceived amount of pain in chronic pain patients (Dahl, Wilson, & Nilsson, 2004). A number of studies have shown that the changes in perception that follow the successful completion of ACT can be very helpful in managing chronic pain. ACT has been shown to improve both mental and physical functioning of chronic pain patients; it has been shown to improve their mood, stability, and emotional flexibility and, therefore, it is comparable to the efficient CBT (Bach & Hayes, 2000; Vowles & McCracken, 2008; Wetherell et al., 2011).

Graded Exercise Therapy

Oftentimes, pain flares up because of overexertion or because of going without rest for long periods of time. In this way, the body's comfort zone is exercised, leading to hypersensitization, in which even small amounts of exertion lead to heightened levels of pain. When patients experience pain, their natural response is to stop the activity they are doing and rest. In many patients, negative cognitions about physical activity and movement are developed. These are often accompanied by stress and shame and frustration. Avoiding and dreading physical movement because of the anticipated pain leads to an unfortunate cycle, in which long periods of inactivity are common.

Inactivity is among the main behavioral issues seen in chronic pain patients. As much as half of the waking hours of a chronic pain patient can be spent passively resting (Keefe & Lefebvre, 1994). Such long periods of inactivity are highly detrimental to the patient's mental and physical well-being. In addition, they become progressively more dependent on their caregivers and family members, and their tolerance for physical movement and for daily challenges dramatically decreases. Patients become stressed, often bitter, and the hope of recovery seems distant. It is difficult for them to increase their activity levels, and efforts often result in unsuccessful attempts that are too painful and strenuous.

Graded exercise therapy encourages patients who have developed a sedentary lifestyle to start moving more. This is done in a highly controlled, gradual manner. Clear short-term goals are set and reinforcement of the patient's efforts is frequent, to boost and sustain motivation. The goal of graded exercise therapy is to break the cycle of inactivity, by very slowly increasing the level of activity during the day. The patient can thus keep progressing in order to rebuild physical strength and tolerance to pain, which leads to alleviation of symptoms.

CONCLUSION

As we have seen, both chronic fatigue and chronic pain syndromes are very complex conditions that scientists are only beginning to understand. Thanks to advances in technology, and to the extensive funding that has been devoted to researching these conditions, an emerging picture is starting to unfold—that the neuropathologies of these syndromes have certain common variables. Interestingly, neuroimmunological dysfunctions, changes in the major components of the central nervous system, abnormalities of the HPA axis, and structural changes in white matter structures, as well as flaws in the functioning of cytokines and cortisol, have been implicated in both of these conditions. Figure 1 shows an overview of the identified

Pathophysiology	Chronic fatigue	Chronic pain
Neurological abnormalities	x	x
• Motor system	x	
• Blood-brain-barrier	x	
• Sodium channels		x
• Nociceptors		x
Psychoneuroimmunological interactions	x	x
Neuroinflammation	x	x
White matter abnormalities	x	x
Infectious causes	x	
Peripheral nervous system dysfunction		x

Figure 1 Overview of the pathophysiology of chronic pain and chronic fatigue.

pathophysiology in both syndromes, showing significant overlap in a number of disordered physiological processes associated with chronic pain and chronic fatigue syndromes.

Future research should focus on expanding our knowledge of the pathophysiology present in these syndromes and using this knowledge to develop reliable biomarkers for better, quicker, and well-grounded diagnosis. In both of these syndromes, CBT, which aims to modify these patients' perceptions of and consequent reactions to pain, has proven beneficial. Similar efficiency has been observed for mindfulness programs and ACT. With our knowledge of the pathophysiology expanding, potentially leading to the successful use of biomarkers, there is also great room for improvement in the availability of these therapies to a variety of chronic pain and fatigue patient populations.

REFERENCES

Abu-Saad, H. H. (2010). Chronic Pain : A review. *Journal Medical Libanais, 58*(1), 21–27.

Aggarwal, V. R., Lovell, K., Peters, S., Javidi, H., Joughin, A., & Goldthorpe, J. (2011). Psychosocial interventions for the management of chronic orofacial pain. *The Cochrane Database of Systematic Reviews, 11*. Article No. CD008456.

Andrasik, F. (2007). What does the evidence show? Efficacy of behavioural treatments for recurrent headaches in adults. *Neurological Sciences, 28*(Suppl. 2), S70–S77.

Bach, P., & Hayes, S. C. (2000). The use of acceptance and commitment therapy to prevent the rehospitalization of psychotic patients: a randomized controlled trial. *Journal of Consulting and Clinical Psychology, 70*(5), 1129–1139.

Baliki, M. N., Schnitzer, T. J., Bauer, W. R., & Apkarian, A. V. (2011). Brain morphological signatures for chronic pain. *PLoS One, 6*, e26010.

Bested, A. C., Saunders, P. R., & Logan, A. C. (2001). Chronic fatigue syndrome: neurological findings may be related to blood–brain barrier permeability. *Medical Hypotheses, 57*(2), 231–237.

Bjørkum, T., Wang, C. E. A., & Waterloo, K. (2009). Pasienterfaringer med ulike tiltak ved kronisk utmattelsessyndrom. *Tidsskr Nor Legeforen, 129*, 1214–1216.

Borsook, D., Maleki, N., Becerra, L., & McEwen, B. (2012). Understanding migraine through the lens of maladaptive stress responses: a model disease of allostatic load. *Neuron, 73*, 219–234.

Brent, E. W., van Driel, M. L., Staines, D. R., Ashton, K. J., Hardcastle, S. L., Keane, J., et al. (2012). Longitudinal investigation of natural killer cells and cytokines in chronic fatigue syndrome/myalgic encephalomyelitis. *Journal of Translational Medicine, 10*(88).

Chambers, D., Bagnall, A. M., Hempel, S., & Forbes, C. (2006). Interventions for the treatment, management and rehabilitation of patients with chronic fatigue syndrome/myalgic encephalomyelitis: an updated systematic review. *Journal of the Royal Society of Medicine, 99*(10), 506–520.

Dahl, J., Wilson, K., & Nilsson, A. (2004). Acceptance and commitment therapy and the treatment of persons at risk for long-term disability resulting from stress and pain symptoms: a randomized control clinical trial. *Behaviour Therapy, 35*, 785–801.

Drenth, J. P. H., te Morsche, R. H. M., Guillet, G., Taiev, A., Kirby, R. L., & Jansen, J. B. M. J. (2005). SCN9S mutations define primary erythermalgia as a neuropathic disorder of voltage gated sodium channels. *The Journal of Investigative Dermatology, 124*, 1333–1338.

Edmonds, M., McGuire, H., & Price, J. (2004). Exercise therapy for chronic fatigue syndrome. *Cochrane Database Systemic Reviews, 3*.

Esmer, G., Blum, J., Rulf, J., & Pier, J. (2010). Mindfulness-based stress reduction for failed back surgery syndrome: a randomized controlled trial. *The Journal of American Osteopathic Association, 110*, 646–652.

Fertleman, C. R., Baker, M. D., Parker, K. A., et al. (2006). SNC9A mutations in paroxysmal extreme pain disorder: allelic variants underlie distinct channel defects and phenotypes. *Neuron, 52*, 767–774.

Fertleman, C. R., & Ferrie, C. D. (2006). What's in a name—familial rectal pain syndrome becomes paroxysmal extreme pain disorder. *Journal of Neurology, Neurosurgery and Psychiatry, 77*(11), 1294–1295.

Fjorback, L. O., Arendt, M., Ørnbøl, E., Walach, H., Rehfeld, E., Schröder, A., et al. (2013). Mindfulness therapy for somatization disorder and functional somatic syndromes — Randomized trial with one-year follow-up. *Journal of Psychosomatic Research, 74*, 31–40.

Gardner-Nix, J., & Costin-Hall, L. (2009). The Mindfulness Solution to Pain: Step-by-step Techniques for Chronic Pain Management. Oakland, CA: New Harbinger Publications.

Gatchel, R. J., Peng, Y. B., Peters, M. L., Fuchs, P. N., & Turk, D. C. (2007). The biopsychosocial approach to chronic pain: scientific advances and future directions. *Psychological Bulletin, 133*, 581–624.

Hains, B. C., & Waxman, S. G. (1994). Activated microglia contribute to the maintenance of chronic pain after spinal cord injury. *The Journal of Neuroscience, 26*(16), 4308–4317.

Hall, D. L., Lattie, E. G., Antoni, M. H., Fletcher, M. A., Czaja, S., Perdomo, D., et al. (2014). Stress management skills, cortisol awakening response, and post-exertional malaise in chronic fatigue syndrome. *Psychoneuroendocrinology, 49*, 26–31.

Heins, M. J., Knoop, H., & Bleijenberg, G. (2013). The role of the therapeutic relationship in cognitive behaviour therapy for chronic fatigue syndrome. *Behaviour Research and Therapy, 51*, 368–376.

Hickie, I., Davenport, T., Wakefield, D., Vollmer-Conna, U., Cameron, B., Vernon, S. D., et al. (2006). Post-infective and chronic fatigue syndromes precipitated by viral and non-viral pathogens: prospective cohort study. *BMJ, 333*(7568), 575.

Hilty, L., Langer, N., Pascual-Marqui, R., Boutellier, U., & Lutz, K. (2011). Fatigue-induced increase in intracortical communication between mid/anterior insular and motor cortex during cycling exercise. *European Journal of Neuroscience, 34*(12), 2035–2042.

Hoffman, B. M., Papas, R. K., Chatkoff, D. K., & Kerns, R. D. (2007). Meta-analysis of psychological interventions for chronic low back pain. *Health Psychology, 26*(1), 1–9.

Katz, B. Z., Shiraishi, Y., Mears, C. J., Binns, H. J., & Taylor, R. (2009). Chronic fatigue syndrome after infectious mononucleosis in adolescents. *Pediatrics, 124*(1), 189–193.

Keefe, F. J., & Lefebvre, J. C. (1994). Behaviour therapy. In P. D. Wall, & R. Melzack (Eds.), *Textbook of pain* (pp. 1367–1380). Edinburgh: Churchill Livingstone.

Lloyd, S., Chalder, T., & Rimes, K. A. (2012). Family-focused cognitive behaviour therapy versus psycho-education for adolescents with chronic fatigue syndrome: long-term follow-up of an RCT. *Behaviour Research and Therapy, 50*, 719–725.

Mansour, A. R., Baliki, M. N., Huang, L., Torbey, S., Herrmann, K. M., Schnitzer, T. J., et al. (2013). Brain white matter structural properties predict transition to chronic pain. *Pain, 154*(10), 2160–2168.

McCracken, L. M., & Eccleston, C. (2004). Acceptance of chronic pain: component analysis and a revised assessment method. *Pain, 107*(1–2), 159–166.

McCracken, L. M., & Thompson, M. (2009). Components of mindfulness in patients with chronic pain. *Journal of Psychopathology and Behavioral Assessment, 31*, 75–82.

McEwen, B. S. (1998). Stress, adaptation, and disease. Allostasis and allostatic load. *Annals of the New York Academy of Sciences, 840*, 33–44.

McEwen, B. S., & Kalia, M. (2010). The role of corticosteroids and stress in chronic pain conditions. *Metabolism, 59*(Suppl. 1), S9–S15.

Mirescu, C., & Gould, E. (2006). Stress and adult neurogenesis. *Hippocampus, 16*, 233–238.

Montoya, J. G., Kogelnik, A. M., Bhangoo, M., Lunn, M. R., Flamand, L., Merrihew, L. E., et al. (2013). Randomized clinical trial to evaluate the efficacy and safety of valganciclovir in a subset of patients with chronic fatigue syndrome. *Journal of Medical Virology, 85*(12), 2101–2109.

Morris, G., & Maes, M. (2014). Oxidative and nitrosative stress and immune inflammatory pathways in patients with myalgic encephalomyelitis (ME)/Chronic fatigue syndrome (CFS). *Current Neuropharmacology, 12*, 168–185.

Moss-Morris, R., Sharon, C., Tobin, R., & Baldi, J. C. (2005). A randomized controlled graded exercise trial for chronic fatigue syndrome: outcomes and mechanisms of change. *Journal of Health Psychology, 10*(2), 245–259.

Nakatomi, Y., Mizuno, K., Ishii, A., Wada, Y., Tanaka, M., Tazawa, S., et al. (2014). Neuroinflammation in patients with chronic fatigue Syndrome/Myalgic encephalomyelitis: an [11]C-(R)-PK11195 PET study. *Journal of Nuclear Medicine: Official Publication Society of Nuclear Medicine, 55*(6), 945–950.

Nielsen, C. S., Steingrímsdóttir, Ó. A., Berg, C., & Hånes, H. (2011). Chronic pain prevalence in Norway – fact sheet. Norwegian Institute of Public Health. Source reference: http://www.fhi.no/artikler/?id=88781.

Nijs, J., Paul, L., & Wallman, K. (2008). Chronic fatigue syndrome: an approach combining self-management with graded exercise to avoid exacerbations. *Journal of Rehabilitation Medicine, 40*(4), 241–247.

Nordqvist, C. (2015, September 28). "Fatigue: Why Am I So Tired?." *Medical News Today.* Retrieved from http://www.medicalnewstoday.com/articles/248002.php.

O'Dowd, H., Gladwell, P., Rogers, C. A., Hollinghurst, S., & Gregory, A. (2006). Cognitive behavioural therapy in chronic fatigue syndrome: a randomised controlled trial of an outpatient group programme. *Health Technology Assessment, 10*(37).

Powell, D. J. H., Liossi, C., Moss-Morris, R., & Schlotz, W. (2013). Unstimulated cortisol secretory activity in everyday life and its relationship with fatigue and chronic fatigue syndrome: a systematic review and subset meta-analysis. *Psychoneuroendocrinology, 38*, 2405–2422.

Price, J. R., Mitchell, E., Tidy, E., & Hunot, V. (2008). Cognitive behaviour therapy for chronic fatigue syndrome in adults. *Cochrane Database of Systematic Reviews, 16*(3).

Rimes, K. A., & Wingrove, J. (2013). Mindfulness based cognitive therapy for people with chronic fatigue syndrome still experiencing excessive fatigue after cognitive behaviour therapy: a pilot randomized study. *Clinical Psychology & Psychotherapy, 20,* 107–117.

Schutzer, S. E., Angel, T. E., Liu, T., Schepmoes, A. A., Clauss, T. R., Adkins, J. N., et al. (2011). Distinct cerebrospinal fluid proteomes differentiate post-treatment lyme disease from chronic fatigue syndrome. *PLoS ONE, 6*(2), e17287. http://dx.doi.org/10.1371/journal.pone.0017287.

Sherman, S. E., & Loomis, C. W. (1994). Morphine insensitive allodynia is produced by intrathecal strychnine in the lightly anesthetized rat. *Pain, 56,* 17–29.

Siemonsma, P. C., Stuive, I., Roorda, L. D., et al. (2013). Cognitive treatment of illness perceptions in patients with chronic low back pain: a randomized controlled trial. *Physical Therapy, 93,* 435–448.

Stringer, E. A., Baker, K. S., Carroll, I. R., Montoya, J. G., Chu, L., Maecker, H. T., et al. (2013). Daily cytokine fluctuations, driven by leptin, are associated with fatigue severity in chronic fatigue syndrome: evidence of inflammatory pathology. *Journal of Translational Medicine, 11*(93).

Tsuda, M., Inoue, K., & Salter, M. W. (2005). Neuropathic pain and spinal microglia: a big problem from molecules in "small" glia. *Trends in Neurosciences, 28,* 101–107.

US Department of Health & Human Services (Eds.). (2006). *Health, United States, 2005: With chartbook on trends in the health of Americans.* Claitor's Law Books and Publishing Division.

Vachon-Presseau, E., Roy, M., Martel, M. O., Caron, E., Marin, M. F., Chen, J., et al. (2013). The stress model of chronic pain: evidence from basal cortisol and hippocampal structure and function in humans. *Brain, 136,* 815–827.

Vowles, K. E., & McCracken, L. M. (2008). Acceptance and values-based action in chronic pain: a study of effectiveness and treatment process. *Journal of Clinical and Consulting Psychology, 76,* 397–407.

Wetherell, J. L., Afari, N., Rutledge, T., Sorrell, J. T., Stoddard, J. A., Petkus, A. J., et al. (2011). A randomized, controlled trial of acceptance and commitment therapy and cognitive-behavioral therapy for chronic pain. *Pain, 152,* 2098–2107.

Williams, A. C., Eccleston, C., & Morley, S. (2012). Psychological therapies for the management of chronic pain (excluding headache) in adults. *Cochrane Database of Systematic Reviews, 11.*

Zeineh, M. M., Kang, J., Atlas, S. W., Raman, M. M., Reiss, A. L., Norris, J. L., et al. (2014). Right arcuate fasciculus abnormality in chronic fatigue syndrome. *Radiology, 29,* 141079.

Zhang, J. M., & An, J. (2007). Cytokines, inflammation and pain. *International Anesthesiology Clinics, 45*(2), 27–37.

CHAPTER 13

Stress and Pain: Conclusions and Future Directions

Mustafa al'Absi[1], Magne Arve Flaten[2]

[1]University of Minnesota Medical School, Minneapolis, Duluth, MN, USA; [2]Department of Psychology, Norwegian University of Science and Technology, Trondheim, Norway

INTRODUCTION

This book was set out to address the connection between emotions, stress, and pain, an important research and clinical issue that needed an organized synthesis and research agenda. Pain is the most common complaint among people seeking treatment from physicians or practitioners of alternative and complementary medicine. We also know that stress has various physiological and psychological effects that help explain many of the factors that exacerbate and maintain pain. A better understanding of how emotions, stress, and pain interact and a better understanding of how such interactions can worsen or improve painful conditions would be valuable to pain clinicians and to others working in the field of psychosomatic and behavioral medicine.

Throughout this book, leaders in the field provided comprehensive, thoughtfully developed, integrative reviews of the literature and proposed future directions for the field. The chapters thoroughly described many facets of the interactions among stress, emotions, and pain (acute and chronic); and they discussed these facets using a unique approach by focusing on the interaction of factors that influence pain regulation in basic and clinical contexts. The chapters included reviews of the neuroscience of pain and stress; reviews of the neurobiological mechanisms involved in the interaction of stress, emotions, and pain; and integration of basic science to highlight the translational flavor of this work.

Because stress is closely related to the concept of emotion, the chapters covered the role of various emotions in pain. The importance of individual differences in stress regulation, emotion, and pain perception is also apparent throughout the chapters presented in this book. For example, individual differences in fear of pain, anxiety, depression, and other addictive or chronic

The Neuroscience of Pain, Stress, and Emotion
http://dx.doi.org/10.1016/B978-0-12-800538-5.00013-3

conditions were discussed. The chapters also focused on cognitive factors that mediate the effects of stress and emotion on pain. For example, two chapters discussed the role of patients' expectations during treatment and the so-called placebo and nocebo responses in the context of stress modulation.

Fundamental Processes Linking Stress, Emotions, and Pain

In the first chapter, Wieser and Pauli provided an overview of the neural and cognitive processes that underlie acute pain and they elucidated how emotions can modulate these processes. Wieser and Pauli introduced the neural substrates of pain perception and emotions, and they discussed how these phenomena are related. Wieser and Pauli paid special attention to how facial expressions of emotion can affect pain; they highlighted the emotional priming hypothesis, which states that facial expressions of others induce emotional states that facilitate processing of stimuli that are of the same valence and that inhibit processing of stimuli that are of opposite valence. Hence, sad and painful facial expressions should induce negative affect that, in turn, increases pain processing. Their chapter provides basic information that creates a foundation for subsequent chapters.

In addition, Wieser and Pauli discussed the Perception—Action Model, which states that when a person feels the internal state of another person, this activates the corresponding representations in the observer. The theoretical view presented by the authors is that emotion can modulate pain at different levels of pain transmission and at different levels of the processing system, i.e., at both spinal and supraspinal levels. Furthermore, studies on placebo analgesia support this hypothesis. Pain may also affect emotional perception, although the field needs more research and is a promising area for future studies.

In the second chapter, Murison presented a detailed overview and background of the effects of stress, with a particular focus on the neurobiology of stress. Murison carefully discussed definitions of stress and how the stress response has been evaluated both in animal and in human experiments. The context of this work is defining the deleterious effects of stress on response systems that are critical to health and adaptation. Factors that influence the stress response include situational attributes that influence perception of stress. Hence, stress impacts on the biological and behavioral response are integrated into the presented literature within this chapter. Complementing this is an examination of the neurobiological correlates, both central (cortical, limbic, and brain-stem structures) and peripheral (hypothalamopituitary—adrenal response, the sympathetic nervous system, and the sympathoadrenal system), that may mediate the effects of these processes on the stress response.

Murison's review provides an interesting perspective that guides the reader to understanding how stress, emotions, and individual difference factors have neurobiological signatures, and how these signatures may mediate the effects of stress on pain perception in basic and clinical contexts. Addressing the link between these stress-response patterns and pain regulation represents an exciting area for future investigation. Furthermore, to capitalize on relevant evidence of the importance of efficient regulation of the stress response in terms of activation and cessation of the response, future research is needed to understand how the lingering effects of stress (i.e., delayed recovery after exposure to acute stress) may reduce risk and/or manage pain perception. Indeed, this is a significant area of investigation that requires researchers to account for various types of stressors, including biological, cognitive, psychological, and social factors.

In the third chapter, Rhudy provided a thoughtful review and discussion of emotional modulations of pain, making a clear case for factors that make pain a malleable experience that is responsive to various emotional states. The motivational framework described by Rhudy presents a clear conceptual model to understand the interactive connections between emotions and pain. Features that influence these associations are defined with a focus on valence and related arousal. For example, positively valenced emotions, which are associated with reduced pain, are also related to greater arousal, while emotions with negative valence and low-to-moderate arousal are associated with enhanced pain. Yet the author presented evidence indicating that high arousal connected with negatively valenced emotions may inhibit pain. The importance of this framework is its relevance to evidence demonstrating that poor modulation of emotions is related to risk for chronic pain. The clear implication of this model is the need to better define the dynamic processes and moderators that are involved in poor emotion regulation and the nature of the link between these processes and pain. Clear definitions of such processes and relations will set the stage for targeted efforts that address emotion-related risk factors to prevent chronic pain.

In the fourth chapter, Bartley and Fillingim focused on sex differences in the experience of clinical and experimental pain. The literature examining these differences has demonstrated a greater frequency of chronic pain conditions among women than among men; and laboratory studies have shown that females, compared to males, exhibit greater sensitivity to painful stimuli. Bartley and Fillingim carefully discussed some of the mechanisms that may be responsible for these sex differences, including multiple biological and psychological factors, and they discussed how these sex differences relate to stress-response regulation. This is an area that is ripe for more research focusing also on sex-specific psychosocial factors that could translate to clinical practice. Indeed, better understanding of the differential role of stress in pain exacerbation among men and women could enhance both diagnoses and treatment of pain.

Mechanisms Mediating the Influence of Psychological Factors on Pain

One of the primary thrusts of this book was to account for the psychological factors that mediate the effects of stress on pain. Two issues related to psychological and cognitive processes that influence pain were addressed in three chapters related to placebo, nocebo, and interactions with other cognitive processes (Chapters 5, 6, and 8). The placebo and nocebo effects result from expectations that symptoms will either improve or worsen, respectively. These expectations can be induced via verbal information, through personal experience (e.g., classical conditioning), or by watching others receive treatment (social observational learning).

The chapter by Vase and Price focused on memory and meaning related to the placebo and nocebo effects, whereas the chapter by Flaten and al'Absi focused on the emotional consequences of receiving a placebo. In line with findings presented by Rhudy (Chapter 3), it is indicated that placebo effects can be partly explained by a reduction in negative emotions, with a consequent reduction in pain. This idea also fits well with the chapter on nocebo by Benedetti et al., in which it was proposed that nocebo effects are due to an increase in anxiety or fear. Pain-inhibiting and -facilitating mechanisms have been identified from both biochemical and anatomical points of view; thus, it makes sense to think of placebo and nocebo effects as psychobiological processes that may influence the treatment of conditions involving pain.

Benedetti et al. also discussed the difference between anxiety-induced hyperalgesia and stress-induced analgesia; and they proposed the idea that negative emotions sometimes inhibit and sometimes facilitate pain. These effects may be explained by the direction of one's attention, either away from or toward the pain. This pattern of effects has important clinical implications, and managing the direction of attention is already used in some psychological therapies against pain.

One goal for further research and clinical applications is to understand how placebo effects may be strengthened and how nocebo effects may be avoided. Additional research is needed to better understand the clinical significance of placebo and nocebo effects and the robustness of such effects in patients receiving medical or other therapeutic treatments for pain maintenance or reduction. This is a difficult, yet important, field to study because of its implications in clinical work.

As noted by Vase and Price, placebo and nocebo effects are not static; rather, they result from cognitive and emotional processes that change over time. Closely tied to this idea is the hypothesis that placebo effects can be modulated by somatic feedback, in the form of autonomic or other interoceptive reactions to treatment. These interesting notions have also received little attention, but they warrant attention given their potential to enhance the efficacy of treatments and medications and to diminish nocebo effects.

The chapter by Biggs, Meulders, and Vlaeyen nicely complements other chapters by discussing the interaction of fear and pain perception. The authors presented data to explain the complex nature of the association between fear and pain, including their bidirectional influences. They also reviewed work related to the emotional, cognitive, behavioral, and psychophysiological factors that facilitate the influence of fear on the experience of pain. Biggs et al. also discussed cognitive factors, such as expectancy and pain beliefs, which may contribute to enhanced fear and, thus, increased pain. One important facet of their discussion is the evidence they presented regarding the potential for individual differences in fear of pain to serve as a risk factor for developing chronic pain. Given its potential as a risk factor, it is important to carefully define and understand the nature of fear of pain. Understanding how fear of pain is acquired, generalized, and extinguished could prove useful in developing clinical studies to test novel interventions that target fear of pain in groups that are at high risk of developing chronic pain.

Clinical Implications

Considering the prevalence and impact of chronic pain, several chapters of this book focused on psychological conditions that may increase vulnerability to chronic pain and on conditions that may sustain such pain. Okifuji and Turk presented (Chapter 9) a nicely developed review in which they examined the association between chronic pain and depression and the vulnerability and resilience factors that modify this association. In addition to addressing the epidemiology of pain and discussing factors that moderate the relationship between pain and depression, Okifuji and Turk provided insight into the nonlinear nature of the pain–depression relationship. Okifuji and Turk also reviewed a range of factors that may mediate the link between depression and pain; and they articulated a case for how targeting these factors may provide therapeutic benefits for individuals who experience chronic pain.

In Chapter 10, Nakajima and al'Absi discussed the interaction between stress and pain as well as the impact of substance use on the regulation of the stress response and pain perception. The complex nature of these associations remains an open area for research at both preclinical and clinical levels; and addressing the influence of genetic, biological, cognitive, behavioral, and social factors on these associations will be critical. The role of a substance-use disorder in the relationship between stress and pain is likely to be complicated by the motivations that drive substance use (e.g., as a way to cope with pain), although the nature of motivational influence has not been clearly delineated.

In Chapter 11, Ditto, Horsley, and Tavis focused on the connection between hypertension risk and hypoalgesia, an interesting relationship that has been observed over the past few decades. Ditto et al. carefully addressed the literature and defined the effects of pain on sympathetic nervous system activity. They also reviewed literature demonstrating that increases in blood pressure can decrease pain, an association that is evidenced in both acute and sustained elevations of blood pressure observed in studies with animals and in studies with humans. This observation has been replicated across laboratories and across populations, even though the mechanisms mediating this connection remain not well understood. In their chapter, Ditto and colleagues provided an excellent empirical and theoretical framework to explain these associations and they discussed the psychological and biological processes involved. They also provided a discussion of the clinical implications of this phenomenon, such as unrecognized (silent) myocardial ischemia and the development of chronic pain.

Future work must better define the mechanisms mediating the hypoalgesic effects of blood pressure; and future work must also address the role of central processes (psychological/cognitive and neurobiological) that regulate pain and blood pressure. Such work could lead to translational steps that improve diagnostics and that fuel the development of intervention strategies related to both blood pressure and pain regulation.

In Chapter 12, Stiles presented the syndromes of chronic fatigue and chronic pain, i.e., their diagnosis, underlying pathophysiology, and treatment. The syndromes are similar in that they have unknown origins, can be severely debilitating, and are not yet managed with effective treatments. Furthermore, a number of pathophysiological mechanisms seem to be similar across the two syndromes, including dysregulation at the cortical level, abnormalities of the hypothalamic–pituitary–adrenal axis, structural changes in white matter, and abnormal functioning of cytokines and cortisol. Thus, Stiles recommended that future research focus on these pathophysiologies to develop reliable biomarkers that improve diagnosis.

Taken together, the chapters in this book provide a comprehensive and integrative account of existing literature on the interaction among stress, emotions, and pain regulation in multiple contexts. Furthermore, the authors challenge the field to bridge gaps in existing knowledge by defining the manner by which various emotional and psychosocial factors influence pain and by suggesting how to translate this knowledge into clinically useful information and practices.

INDEX

Note: Page numbers followed by "f" indicate figures and "t" indicate tables.

Printed and bound by CPI Group (UK) Ltd, Croydon, CR0 4YY

08/06/2025

01896870-0006